THE ULTIMATE VEGAN MEAL PREP

The Ultimate Guide to High-Protein & Plant-Based Diet For Athletes With Diet Plan, Meal Plan, Meal Prep And Whole Foods Coobook With Tasty Recipes

Table of Contents

VEGAN COOKBOOK FOR ATHLETES

4

Table of Contents
VEGAN COOKBOOK FOR ATHLETES

Table of Contents
VEGAN MEAL PREP

Table of Contents
VEGAN MEAL PREP

VEGAN COOKBOOK FOR ATHLETES

101 high-protein delicious recipes for a plant-based diet plan and For a Strong Body While Maintaining Health, Vitality and Energy

Description

As an athlete, it may sound like the vegan diet may not provide you the right Nutrition. But I am sure after reading these recipes; you can very well debunk that myth.

Inside this guide, there is a bunch of tasty and easy to cook recipes which will make sure that you get your share of protein and carbs. Remember that while being a meat free athlete ain't easy, this is hardly a reason to quit!

One of the greatest benefits of going vegan is the increased level of health you will experience and this manifests well beyond just your physique. Add to this the potent combination of healthy plant-based protein and you have a winner! You can also choose to supplement with vegan protein powder.

Remember to prep your meals ahead of time for maximum convenience. This guide covers the following recipes:

- Breakfast
- Lunch
- Dessert
- Desserts and snacks
- Sauces and dips

Happy Cooking!!

INTRODUCTION TO THE VEGAN DIET

A lot of people seeking to avoid a lifestyle that contributes to disorders and diseases such as heart attacks, type II diabetes and even cancer go Vegan. These people usually go vegan in order to reduce the intake of animal products and the harmful effects they can have on the body.

Most vegan products are plant based and they reduce the risk of these terrible diseases as well as lowering the risk of developing Alzheimer's disease and many others.

A Vegan diet also contributes to weight loss, not only is a plant-based diet less calorie dense, but provides the right nutrients to slim down quickly. A Vegan diet lowers cholesterol levels, LDLs and blood pressure - this will make you not only feel great, but look great too. In fact, people on a vegan diet typically have their blood pressure 25-75% lower than a person with an animal product diet. This also puts Vegans at a far lower risk of dementia.

Essentially, a Vegan diet will create a healthy lifestyle without even needing to work out. If you do work out as well though, that can produce some incredible results in terms of both weight loss and health! I will explore some of these benefits further later on in the book.

In addition, a lot of the antibiotics used in the modern animal farming system cause a lot of terrible side effects, and by going Vegan people are avoiding these.

For example, excess oestrogen, which is used in order to make animals more 'plump' to increase the meat industries 'yield', can contribute to weight gain when consumed by humans. In addition, high levels of oestrogen have been linked to gynecomastia (colloqually referred to as 'man boobs') in men.

BREAKFAST RECIPES
1. Chocolate PB Smoothie

Preparation time: 5 minutes

Cooking time: 0 minutes

Servings: 4

Ingredients

1 banana

¼ cup rolled oats, or 1 scoop plant protein powder

1 tablespoon flaxseed, or chia seeds

1 tablespoon unsweetened cocoa powder

1 tablespoon peanut butter, or almond or sunflower seed butter

1 tablespoon maple syrup (optional)

1 cup alfalfa sprouts, or spinach, chopped (optional)

½ cup non-dairy milk (optional)

1 cup water

Optional

1 teaspoon maca powder

1 teaspoon cocoa nibs

Directions

Purée everything in a blender until smooth, adding more water (or non-dairy milk) if needed. Add bonus boosters, as desired. Purée until blended.

Nutrition: calories: 474; protein: 13g; total fat: 16g; carbohydrates: 79g; fiber: 18g

2. Orange french toast

Preparation time: 15 minutes
Cooking time: 10 minutes

Servings: 4

Ingredients

3 very ripe bananas

1 cup unsweetened nondairy milk

Zest and juice of 1 orange

1 teaspoon ground cinnamon

¼ Teaspoon grated nutmeg

4 slices french bread

1 tablespoon coconut oil

Directions

In a blender, combine the bananas, almond milk, orange juice and zest, cinnamon, and nutmeg and blend until smooth. Pour the mixture into a 9-by-13-inch baking dish. Soak the bread in the mixture for 5 minutes on each side.

While the bread soaks, heat a griddle or sauté pan over medium-high heat. Melt the coconut oil in the pan and swirl to coat. Cook the bread slices until golden brown on both sides, about 5 minutes each. Serve immediately.

3. Oatmeal Raisin Breakfast Cookie

Preparation time: 5 minutes
Cooking time: 15 minutes

Servings: 2 cookies

Ingredients

½ Cup rolled oats

1 tablespoon whole-grain flour

½ Teaspoon baking powder

1 to 2 tablespoons brown sugar

½ Teaspoon pumpkin pie spice or ground cinnamon (optional)

¼ Cup unsweetened applesauce, plus more as needed

2 tablespoons raisins, dried cranberries, or vegan chocolate chips

Directions

In a medium bowl, stir together the oats, flour, baking powder, sugar, and pumpkin pie spice (if using). Stir in the applesauce until thoroughly combined. Add another 1 to 2 tablespoons of applesauce if the mixture looks too dry (this will depend on the type of oats used).

Shape the mixture into 2 cookies. Put them on a microwave-safe plate and heat on high power for 90 seconds. Alternatively, bake on a small tray in a 350°f oven or toaster oven for 15 minutes. Let cool slightly before eating.

Nutrition (2 cookies): calories: 175; protein: 74g; total fat: 2g; saturated fat:0g; carbohydrates: 39g; fiber: 4g

4. Berry Beetsicle Smoothie

Preparation time: 3 minutes
Cooking time: 0minutes

Servings: 1

Ingredients

½ Cup peeled and diced beets

½ Cup frozen raspberries

1 frozen banana

1 tablespoon maple syrup

1 cup unsweetened soy or almond milk

Directions

Combine all the Ingredients in a blender and blend until smooth.

5. Blueberry Oat Muffins

Preparation time: 10 minutes
Cooking time: 20 minutes

Servings: 12 mufins

Ingredients

2 tablespoons coconut oil or vegan margarine, melted, plus more for preparing the muffin tin

1 cup quick-cooking oats or instant oats

1 cup boiling water

½ Cup nondairy milk

¼ Cup ground flaxseed

1 teaspoon vanilla extract

1 teaspoon apple cider vinegar

1½ cups whole-grain flour

½ Cup brown sugar

2 teaspoons baking soda

Pinch salt

1 cup blueberries

Directions

Preheat the oven to 400°f.

Coat a muffin tin with coconut oil, line with paper muffin cups, or use a nonstick tin.

In a large bowl, combine the oats and boiling water. Stir so the oats soften. Add the coconut oil, milk, flaxseed, vanilla, and vinegar and stir to combine. Add the flour, sugar, baking soda, and salt. Stir until just combined. Gently fold in the blueberries. Scoop the muffin mixture into the prepared tin, about ⅓ cup for each muffin.

Bake for 20 to 25 minutes, until slightly browned on top and springy to the touch. Let cool for about 10 minutes. Run a dinner knife around the inside of each cup to loosen, then tilt the muffins on their sides in the muffin wells so air gets underneath. These keep in an airtight container in the refrigerator for up to 1 week or in the freezer indefinitely.

Nutrition (1muffin): calories: 174; protein: 5g; total fat: 3g; saturated fat:2g; carbohydrates: 33g; fiber: 4g

6. Quinoa Applesauce Muffins

Preparation time: 10 minutes
Cooking time: 15 minutes

Servings: 5

Ingredients

2 tablespoons coconut oil or margarine, melted, plus more for coating the muffin tin

¼ Cup ground flaxseed

½ Cup water

2 cups unsweetened applesauce

½ Cup brown sugar

1 teaspoon apple cider vinegar

2½ cups whole-grain flour

1½ cups cooked quinoa

2 teaspoons baking soda

Pinch salt

½ Cup dried cranberries or raisins

Directions

Preheat the oven to 400°f.

Coat a muffin tin with coconut oil, line with paper muffin cups, or use a nonstick tin. In a large bowl, stir together the flaxseed and water. Add the applesauce, sugar, coconut oil, and vinegar. Stir to combine. Add the flour, quinoa, baking soda, and salt, stirring until just combined. Gently fold in the cranberries without stirring too much. Scoop the muffin mixture into the prepared tin, about ⅓ cup for each muffin.

Bake for 15 to 20 minutes, until slightly browned on top and springy to the touch. Let cool for about 10 minutes. Run a dinner knife around the inside of each cup to loosen, then tilt the muffins on their sides in the muffin wells so air gets underneath. These keep in an airtight container in the refrigerator for up to 1 week or in the freezer indefinitely.

Per serving(1muffin): calories: 387; protein: 7g; total fat: 5g; saturated fat: 2g; carbohydrates: 57g; fiber: 8g

Pumpkin pancakes

Preparation time: 15 minutes
Cooking time: 15 minutes

Servings: 4

Ingredients

2 cups unsweetened almond milk

1 teaspoon apple cider vinegar

2½ cups whole-wheat flour

2 tablespoons baking powder

½ Teaspoon baking soda

1 teaspoon sea salt

1 teaspoon pumpkin pie spice or ½ teaspoon ground -cinnamon plus ¼ teaspoon grated -nutmeg plus ¼ teaspoon ground allspice

½ Cup canned pumpkin purée

1 cup water

1 tablespoon coconut oil

Directions

In a small bowl, combine the almond milk and apple cider vinegar. Set aside.

In a bowl, whisk together the flour, baking powder, baking soda, salt, and pumpkin pie spice. In bowl, combine the almond milk mixture, pumpkin purée, and water, whisking to mix well. Mix the wet Ingredients to the dry Ingredients and fold together until the dry -Ingredients are just moistened.

In a nonstick pan or griddle over medium-high heat, melt the coconut oil and swirl to coat. Pour the batter into the pan ¼ cup at a time and cook until the pancakes are browned, about 5 minutes per side. Serve immediately.

Green breakfast smoothie

Preparation time: 10 minutes
Cooking time: 0 minutes

Servings: 2

Ingredients

½ Banana, sliced

2 cups spinach or other greens, such as kale

1 cup sliced berries of your choosing, fresh or frozen

1 orange, peeled and cut into segments

1 cup unsweetened nondairy milk

1 cup ice

Directions

In a blender, combine all the Ingredients.

Starting with the blender on low speed, begin blending the smoothie, gradually increasing blender speed until smooth. Serve immediately.

7. Blueberry Lemonade Smoothie

Preparation time: 5 minutes
Cooking time: 0 minutes

Servings: 1

Ingredients

1 cup roughly chopped kale

¾ Cup frozen blueberries

1 cup unsweetened soy or almond milk

Juice of 1 lemon

1 tablespoon maple syrup

Directions

Combine all the Ingredients in a blender and blend until smooth. Enjoy immediately.

8. Berry Protein Smoothie

Preparation time: 5 minutes
Cooking time: 0 minutes
Servings: 1
Ingredients

1 banana

1 cup fresh or frozen berries

¾ Cup water or nondairy milk, plus more as needed

1 scoop plant-based protein powder, 3 ounces silken tofu, ¼ cup rolled oats, or ½ cup cooked quinoa

Additions

 1 tablespoon ground flaxseed or chia seeds

 1 handful fresh spinach or lettuce, or 1 chunk cucumber

Coconut water to replace some of the liquid

Directions:

In a blender, combine the banana, berries, water, and your choice of protein.

Add any addition Ingredients as desired. Purée until smooth and creamy, about 50 seconds.

Add a bit more water if you like a thinner smoothie.

Nutrition: calories: 332; protein: 7g; total fat: 5g; saturated fat: 1g; carbohydrates: 72g; fiber: 11g

Blueberry and chia smoothie

Preparation time: 10 minutes
Cooking time: 0 minutes

Servings: 2

Ingredients

2 tablespoons chia seeds

2 cups unsweetened nondairy milk

2 cups blueberries, fresh or frozen

2 tablespoons pure maple syrup or agave

2 tablespoons cocoa powder

Directions:

Soak the chia seeds in the almond milk for 5 minutes.

In a blender, combine the soaked chia seeds, almond milk, blueberries, maple syrup, and cocoa powder and blend until smooth. Serve immediately.

9. Green Kickstart Smoothie

Preparation time: 5 minutes
Cooking time: 0 minutes
Servings: 1
Ingredients

½ Avocado or 1 banana

½ Cup chopped cucumber, peeled if desired

1 handful fresh spinach or chopped lettuce

1 pear or apple, peeled and cored, or 1 cup unsweetened applesauce

2 tablespoons freshly squeezed lime juice

1 cup water or nondairy milk, plus more as needed

Additions

½-Inch piece peeled fresh ginger

1 tablespoon ground flaxseed or chia seeds

½ Cup soy yogurt or 3 ounces silken tofu

Coconut water to replace some of the liquid

2 tablespoons chopped fresh mint or ½ cup chopped mango

Directions:

In a blender, combine the avocado, cucumber, spinach, pear, lime juice, and water.

Add any Additions Ingredients as desired. Purée until smooth and creamy, about 50 seconds. Add a bit more water if you like a thinner smoothie.

Nutrition: calories: 263; protein: 4g; total fat: 14g; saturated fat: 2g; carbohydrates: 36g; fiber: 10g

10. Warm Maple and Cinnamon Quinoa

Preparation time: 5 minutes
Cooking time: 15 minutes

Servings: 4

Ingredients

1 cup unsweetened nondairy milk

1 cup water

1 cup quinoa, rinsed

1 teaspoon cinnamon

¼ Cup chopped pecans or other nuts or seeds, such as chia, sunflower seeds, or almonds

2 tablespoons pure maple syrup or agave

Directions:

In a medium saucepan over medium-high heat, bring the almond milk, water, and quinoa to a boil. Lower the heat to medium-low and cover. Simmer until the liquid is mostly absorbed and the quinoa softens, about 15 minutes.

Turn off the heat and allow to sit, covered, for 5 minutes. Stir in the cinnamon, pecans, and syrup. Serve hot.

11. Warm Quinoa Breakfast Bowl

Preparation time: 5 minutes
Cooking time: 0 minutes

Servings: 4

Ingredients

3 cups freshly cooked quinoa

1⅓ cups unsweetened soy or almond milk

2 bananas, sliced

1 cup raspberries

1 cup blueberries

½ Cup chopped raw walnuts

¼ Cup maple syrup

Directions:

Divide the Ingredients among 4 bowls, starting with a base of ¾ cup quinoa, ⅓ cup milk, ½ banana, ¼ cup raspberries, ¼ cup blueberries, and 2 tablespoons walnuts.

Drizzle 1 tablespoon of maple syrup over the top of each bowl.

12. Banana Bread Rice Pudding

Preparation time: 5 minutes
Cooking time: 50 minutes

Servings: 4

Ingredients

1cup brown rice

1½ cups water

1½ cups nondairy milk

3 tablespoons sugar (omit if using a sweetened nondairy milk)

2 teaspoons pumpkin pie spice or ground cinnamon

2 bananas

3 tablespoons chopped walnuts or sunflower seeds (optional)

Directions

In a medium pot, combine the rice, water, milk, sugar, and pumpkin pie spice. Bring to a boil over high heat, turn the heat to low, and cover the pot. Simmer, stirring occasionally, until the rice is soft and the liquid is absorbed. White rice takes about 20 minutes; brown rice takes about 50 minutes.

Smash the bananas and stir them into the cooked rice. Serve topped with walnuts (if using). Leftovers will keep refrigerated in an airtight container for up to 5 days.

Nutrition: calories: 479; protein: 9g; total fat: 13g; saturated fat: 1g; carbohydrates: 86g; fiber: 7g

Apple and cinnamon oatmeal

Preparation time: 10 minutes
Cooking time:10 minutes

Servings: 2

Ingredients

1¼ cups apple cider

1 apple, peeled, cored, and chopped

⅔ Cup rolled oats

1 teaspoon ground cinnamon

1 tablespoon pure maple syrup or agave (optional)

Directions

In a medium saucepan, bring the apple cider to a boil over medium-high heat. Stir in the apple, oats, and cinnamon.

Bring the cereal to a boil and turn down heat to low. Simmer until the oatmeal thickens, 3 to 4 minutes. Spoon into two bowls and sweeten with maple syrup, if using. Serve hot.

13. Mango Key Lime Pie Smoothie

Preparation time: 5 minutes
Cooking time: 0 minutes

Servings: 1

Ingredients

¼ Avocado

1 cup baby spinach

½ Cup frozen mango chunks

1 cup unsweetened soy or almond milk

Juice of 1 lime (preferably a key lime).

1 tablespoon maple syrup

Directions

Combine all the **Ingredients** in a blender and blend until smooth. Enjoy immediately.

Spiced orange breakfast couscous

Preparation time: 10 minutes
Cooking time: 10 minutes

Servings: 4

Ingredients

3 cups orange juice

1½ cups couscous

1 teaspoon ground cinnamon

¼ Teaspoon ground cloves

½ Cup dried fruit, such as raisins or apricots

½ Cup chopped almonds or other nuts or seeds

Directions

In a small saucepan, bring the orange juice to a boil. Add the couscous, cinnamon, and cloves and remove from heat. Cover the pan with a lid and allow to sit until the -couscous softens, about 5 minutes.

Fluff the couscous with a fork and stir in the dried fruit and nuts. Serve -immediately.

Breakfast parfaits

Preparation time: 15 minutes
Cooking time: 0 minutes

Servings: 2

Ingredients

One 14-ounce can coconut milk, refrigerated overnight

1 cup granola

½ Cup walnuts

1 cup sliced strawberries or other seasonal berries

Directions

Pour off the canned coconut-milk liquid and retain the solids.

In two parfait glasses, layer the coconut-milk solids, granola, walnuts, and -strawberries. Serve immediately.

Sweet potato and kale hash

Preparation time: 10 minutes
Cooking time: 15 minutes

Servings: 2

Ingredients

1 sweet potato

2 tablespoons olive oil

½ Onion, chopped

1 carrot, peeled and chopped

2 garlic cloves, minced

½ Teaspoon dried thyme

1 cup chopped kale

Sea salt

Freshly ground black pepper

Directions

Prick the sweet potato with a fork and microwave on high until soft, about 5 minutes. Remove from the microwave and cut into ¼-inch cubes.

In a large nonstick sauté pan, heat the olive oil over medium-high heat. Add the onion and carrot and cook until softened, about 5 minutes. Add the garlic and thyme and cook until the garlic is fragrant, about 30 seconds.

Add the sweet potatoes and cook until the potatoes begin to brown, about 7 -minutes. Add the kale and cook just until it wilts, 1 to 2 minutes. Season with salt and pepper. Serve immediately.

14.Delicious Oat Meal

Preparation time: 10 minutes

Cooking time: 6 hours

Servings: 4

Ingredients:

3 cups water

3 cups almond milk

1 and ½ cups steel oats

4 dates, pitted and chopped

1 teaspoon cinnamon, ground

2 tablespoons coconut sugar

½ Teaspoon ginger powder

A pinch of nutmeg, ground

A pinch of cloves, ground

1 teaspoon vanilla extract

Directions:

Put water and milk in your slow cooker and stir.

Add oats, dates, cinnamon, sugar, ginger, nutmeg, cloves and vanilla extract, stir, cover and cook on low for 6 hours.

Divide into bowls and serve for breakfast.

Enjoy!

Nutrition: calories 120, fat 1, fiber 2, carbs 3, protein 5

15.Breakfast Cherry Delight

Preparation time: 10 minutes
Cooking time: 8 hours and 10 minutes
Servings: 4
Ingredients:
2 cups almond milk
2 cups water
1 cup steel cut oats
2 tablespoons cocoa powder
1/3 cup cherries, pitted
¼ Cup maple syrup
½ Teaspoon almond extract
For the sauce:
2 tablespoons water
1 and ½ cups cherries, pitted and chopped
¼ Teaspoon almond extract

Directions:
Put the almond milk in your slow cooker.

Add 2 cups water, oats, cocoa powder, 1/3 cup cherries, maples syrup and ½ teaspoon almond extract.

Stir, cover and cook on low for 8 hours.

In a small pan, mix 2 tablespoons water with 1 and ½ cups cherries and ¼ teaspoon almond extract, stir well, bring to a simmer over medium heat and cook for 10 minutes until it thickens.

Divide oatmeal into breakfast bowls, top with the cherries sauce and serve.

Enjoy!

Nutrition: calories 150, fat 1, fiber 2, carbs 6, protein 5

16. Crazy Maple and Pear Breakfast

Preparation time: 10 minutes

Cooking time: 9 hours

Servings: 2

Ingredients:

1 pear, cored and chopped

½ Teaspoon maple extract

2 cups coconut milk

½ Cup steel cut oats

½ Teaspoon vanilla extract

1 tablespoon stevia

¼ Cup walnuts, chopped for serving

Cooking spray

Directions:

Spray your slow cooker with some cooking spray and add coconut milk.

Also, add maple extract, oats, pear, stevia and vanilla extract, stir, cover and cook on low for 9 hours.

Stir your oatmeal again, divide it into breakfast bowls and serve with chopped walnuts on top.

Enjoy!

Nutrition: calories 150, fat 3, fiber 2, carbs 6, protein 6

17.Hearty French Toast Bowls

Preparation time: 10 minutes

Cooking time: 5 hours

Servings: 4

Ingredients:

1 and ½ cups almond milk

1 cup coconut cream

1 tablespoon vanilla extract

½ Tablespoon cinnamon powder

2 tablespoons maple syrup

¼ Cup spenda

2 apples, cored and cubed

½ Cup cranberries, dried

1 pound vegan bread, cubed

Cooking spray

Directions:

Spray your slow cooker with some cooking spray and add the bread.

Also, add cranberries and apples and stir gently.

Add milk, coconut cream, maple syrup, vanilla extract, cinnamon powder and splenda.

Stir, cover and cook on low for 5 hours.

Divide into bowls and serve right away.

Enjoy!

Nutrition: calories 140, fat 2, fiber 3, carbs 6, protein 2

18. Tofu Burrito

Preparation time: 10 minutes
Cooking time: 8 hours
Servings: 4
Ingredients:

15 ounces canned black beans, drained
2 tablespoons onions, chopped
7 ounces tofu, drained and crumbled
2 tablespoons green bell pepper, chopped
½ Teaspoon turmeric
¾ Cup water
¼ Teaspoon smoked paprika
¼ Teaspoon cumin, ground
¼ Teaspoon chili powder
A pinch of salt and black pepper
4 gluten free whole wheat tortillas
Avocado, chopped for serving
Salsa for serving

Directions:

Put black beans in your slow cooker.

Add onions, tofu, bell pepper, turmeric, water, paprika, cumin, chili powder, a pinch of salt and pepper, stir, cover and cook on low for 8 hours.

Divide this on each tortilla, add avocado and salsa, wrap, arrange on plates and serve.

Enjoy!

Nutrition: calories 130, fat 4, fiber 2, carbs 5, protein 4

19. Tasty Mexican Breakfast

Preparation time: 10 minutes

Cooking time: 2 hours

Servings: 4

Ingredients:

1 cup brown rice

1 cup onion, chopped

2 cups veggie stock

1 red bell pepper, chopped

1 green bell pepper, chopped

4 ounces canned green chilies, chopped

15 ounces canned black beans, drained

A pinch of salt

Black pepper to the taste

For the salsa:

3 tablespoons lime juice

1 avocado, pitted, peeled and cubed

½ Cup cilantro, chopped

½ Cup green onions, chopped

½ Cup tomato, chopped

1 poblano pepper, chopped

2 tablespoons olive oil

½ Teaspoon cumin

Directions:

Put the stock in your slow cooker.
Add rice, onions and beans, stir, cover and cook on high for 1 hour and 30 minutes.

Add chilies, red and green bell peppers, a pinch of salt and black pepper, stir, cover again and cook on high for 30 minutes more.

Meanwhile, in a bowl, mix avocado with green onions, tomato, poblano pepper, cilantro, oil, cumin, a pinch of salt, black pepper and lime juice and stir really well.

Divide rice mix into bowls; top each with the salsa you've just made and serve.

Enjoy!

Nutrition: calories 140, fat 2, fiber 2, carbs 5, protein 5

20. Divine Carrot Oatmeal

Preparation time: 10 minutes

Cooking time: 7 hours

Servings: 3

Ingredients:

2 cups coconut milk

½ Cup old fashioned rolled oats

1 cup carrots, chopped

2 tablespoons agave nectar

1 teaspoon cardamom, ground

A pinch of saffron

Some chopped pistachios

Cooking spray

Directions:

Spray your slow cooker with some cooking spray and add coconut milk.

Also, add oats, carrots, agave nectar, cardamom and saffron.

Stir, cover and cook on Low for 7 hours.

Stir oatmeal again, divide into bowls and serve with chopped pistachios on top.

Enjoy!

Nutrition: calories 140, fat 2, fiber 2, carbs 4, protein 5

21. Wonderful Blueberry Butter

Preparation time: 10 minutes

Cooking time: 6 hours

Servings: 12

Ingredients:

5 cups blueberries puree

2 teaspoons cinnamon powder

Zest from 1 lemon

1 cup coconut sugar

½ Teaspoon nutmeg, ground

¼ Teaspoon ginger, ground

Directions:

Put blueberries in your slow cooker, cover and cook on low for 1 hour.

Stir your berries puree, cover and cook on low for 4 hours more.

Add sugar, ginger, nutmeg and lemon zest, stir and cook on high uncovered for 1 hour more.

Divide into jars, cover them and keep in a cold place until you serve it for breakfast.

Enjoy!

Nutrition: calories 143, fat 2, fiber 3, carbs 3, protein 4

22. Delicious Pumpkin Butter

Preparation time: 10 minutes
Cooking time: 4 hours
Servings: 5
Ingredients:
2 teaspoons cinnamon powder
4 cups pumpkin puree
1 and ¼ cup maple syrup
½ Teaspoon nutmeg
1 teaspoon vanilla extract
Directions:
In your slow cooker, mix pumpkin puree with maple syrup and vanilla extract, stir, cover and cook on high for 4 hours.

Add cinnamon and nutmeg, stir, divide into jars and serve for breakfast!

Enjoy!
Nutrition: calories 120, fat 2, fiber 2, carbs 4, protein 2

LUNCH RECIPES

Preparation time: 10 minutes

Cooking time: 3 hours

Servings: 4

Ingredients:

½ Cup quinoa

2 and ½ cups veggie stock

14 ounces canned tomatoes, chopped

15 ounces canned black beans, drained

¼ Cup green bell pepper, chopped

¼ Cup red bell pepper, chopped

A pinch of salt and black pepper

2 garlic cloves, minced

1 carrots, shredded

1 small chili pepper, chopped

2 teaspoons chili powder

1 teaspoon cumin, ground

A pinch of cayenne pepper

½ Cup corn

1 teaspoon oregano, dried

For the vegan sour cream:

A drizzle of apple cider vinegar

4 tablespoons water

½ Cup cashews, soaked overnight and drained

1 teaspoon lime juice

Directions:

Put the stock in your slow cooker.

Add quinoa, tomatoes, beans, red and green bell pepper, garlic, carrot, salt, pepper, corn, cumin, cayenne, chili powder, chili pepper and oregano, stir, cover and cook on High for 3 hours.

Meanwhile, put the cashews in your blender.

Add water, vinegar and lime juice and pulse really well.

Divide beans chili into bowls, top with vegan sour cream and serve.

Enjoy!

Nutrition: calories 300, fat 4, fiber 4, carbs 10, protein 7

23. Amazing Potato Dish

Preparation time: 10 minutes

Cooking time: 3 hours

Servings: 4

Ingredients:

1 and ½ pounds potatoes, peeled and roughly chopped

1 tablespoon olive oil

3 tablespoons water

1 small yellow onion, chopped

½ Cup veggie stock cube, crumbled

½ Teaspoon coriander, ground

½ Teaspoon cumin, ground

½ Teaspoon garam masala

½ Teaspoon chili powder

Black pepper to the taste

½ Pound spinach, roughly torn

Directions:

Put the potatoes in your slow cooker.

Add oil, water, onion, stock cube, coriander, cumin, garam masala, chili powder, black pepper and spinach.

Stir, cover and cook on High for 3 hours.

Divide into bowls and serve.

Enjoy!

Nutrition: calories 270, fat 4, fiber 6, carbs 8, protein 12

24. Textured Sweet Potatoes and Lentils Delight

Preparation time: 10 minutes

Cooking time: 4 hours and 30 minutes

Servings: 6

Ingredients:

6 cups sweet potatoes, peeled and cubed

2 teaspoons coriander, ground

2 teaspoons chili powder

1 yellow onion, chopped

3 cups veggie stock

4 garlic cloves, minced

A pinch of sea salt and black pepper

10 ounces canned coconut milk

1 cup water

1 and ½ cups red lentils

Directions:

Put sweet potatoes in your slow cooker.

Add coriander, chili powder, onion, stock, garlic, salt and pepper, stir, cover and cook on high for 3 hours.

Add lentils, stir, cover and cook for 1 hour and 30 minutes.

Add water and coconut milk, stir well, divide into bowls and serve right away.

Enjoy!

Nutrition: calories 300, fat 10, fiber 8, carbs 16, protein 10

25. Incredibly Tasty Pizza

Preparation time: 1 hour and 10 minutes

Cooking time: 1 hour and 45 minutes

Servings: 3

Ingredients:

For the dough:

½ Teaspoon italian seasoning

1 and ½ cups whole wheat flour

1 and ½ teaspoons instant yeast

1 tablespoon olive oil

A pinch of salt

½ Cup warm water

Cooking spray

For the sauce:

¼ Cup green olives, pitted and sliced

¼ Cup kalamata olives, pitted and sliced

½ Cup tomatoes, crushed

1 tablespoon parsley, chopped

1 tablespoon capers, rinsed

¼ Teaspoon garlic powder

¼ Teaspoon basil, dried

¼ Teaspoon oregano, dried

¼ Teaspoon palm sugar

¼ Teaspoon red pepper flakes

A pinch of salt and black pepper

½ Cup cashew mozzarella, shredded

Directions:

In your food processor, mix yeast with italian seasoning, a pinch of salt and flour.

Add oil and the water and blend well until you obtain a dough.

Transfer dough to a floured working surface, knead well, transfer to a greased bowl, cover and leave aside for 1 hour.

Meanwhile, in a bowl, mix green olives with kalamata olives, tomatoes, parsley, capers, garlic powder, oregano, sugar, salt, pepper and pepper flakes and stir well.

Transfer pizza dough to a working surface again and flatten it.

Shape so it will fit your slow cooker.

Grease your slow cooker with cooking spray and add dough.

Press well on the bottom.

Spread the sauce mix all over, cover and cook on high for 1 hour and 15 minutes.

Spread vegan mozzarella all over, cover again and cook on high for 30 minutes more.

Leave your pizza to cool down before slicing and serving it.

Nutrition: calories 340, fat 5, fiber 7, carbs 13, protein 15

26. Rich Beans Soup

Preparation time: 10 minutes

Cooking time: 7 hours

Servings: 4

Ingredients:

1 pound navy beans

1 yellow onion, chopped

4 garlic cloves, crushed

2 quarts veggie stock

A pinch of sea salt

Black pepper to the taste

2 potatoes, peeled and cubed

2 teaspoons dill, dried

1 cup sun-dried tomatoes, chopped

1 pound carrots, sliced

4 tablespoons parsley, minced

Directions:

Put the stock in your slow cooker.

Add beans, onion, garlic, potatoes, tomatoes, carrots, dill, salt and pepper, stir, cover and cook on low for 7 hours.

Stir your soup, add parsley, divide into bowls and serve.

Enjoy!

Nutrition: calories 250, fat 4, fiber 3, carbs 9, protein 10

27. Delicious Baked Beans

Preparation time: 10 minutes

Cooking time: 12 hours

Servings: 8

Ingredients:

1 pound navy beans, soaked overnight and drained

1 cup maple syrup

1 cup bourbon

1 cup vegan bbq sauce

1 cup palm sugar

¼ Cup ketchup

1 cup water

¼ Cup mustard

¼ Cup blackstrap molasses

¼ Cup apple cider vinegar

¼ Cup olive oil

2 tablespoons coconut aminos

Directions:

Put the beans in your slow cooker.

Add maple syrup, bourbon, bbq sauce, sugar, ketchup, water, mustard, molasses, vinegar, oil and coconut aminos.

Stir everything, cover and cook on Low for 12 hours.

Divide into bowls and serve.

Enjoy!

Nutrition: calories 430, fat 7, fiber 8, carbs 15, protein 19

28. Indian Lentils

Preparation time: 10 minutes
Cooking time: 3 hours
Servings: 4
Ingredients:
1 yellow bell pepper, chopped
1 sweet potato, chopped
2 and ½ cups lentils, already cooked
4 garlic cloves, minced
1 yellow onion, chopped
2 teaspoons cumin, ground
15 ounces canned tomato sauce
½ Teaspoon ginger, ground
A pinch of cayenne pepper
1 tablespoons coriander, ground
1 teaspoon turmeric, ground
2 teaspoons paprika
2/3 cup veggie stock
1 teaspoon garam masala
A pinch of sea salt
Black pepper to the taste
Juice of 1 lemon

Directions:
Put the stock in your slow cooker.
Add potato, lentils, onion, garlic, cumin, bell pepper, tomato sauce, salt, pepper, ginger, coriander, turmeric, paprika, cayenne, garam masala and lemon juice.
Stir, cover and cook on high for 3 hours.
Stir your lentils mix again, divide into bowls and serve.

Enjoy!
Nutrition: calories 300, fat 6, fiber 5, carbs 9, protein 12

29.   Delicious Butternut Squash Soup

Preparation time: 10 minutes
Cooking time: 6 hours
Servings: 8
Ingredients:
1 apple, cored, peeled and chopped
½ Pound carrots, chopped
1 pound butternut squash, peeled and cubed
1 yellow onion, chopped
A pinch of sea salt
Black pepper to the taste
1 bay leaf
3 cups veggie stock
14 ounces canned coconut milk
¼ Teaspoon sage, dried
Directions:
Put the stock in your slow cooker.
Add apple squash, carrots, onion, salt, pepper and bay leaf.
Stir, cover and cook on low for 6 hours.
Transfer to your blender, add coconut milk and sage and pulse really well.
Ladle into bowls and serve right away.
Enjoy!
Nutrition: calories 200, fat 3, fiber 6, carbs 8, protein 10

30. Amazing Mushroom Stew

Preparation time: 10 minutes

Cooking time: 8 hours

Servings: 4

Ingredients:

2 garlic cloves, minced

1 celery stalk, chopped

1 yellow onion, chopped

1 and ½ cups firm tofu, pressed and cubed

1 cup water

10 ounces mushrooms, chopped

1 pound mixed peas, corn and carrots

2 and ½ cups veggie stock

1 teaspoon thyme, dried

2 tablespoons coconut flour

A pinch of sea salt

Black pepper to the taste

Directions:

Put the water and stock in your slow cooker.

Add garlic, onion, celery, mushrooms, mixed veggies, tofu, thyme, salt, pepper and flour.

Stir everything, cover and cook on low for 8 hours.

Divide into bowls and serve hot.

Enjoy!

Nutrition: calories 230, fat 4, fiber 6, carbs 10, protein 7

31. Simple Tofu Dish

Preparation time: 10 minutes
Cooking time: 3 hours
Servings: 6
Ingredients:

1 big tofu package, cubed
1 tablespoon sesame oil
¼ Cup pineapple, cubed
1 tablespoon olive oil
2 garlic cloves, minced
1 tablespoons brown rice vinegar
2 teaspoon ginger, grated
¼ Cup soy sauce
5 big zucchinis, cubed
¼ Cup sesame seeds

Directions:

In your food processor, mix sesame oil with pineapple, olive oil, garlic, ginger, soy sauce and vinegar and whisk well.

Add this to your slow cooker and mix with tofu cubes.

Cover and cook on High for 2 hours and 45 minutes.

Add sesame seeds and zucchinis, stir gently, cover and cook on High for 15 minutes.

Divide between plates and serve.

Enjoy!

Nutrition: calories 200, fat 3, fiber 4, carbs 9, protein 10

32. Special Jambalaya

Preparation time: 10 minutes
Cooking time: 6 hours
Servings: 4
Ingredients:

6 ounces soy chorizo, chopped

1 and ½ cups celery ribs, chopped

1 cup okra

1 green bell pepper, chopped

16 ounces canned tomatoes and green chilies, chopped

2 garlic cloves, minced

½ Teaspoon paprika

1 and ½ cups veggie stock

A pinch of cayenne pepper

Black pepper to the taste

A pinch of salt

3 cups already cooked wild rice for serving

Directions:

Heat up a pan over medium high heat, add soy chorizo, stir, brown for a few minutes and transfer to your slow cooker.

Also, add celery, bell pepper, okra, tomatoes and chilies, garlic, paprika, salt, pepper and cayenne to your slow cooker.

Stir everything, add veggie stock, cover the slow cooker and cook on low for 6 hours.

Divide rice on plates, top each serving with your vegan jambalaya and serve hot.

Enjoy!

Nutrition: calories 150, fat 3, fiber 7, carbs 15, protein 9

33. Delicious Chard Soup

Preparation time: 10 minutes
Cooking time: 8 hours
Servings: 6
Ingredients:

1 yellow onion, chopped

1 tablespoon olive oil

1 celery stalk, chopped

2 garlic cloves, minced

1 carrot, chopped

1 bunch swiss chard, torn

1 cup brown lentils, dried

5 potatoes, peeled and cubed

1 tablespoon soy sauce

Black pepper to the taste

A pinch of sea salt

6 cups veggie stock

Directions:

Heat up a big pan with the oil over medium high heat, add onion, celery, garlic, carrot and Swiss chard, stir, cook for a few minutes and transfer to your slow cooker.

Also, add lentils, potatoes, soy sauce, salt, pepper and stock to the slow cooker, stir, cover and cook on Low for 8 hours.

Divide into bowls and serve hot.

Enjoy!

Nutrition: calories 200, fat 4, fiber 5, carbs 9, protein 12

34. Chinese Tofu and Veggies

Preparation time: 10 minutes

Cooking time: 4 hours

Servings: 4

Ingredients:

14 ounces extra firm tofu, pressed and cut into medium triangles

Cooking spray

2 teaspoons ginger, grated

1 yellow onion, chopped

3 garlic cloves, minced

8 ounces tomato sauce

¼ Cup hoisin sauce

¼ Teaspoon coconut aminos

2 tablespoons rice wine vinegar

1 tablespoon soy sauce

1 tablespoon spicy mustard

¼ Teaspoon red pepper, crushed

2 teaspoons molasses

2 tablespoons water

A pinch of black pepper

3 broccoli stalks

1 green bell pepper, cut into squares

2 zucchinis, cubed

Directions:

Heat up a pan over medium high heat, add tofu pieces, brown them for a few minutes and transfer to your slow cooker.

Heat up the pan again over medium high heat, add ginger, onion, garlic and tomato sauce, stir, sauté for a few minutes and transfer to your slow cooker as well.

Add hoisin sauce, aminos, vinegar, soy sauce, mustard, red pepper, molasses, water and black pepper, stir gently, cover and cook on high for 3 hours.

Add zucchinis, bell pepper and broccoli, cover and cook on high for 1 more hour.

Divide between plates and serve right away.

Enjoy!

Nutrition: calories 300, fat 4, fiber 8, carbs 14, protein 13

35. Wonderful Corn Chowder

Preparation time: 10 minutes
Cooking time: 8 hours and 30 minutes
Servings: 6
Ingredients:

2 cups yellow onion, chopped

2 tablespoons olive oil

1 red bell pepper, chopped

1 pound gold potatoes, cubed

1 teaspoon cumin, ground

4 cups corn kernels

4 cups veggie stock

1 cup almond milk

A pinch of salt

A pinch of cayenne pepper

½ Teaspoon smoked paprika

Chopped scallions for serving

Directions:

Heat up a pan with the oil over medium heat, add onion, stir and sauté for 5 minutes and then transfer to your slow cooker.

Add bell pepper, 1 cup corn, potatoes, paprika, cumin, salt and cayenne, stir, cover and cook on low for 8 hours.

Blend this using an immersion blender and then mix with almond milk and the rest of the corn.

Stir chowder, cover and cook on low for 30 minutes more.

Ladle into bowls and serve with chopped scallions on top.

Enjoy!

Nutrition: calories 200, fat 4, fiber 7, carbs 13, protein 16

36. Black Eyed Peas Stew

Preparation time: 10 minutes
Cooking time: 4 hours
Servings: 8
Ingredients:
3 celery stalks, chopped
2 carrots, sliced
1 yellow onion, chopped
1 sweet potato, cubed
1 green bell pepper, chopped
3 cups black-eyed peas, soaked for 8 hours and drained
1 cup tomato puree
4 cups veggie stock
A pinch of salt
Black pepper to the taste
1 chipotle chile, minced
1 teaspoon ancho chili powder
1 teaspoons sage, dried and crumbled
2 teaspoons cumin, ground
Chopped coriander for serving

Directions:
Put celery in your slow cooker.
Add carrots, onion, potato, bell pepper, black-eyed peas, tomato puree, salt, pepper, chili powder, sage, chili, cumin and stock.
Stir, cover and cook on High for 4 hours.
Stir stew again, divide into bowls and serve with chopped coriander on top.

Enjoy!
Nutrition: calories 200, fat 4, fiber 7, carbs 9, protein 16

37.   White Bean Cassoulet

Preparation time: 10 minutes
Cooking time: 6 hours
Servings: 4
Ingredients:
2 celery stalks, chopped
3 leeks, sliced
4 garlic cloves, minced
2 carrots, chopped
2 cups veggie stock
15 ounces canned tomatoes, chopped
1 bay leaf
1 tablespoon italian seasoning
30 ounces canned white beans, drained
For the breadcrumbs:
Zest from 1 lemon, grated
1 garlic clove, minced
2 tablespoons olive oil
1 cup vegan bread crumbs
¼ Cup parsley, chopped

Directions:
Heat up a pan with a splash of the veggie stock over medium heat, add celery and leeks, stir and cook for 2 minutes.

Add carrots and garlic, stir and cook for 1 minute more.

Add this to your slow cooker and mix with stock, tomatoes, bay leaf, italian seasoning and beans.

Stir, cover and cook on low for 6 hours.

Meanwhile, heat up a pan with the oil over medium high heat, add bread crumbs, lemon zest, 1 garlic clove and parsley, stir and toast for a couple of minutes.

Divide your white beans mix into bowls, sprinkle bread crumbs mix on top and serve.

Enjoy!
Nutrition: calories 223, fat 3, fiber 7, carbs 10, protein 7

38. Light Jackfruit Dish

Preparation time: 10 minutes

Cooking time: 6 hours

Servings: 4

Ingredients:

40 ounces green jackfruit in brine, drained

½ Cup agave nectar

½ Cup gluten free tamari sauce

¼ Cup soy sauce

1 cup white wine

2 tablespoons ginger, grated

8 garlic cloves, minced

1 pear, cored and chopped

1 yellow onion, chopped

½ Cup water

4 tablespoons sesame oil

Directions:

Put jackfruit in your slow cooker.

Add agave nectar, tamari sauce, soy sauce, wine, ginger, garlic, pear, onion, water and oil.

Stir well, cover and cook on low for 6 hours.

Divide jackfruit mix into bowls and serve.

Enjoy!

Nutrition: calories 160, fat 4, fiber 1, carbs 10, protein 3

39. Veggie Curry

Preparation time: 10 minutes
Cooking time: 4 hours
Servings: 4
Ingredients:

1 tablespoon ginger, grated

14 ounces canned coconut milk

Cooking spray

16 ounces firm tofu, pressed and cubed

1 cup veggie stock

¼ Cup green curry paste

½ Teaspoon turmeric

1 tablespoon coconut sugar

1 yellow onion, chopped

1 and ½ cup red bell pepper, chopped

A pinch of salt

¾ Cup peas

1 eggplant, chopped

Directions:

Put the coconut milk in your slow cooker.

Add ginger, stock, curry paste, turmeric, sugar, onion, bell pepper, salt, peas and eggplant pieces, stir, cover and cook on high for 4 hours.

Meanwhile, spray a pan with cooking spray and heat up over medium high heat.

Add tofu pieces and brown them for a few minutes on each side.

Divide tofu into bowls, add slowly cooked curry mix on top and serve.

Enjoy!

Nutrition: calories 200, fat 4, fiber 6, carbs 10, protein 9

DINNER RECIPES
40. Low Carb Peanut Dip (Instant Pot)

Servings: 6
Preparation time: 10 minutes
Nutrition
Calories: 451 kcal
Carbs: 18.9g
Fat: 37.7g
Protein: 9.8g
Fiber: 4.9g
Sugar: 3.7g

Ingredients:

2 tbsp. Peanut oil
1 cup peanut cheese spread
1 low carb crust
1 cup onion (chopped)
1 tbsp. Garlic (minced)
1 cup fire roasted tomatoes
1 tbsp. Chipotle pepper (chopped)
½ Cup water
1 tbsp. Chili powder
2 tsp. Ground cumin
2 tsp. Salt
1 tsp. Dried oregano
Total number of **Ingredients**: 12

Directions:

Select the "sauté" option on the instant pot, waiting till it reads "hot" to add the onions and garlic with olive oil, stirring for about 30 minutes.

Blend the canned tomatoes and the peanut butter until it is relatively smooth.

Mix the cumin, salt, chili powder, and oregano; then mix with the onions and garlic for 30 seconds, allowing them to soak in the flavor.

Pour the blender mix into the pot along with the water. Close the pot and cook on instant pressure for 10 minutes, allowing natural pressure release for 10 minutes after that.

Mix well, and serve with a low carb crust for dipping!

41. Spice-Rubbed Cauliflower (Instant Pot)

Servings: 4
Preparation time: 10 minutes
Nutrition
Calories: 86 kcal
Carbs: 12.3g
Fat: 2.7g
Protein: 3.3g
Fiber: 7.5g
Sugar: 5.6g

Ingredients:
2 lbs. Cauliflower
2 tbsp. Olive oil
2 tsp. Paprika
2 tsp. Ground cumin
Salt to taste
1 cup cilantro (fresh, chopped)
1 lemon (quartered)
Total number of **Ingredients**: 7

Directions:
Insert the steam rack in the instant pot, adding 1 ½ cups of water.

Remove the leaves of the cauliflower, cut the end from the base, and place on the steam rack.

Combine the oil, salt, paprika, and cumin in a bowl; then pour over the cauliflower to coat.

Lock the lid and cook under pressure for 4 minutes; use the quick release to let out the steam, and open the lid.

Take the cauliflower out and cut it into 1 inch sized "steaks."

Divide onto plates, sprinkle the cilantro on top, and place a quartered lemon on each plate.

42. Satay Veggie Bowl

Servings: 4
Preparation time: 15 minutes
Nutrition
Calories: 605 kcal

Carbs: 16g

Fat: 53.1g

Protein: 15.9g

Fiber: 9.8g

Sugar: 4.7g

Ingredients:
Handful of olives

Olive oil, garlic powder, and salt to taste

1 cup broccoli (florets)

1 cup spinach (frozen)

3 cups peanut butter or cashew cheese

Total number of **Ingredients:** 5

Directions:
In a greased skillet, add broccoli, and frozen spinach.

Adding salt and garlic powder to taste, mix well and wait until the spinach has softened and the tempeh is cooked.

Transfer to a bowl, and add olive oil, garlic powder, and salt to taste. Garnish with olives.

43. Shiritaki Noodles and Veggies

Servings: 1
Preparation time: 15 minutes
Nutrition
Calories: 279 kcal
Carbs: 13.5g
Fat: 28.2g
Protein: 3.0g
Fiber: 4.6g
Sugar: 5.2g

Ingredients:

1 package shiritaki noodles (rinsed, drained)
2 tbsp. Peanut oil
¼ Cup marinara sauce
½ Cup mixed veggies (of choice)
Total number of **Ingredients:** 4

Directions:

Boil the noodles until soft.

Once done, transfer to a skillet and add the marinara sauce, oil, and mixed veggies.

Keep mixing, letting the mixture heat until the veggies are warm and incorporated.

44. Shiritaki Alfredo

Servings: 1
Preparation time: 10 minutes
Nutrition
Calories: 377 kcal
Carbs: 11.3g
Fat: 34.3g
Protein: 5.6g
Fiber: 5.5g
Sugar: 1.0g

Ingredients:

1 package shiritaki noodles (rinsed, drained)

2 tbsp. Olive oil

¼ Cup vegan cream cheese

1 cup spinach (frozen)

Salt, pepper, and garlic powder (to taste)

Almond milk (to reach desired consistency)

Total number of **Ingredients:** 8

Directions:

Dump all **Ingredients** in a pan with olive oil and slowly add almond milk for a creamy feel.

Once all **Ingredients** are mixed and the milk thickens, turn off the heat and serve.

45.   Taco-Spiced Stir-fry

Servings: 1
Preparation time: 15 minutes
Nutrition
Calories: 293 kcal
Carbs: 18.7g
Fat: 22.5g
Protein: 4.0g
Fiber: 10.5g
Sugar: 3.7g

Ingredients:
1 package cauliflower rice
1 tbsp. Peanut oil
1 tbsp. Taco seasoning
½ Tbsp. Chili powder
2 tbsp. Guacamole
¼ Cup sliced olives
Total number of **Ingredients:** 6

Directions:
Mix all Ingredients, except the guacamole and olives, in a pan on medium heat until the cauliflower rice has softened.

Take off the stove and it cool when rice has softened, before serving.

46.   Green-Glory Soup (Instant Pot)

Servings: 6
Preparation time: 15 minutes

Nutrition

Calories: 284 kcal

Carbs: 9.1g

Fat: 26.3g

Protein: 2.9g

Fiber: 3.1g

Sugar: 5.3g

Ingredients:

1 head cauliflower (florets)

1 onion (diced)

2 cloves garlic (minced)

1 cup spinach (fresh or frozen)

1 bay leaf (crumbled)

1 cup coconut milk

4 cups vegetable stock

Salt and pepper to taste

Herbs for garnish (optional)

½ Cup coconut oil

Total number of **Ingredients:** 11

Directions:

In a pressure pot on "sauté" mode, sauté onions and garlic until onions are browned. Once cooked, add the cauliflower and bay leaf and cook for about 5 minutes, stirring occasionally.

Add the spinach and continue cooking and stirring for 5 minutes.

Pour in the vegetable stock and set the timer for 10 minutes on high pressure to let the mix come to a boil; then allow quick pressure release and add the coconut milk.

Season with garnishes of choice as well as salt and pepper. Turn off the pot and mix the soup until it becomes thick and creamy with a hand blender.

47.   Mediterranean-Style Pasta

Servings: 4
Preparation time: 10 minutes
Nutrition
Calories: 117 kcal
Carbs: 7.9g
Fat: 8.7g
Protein: 1.8g
Fiber: 2.6g
Sugar: 4.2g
Ingredients:
2 zucchinis (large, spiral-sliced)
1 cup spinach
2 tbsp. Olive oil
5 cloves garlic (minced)
Salt and pepper (to taste)
¼ Cup tomatoes (sun dried for added flavor)
2 tbsp. Capers
2 tbsp. Parsley (chopped)
10 kalamata olives (halved)
Total number of **Ingredients:** 10
Directions:
In a lightly oiled pan, add the spinach, zucchini, salt, pepper, and garlic, sautéing until the zucchini is tender; drain the excess liquid.

Add tomatoes, capers, olives, and parsley, mixing for about 3 minutes.

Remove from heat and toss well before serving, adding more or less of any item for preference.

48. Kale-Stuffed Mushroom Caps

Servings: 2
Preparation time: 15 minutes
Nutrition

Calories: 81 kcal

Carbs: 7.3g

Fat: 4.8g

Protein: 3g

Fiber: 2.2g

Sugar: 1.1g

Ingredients:

4 cups kale (fresh, chopped)

2 tbsp. Olive oil

3 tsp. Garlic (minced)

1 tsp. Garlic powder

½ Tsp. Salt

4 portobello mushroom caps (large)

Total number of **Ingredients:** 6

Directions:

Sauté the garlic and olive oil in a pan. Before it burns, add the kale, stirring well for about 7 minutes. Then add the garlic powder and salt, stirring well for 3 more minutes. Turn off the heat.

Mix the other half of the olive oil and garlic, then rub on the mushroom caps.

Place caps on the grill on medium heat, allowing them to cook for about 10 minutes—5 minutes per side—until tender.

Remove from the grill and divide your kale mixture on top of each cap; serve and enjoy.

Check out this recipe for a delicious, unique treat
to spice up any dinner or gathering.

49. Boiled Seasoned Veggies (Instant Pot)

Servings: 1
Preparation time: 15 minutes
Nutrition
Calories: 816 kcal

Carbs: 66.1g

Fat: 55.8g

Protein: 12.5g

Fiber: 26.9g

Sugar: 32.2g

Ingredients:

1 eggplant (cubed, medium)

2 zucchinis (halved and sliced)

8 oz. Mushrooms (of choice, quartered)

6 cloves garlic (minced)

3 sprigs fresh rosemary (chopped)

¼ Cup olive oil

2 tbsp. Balsamic vinegar

2 tbsp. Dried onion flakes

½ Cup water

Salt and pepper to taste

Total number of **Ingredients:** 11

Directions:

Preheat oven to 400°f.

In a bowl, mix all Ingredients, lightly tossing and making sure all the vegetables are coated in spices and olive oil.

Throw mixture in a pressure pot with ½ cup of water and cook on high pressure for about 20 minutes, allowing for natural pressure release once time is up.

Open, and add more or less of the spices you prefer.

If you're a veggie lover, you are sure to love this dish. Vegetables are heart-healthy, filling, and kind alternatives to other non-vegan or ketogenic meals!

50. Cauliflower Soup (Instant Pot)

Servings: 6
Preparation time: 10 minutes
Nutrition

Calories: 43 kcal

Carbs: 4.3g

Fat: 2.2g

Protein: 1.4g

Fiber: 1.3g

Sugar: 2.2g

Ingredients:

3 cups vegetable stock

2 tsp. Thyme powder

½ Tsp. Matcha green tea powder

1 head cauliflower (about 2.5 cups, florets)

1 tbsp. Olive oil

5 garlic cloves (minced)

Salt and pepper to taste

Total number of **Ingredients:** 8

Directions:

In an instant pressure pot, add the vegetable stock, thyme, and matcha powder on medium heat. Bring to a boil.

Add the cauliflower and set timer for 10 minutes on high pressure, allowing for quick pressure release when finished.

In a saucepan, add garlic and olive oil until tender, and you can smell it; then add it to the pot along with salt and cook for 1 to 2 minutes.

Turn off the heat and. Blend the soup until smooth and creamy with a blender.

51. Tahini Covered Eggplant

Servings: 1
Preparation time: 20 minutes
Nutrition
Calories: 474 kcal
Carbs: 41.9g
Fat: 31.2g
Protein: 6.3g
Fiber: 21.9g
Sugar: 17.9g

Ingredients:
1 eggplant (sliced)
1 garlic clove (minced)
1 tbsp. Olive oil
Salt and pepper (to taste)
½ Cup chopped parsley
Sauce:
1 tsp. Olive oil
1 onion (chopped)
½ Garlic clove (chopped)
Handful of parsley (chopped)
⅓ Cup almond milk
1 tsp. Tahini
Salt (to taste)
Total number of **Ingredients:** 12

Directions:
Preheat oven to 350°f.
Mix all Ingredients in a medium bowl with the eggplant.
Place on baking tray, and bake for 30 minutes.
Sauce:
Blend all Ingredients. Add more or less to taste.

DESSERT AND SNACK RECIPES

52. Banana-Nut Bread Bars

Preparation time: 5 minutes
Cooking time: 30 minutes

Servings: 9 bars

Ingredients

Nonstick cooking spray (optional)

2 large ripe bananas

1 tablespoon maple syrup

½ Teaspoon vanilla extract

2 cups old-fashioned rolled oats

½ Teaspoons salt

¼ Cup chopped walnuts

Directions:

Preheat the oven to 350°f. Lightly coat a 9-by-9-inch baking pan with nonstick cooking spray (if using) or line with parchment paper for oil-free baking.

In a medium bowl, mash the bananas with a fork. Add the maple syrup and vanilla extract and mix well. Add the oats, salt, and walnuts, mixing well.

Transfer the batter to the baking pan and bake for 25 to 30 minutes, until the top is crispy. Cool completely before slicing into 9 bars. Transfer to an airtight storage container or a large plastic bag.

Nutrition (1 bar): calories: 73; fat: 1g; protein: 2g; carbohydrates: 15g; fiber: 2g; sugar: 5g; sodium: 129mg

53.   Lemon Coconut Cilantro Rolls

Preparation time: 30 minutes • chill time: 30 minutes
Servings: 16 pieces

Ingredients

½ Cup fresh cilantro, chopped

1 cup sprouts (clover, alfalfa)

1 garlic clove, pressed

2 tablespoons ground brazil nuts or almonds

2 tablespoons flaked coconut

1 tablespoon coconut oil

Pinch cayenne pepper

Pinch sea salt

Pinch freshly ground black pepper

Zest and juice of 1 lemon

2 tablespoons ground flaxseed

1 to 2 tablespoons water

2 whole-wheat wraps, or corn wraps

Directions:

Put everything but the wraps in a food processor and pulse to combine. Or combine the Ingredients in a large bowl. Add the water, if needed, to help the mix come together.

Spread the mixture out over each wrap, roll it up, and place it in the fridge for 30 minutes to set.

Remove the rolls from the fridge and slice each into 8 pieces to serve as appetizers or sides with a soup or stew.

Get the best flavor by buying whole raw brazil nuts or almonds, toasting them lightly in a dry skillet or toaster oven, and then grinding them in a coffee grinder.

Nutrition (1 piece) calories: 66; total fat: 4g; carbs: 6g; fiber: 1g; protein: 2g

54.   Tamari Almonds

Preparation time: 5 minutes
Cooking time: 15 minutes
Servings: 8

Ingredients

1 pound raw almonds

3 tablespoons tamari or soy sauce

2 tablespoons extra-virgin olive oil

1 tablespoon Nutritional yeast

1 to 2 teaspoons chili powder, to taste

Directions:

Preheat the oven to 400ºf.

Line a baking sheet with parchment paper.

In a medium bowl, combine the almonds, tamari, and olive oil until well coated.

Spread the almonds on the prepared baking sheet and roast for 10 to 15 minutes, until browned.

Cool for 10 minutes, then season with the Nutritional yeast and chili powder.

Transfer to a glass jar and close tightly with a lid.

Nutrition: calories: 364; fat: 32g; protein: 13g; carbohydrates: 13g; fiber: 7g; sugar: 3g; sodium: 381mg

55.   Tempeh Taco Bites

Preparation time: 5 minutes
Cooking time: 45 minutes
Servings: 3 dozen

Ingredients

8 ounces tempeh

3 tablespoons soy sauce

2 teaspoons ground cumin

1 teaspoon chili powder

1 teaspoon dried oregano

1 tablespoon olive oil

1/2 cup finely minced onion

2 garlic cloves, minced

Salt and freshly ground black pepper

2 tablespoons tomato paste

1 chipotle chile in adobo, finely minced

1/4 cup hot water or vegetable broth, homemade or store-bought, plus more if needed

36 phyllo pastry cups, thawed

1/2 cup basic guacamole, homemade or store-bought

18 ripe cherry tomatoes, halved

Directions

In a medium saucepan of simmering water, cook the tempeh for 30 minutes. Drain well, then finely mince and place it in a bowl. Add the soy sauce, cumin, chili powder, and oregano. Mix well and set aside.

In a medium skillet, heat the oil over medium heat. Add the onion, cover, and cook for 5 minutes. Stir in the garlic, then add the tempeh mixture and cook, stirring, for 2 to 3 minutes. Season with salt and pepper to taste. Set aside.

In a small bowl, combine the tomato paste, chipotle, and the hot water or broth. Return tempeh mixture to heat and in stir tomato-chile mixture and cook for 10 to 15 minutes, stirring occasionally, until the liquid is absorbed.

The mixture should be fairly dry, but if it begins to stick to the pan, add a little more hot water, 1 tablespoon at a time. Taste, adjusting seasonings if necessary. Remove from the heat.

To assemble, fill the phyllo cups to the top with the tempeh filling, using about 2 teaspoons of filling in each. Top with a dollop of guacamole and a cherry tomato half and serve.

56. Mushroom Croustades

Preparation time: 10 minutes
Cooking time: 10 minutes
Servings: 12 croustades

Ingredients

12 thin slices whole-grain bread

1 tablespoon olive oil, plus more for brushing bread

2 medium shallots, chopped

2 garlic cloves, minced

12 ounces white mushrooms, chopped

1/4 cup chopped fresh parsley

1 teaspoon dried thyme

1 tablespoon soy sauce

Directions

Preheat the oven to 400°f. Using a 3-inch round pastry cutter or a drinking glass, cut a circle from each bread slice. Brush the bread circles with oil and press them firmly but gently into a mini-muffin tin. Bake until the bread is toasted, about 10 minutes.

Meanwhile, in a large skillet, heat the 1 tablespoon oil over medium heat. Add the shallots, garlic, and mushrooms and sauté for 5 minutes to soften the vegetables. Stir in the parsley, thyme, and soy sauce and cook until the liquid is absorbed, about 5 minutes longer. Spoon the mushroom mixture into the croustade cups and return to the oven for 3 to 5 minutes to heat through. Serve warm.

57. Stuffed Cherry Tomatoes

Preparation time: 15 minutes
Cooking time: 0 minutes
Servings: 6

Ingredients

2 pints cherry tomatoes, tops removed and centers scooped out

2 avocados, mashed

Juice of 1 lemon

½ Red bell pepper, minced

4 green onions (white and green parts), finely minced

1 tablespoon minced fresh tarragon

Pinch of sea salt

Directions:

Place the cherry tomatoes open-side up on a platter.

In a small bowl, -combine the avocado, lemon juice, bell pepper, scallions, tarragon, and salt.

Stir until well -combined. Scoop into the cherry tomatoes and serve immediately.

58. Spicy Black Bean Dip

Preparation time: 10 minutes
Cooking time: 0 minutes
Servings: 2 cups

Ingredients

1 (14-ounce) can black beans, drained and rinsed, or 1½ cups cooked

Zest and juice of 1 lime

1 tablespoon tamari, or soy sauce

¼ Cup water

¼ Cup fresh cilantro, chopped

1 teaspoon ground cumin

Pinch cayenne pepper

Directions:

Put the beans in a food processor (best choice) or blender, along with the lime zest and juice, tamari, and about ¼ cup of water.

Blend until smooth, then blend in the cilantro, cumin, and cayenne.

If you don't have a blender or prefer a different consistency, simply transfer it to a bowl once the beans have been puréed and stir in the spices, instead of forcing the blender.

Nutrition (1 cup) calories: 190; total fat: 1g; carbs: 35g; fiber: 12g; protein: 13g

59.   French Onion Pastry Puffs

Preparation time: 10 minutes
Cooking time: 35 minutes - makes 24 puffs

Ingredients

2 tablespoons olive oil

2 medium sweet yellow onions, thinly sliced

1 garlic clove, minced

1 teaspoon chopped fresh rosemary

Salt and freshly ground black pepper

1 tablespoon capers

1 sheet frozen vegan puff pastry, thawed

18 pitted black olives, quartered

Directions

In a medium skillet, heat the oil over medium heat. Add the onions and garlic, season with rosemary and salt and pepper to taste. Cover and cook until very soft, stirring occasionally, about 20 minutes. Stir in the capers and set aside.

Preheat the oven to 400°f. Roll out the puff pastry and cut into 2- to 3-inch circles using a lightly floured pastry cutter or drinking glass. You should get about 2 dozen circles.

Arrange the pastry circles on baking sheets and top each with a heaping teaspoon of onion mixture, patting down to smooth the top.

Top with 3 olive quarters, arranged decoratively—either like flower petals emanating from the center or parallel to each other like 3 bars.

Bake until pastry is puffed and golden brown, about 15 minutes. Serve hot.

60. Cheezy Cashew–Roasted Red Pepper Toasts

Preparation time: 15 minutes
Cooking time: 0 minutes
Servings: 16 to 24 toasts

Ingredients

2 jarred roasted red peppers

1 cup unsalted cashews

1/4 cup water

1 tablespoon soy sauce

2 tablespoons chopped green onions

1/4 cup Nutritional yeast

2 tablespoons balsamic vinegar

2 tablespoons olive oil

Directions

Use canapé or cookie cutters to cut the bread into desired shapes about 2 inches wide. If you don't have a cutter, use a knife to cut the bread into squares, triangles, or rectangles. You should get 2 to 4 pieces out of each slice of bread. Toast the bread and set aside to cool.

Coarsely chop 1 red pepper and set aside. Cut the remaining pepper into thin strips or decorative shapes and set aside for garnish.

In a blender or food processor, grind the cashews to a fine powder. Add the water and soy sauce and process until smooth. Add the chopped red pepper and puree. Add the green onions, Nutritional yeast, vinegar, and oil and process until smooth and well blended.

Spread a spoonful of the pepper mixture onto each of the toasted bread pieces and top decoratively with the reserved pepper strips. Arrange on a platter or tray and serve.

61.Baked Potato Chips

Preparation time: 10 minutes
Cooking time: 30 minutes
Servings: 4

Ingredients

1 large russet potato

1 teaspoon paprika

½ Teaspoon garlic salt

¼ Teaspoon vegan sugar

¼ Teaspoon onion powder

¼ Teaspoon chipotle powder or chili powder

⅛ Teaspoon salt

⅛ Teaspoon ground mustard

⅛ Teaspoon ground cayenne pepper

1 teaspoon canola oil

⅛ Teaspoon liquid smoke

Directions:

Wash and peel the potato. Cut into thin, 1/10-inch slices (a mandoline slicer or the slicer blade in a food processor is helpful for consistently sized slices).

Fill a large bowl with enough very cold water to cover the potato. Transfer the potato slices to the bowl and soak for 20 minutes.

Preheat the oven to 400ºf. Line a baking sheet with parchment paper.

In a small bowl, combine the paprika, garlic salt, sugar, onion powder, chipotle powder, salt, mustard, and cayenne.

Drain and rinse the potato slices and pat dry with a paper towel.

Transfer to a large bowl.

Add the canola oil, liquid smoke, and spice mixture to the bowl. Toss to coat.

Transfer the potatoes to the prepared baking sheet.

Bake for 15 minutes. Flip the chips over and bake for 15 minutes longer, until browned. Transfer the chips to 4 storage containers or large glass jars.

Let cool before closing the lids tightly.

Nutrition: calories: 89; fat: 1g; protein: 2g; carbohydrates: 18g; fiber: 2g; sugar: 1g; sodium: 65mg

62. Mushrooms Stuffed With Spinach And Walnuts

Preparation time: 10 minutes
Cooking time: 6 minutes
Servings: 4 to 6 servings

Ingredients

2 tablespoons olive oil

8 ounces white mushroom, lightly rinsed, patted dry, and stems reserved

1 garlic clove, minced

1 cup cooked spinach

1 cup finely chopped walnuts

1/2 cup unseasoned dry bread crumbs

Salt and freshly ground black pepper

Directions

Preheat the oven to 400°f. Lightly oil a large baking pan and set aside. In a large skillet, heat the oil over medium heat. Add the mushroom caps and cook for 2 minutes to soften slightly. Remove from the skillet and set aside.

Chop the mushroom stems and add to the same skillet. Add the garlic and cook over medium heat until softened, about 2 minutes. Stir in the spinach, walnuts, bread crumbs, and salt and pepper to taste. Cook for 2 minutes, stirring well to combine.

Fill the reserved mushroom caps with the stuffing mixture and arrange in the baking pan. Bake until the mushrooms are tender and the filling is hot, about 10 minutes. Serve hot.

63. Salsa Fresca

Preparation time: 15 minutes
Cooking time: 0 minutes
Servings: 4

Ingredients

3 large heirloom tomatoes or other fresh tomatoes, chopped

½ Red onion, finely chopped

½ Bunch cilantro, chopped

2 garlic cloves, minced

1 jalapeño, minced

Juice of 1 lime, or 1 tablespoon prepared lime juice

¼ Cup olive oil

Sea salt

Whole-grain tortilla chips, for serving

Directions:

In a small bowl, combine the tomatoes, onion, cilantro, garlic, jalapeño, lime juice, and olive oil and mix well. Allow to sit at room temperature for 15 minutes. Season with salt.

Serve with tortilla chips.

The salsa can be stored in an airtight container in the refrigerator for up to 1 week.

64. **Guacamole**

Preparation time: 10 minutes
Cooking time: 0 minutes
Servings: 2

Ingredients

2 ripe avocados

2 garlic cloves, pressed

Zest and juice of 1 lime

1 teaspoon ground cumin

Pinch sea salt

Pinch freshly ground black pepper

Pinch cayenne pepper (optional)

Directions:

Mash the avocados in a large bowl. Add the rest of the Ingredients and stir to combine.

Try adding diced tomatoes (cherry are divine), chopped scallions or chives, chopped fresh cilantro or basil, lemon rather than lime, paprika, or whatever you think would taste good!

Nutrition (1 cup) calories: 258; total fat: 22g; carbs: 18g; fiber: 11g; protein: 4g

65.   Veggie Hummus Pinwheels

Preparation time: 10 minutes
Cooking time: 0 minutes
Servings: 3
Ingredients

3 whole-grain, spinach, flour, or gluten-free tortillas
3 large swiss chard leaves
¾ Cup edamame hummus or prepared hummus
¾ Cup shredded carrots

Directions:

Lay 1 tortilla flat on a cutting board.

Place 1 swiss chard leaf over the tortilla. Spread ¼ cup of hummus over the swiss chard. Spread ¼ cup of carrots over the hummus. Starting at one end of the tortilla, roll tightly toward the opposite side.

Slice each roll up into 6 pieces. Place in a single-serving storage container.

Repeat with the remaining tortillas and filling and seal the lids.

Nutrition: calories: 254; fat: 8g; protein: 10g; carbohydrates: 39g; fiber: 8g; sugar: 4g; sodium: 488mg

66. Asian Lettuce Rolls

Preparation time: 15 minutes
Cooking time: 5 minutes
Servings: 4

Ingredients

2 ounces rice noodles

2 tablespoons chopped thai basil

2 tablespoons chopped cilantro

1 garlic clove, minced

1 tablespoon minced fresh ginger

Juice of ½ lime, or 2 teaspoons prepared lime juice

2 tablespoons soy sauce

1 cucumber, julienned

2 carrots, peeled and julienned

8 leaves butter lettuce

Directions:

Cook the rice noodles according to package Directions.

In a small bowl, whisk together the basil, cilantro, garlic, ginger, lime juice, and soy sauce. Toss with the cooked noodles, cucumber, and carrots.

Divide the mixture evenly among lettuce leaves and roll.

Secure with a toothpick and serve immediately.

67.   Pinto-Pecan Fireballs

Preparation time: 5 minutes
Cooking time: 30 minutes
Servings: about 20 pieces

Ingredients

1-1/2 cups cooked or 1 (15.5-ounce) can pinto beans, drained and rinsed

1/2 cup chopped pecans

1/4 cup minced green onions

1 garlic clove, minced

3 tablespoons wheat gluten flour (vital wheat gluten)

3 tablespoons unseasoned dry bread crumbs

4 tablespoons tabasco or other hot sauce

1/4 teaspoon salt

1/8 teaspoon ground cayenne

1/4 cup vegan margarine

Directions

Preheat the oven to 350°f. Lightly oil a 9 x 13-inch baking pan and set aside. Blot the drained beans well with a paper towel, pressing out any excess liquid. In a food processor, combine the pinto beans, pecans, green onions, garlic, flour, bread crumbs, 2 tablespoons of the tabasco, salt, and cayenne. Pulse until well combined, leaving some texture. Use your hands to roll the mixture firmly into 1-inch balls.

Place the balls in the prepared baking pan and bake until nicely browned, about 25 to 30 minutes, turning halfway through.

Meanwhile, in small saucepan, combine the remaining 2 tablespoons tabasco and the margarine and melt over low heat. Pour the sauce over the fireballs and bake 10 minutes longer. Serve immediately.

68.   Sweet Potato Biscuits

Preparation time: 60 minutes
Cooking time: 10 minutes
Servings: 12 biscuits

Ingredients

1 medium sweet potato

3 tablespoons melted coconut oil, divided

1 tablespoon maple syrup

1 cup whole-wheat flour

2 teaspoons baking powder

Pinch sea salt

Directions:

Bake the sweet potato at 350°F for about 45 minutes, until tender.

Allow it to cool, then remove the flesh and mash.

Turn the oven up to 375°F and line a baking sheet with parchment paper or lightly grease it. Measure out 1 cup potato flesh.

In a medium bowl, combine the mashed sweet potato with 1½ tablespoons of the coconut oil and the maple syrup. Mix together the flour and baking powder in a separate medium bowl, then add the flour mixture to the potato mixture and blend well with a fork.

On a floured board, pat the mixture out into a ½-inch-thick circle and cut out 1-inch rounds, or simply drop spoonfuls of dough and pat them into rounds.

Put the rounds onto the prepared baking sheet. Brush the top of each with some of the remaining 1½ tablespoons melted coconut oil. Bake 10 minutes, or until lightly golden on top. Serve hot.

Nutrition (1 biscuit) calories: 116; total fat: 4g; carbs: 19g; fiber: 3g; protein: 3g

69. Lemon And Garlic Marinated Mushrooms

Preparation time: 15 minutes
Cooking time: 0 minutes
Servings: 4 servings

Ingredients

3 tablespoons olive oil

2 tablespoons fresh lemon juice

2 garlic cloves, crushed

1 teaspoon dried marjoram

1/2 teaspoon coarsely ground fennel seed

1/2 teaspoon salt

1/4 teaspoon freshly ground black pepper

8 ounces small white mushrooms, lightly rinsed, patted dry, and stemmed

1 tablespoon minced fresh parsley

Directions

In a medium bowl, whisk together the oil, lemon juice, garlic, marjoram, fennel seed, salt, and pepper. Add the mushrooms and parsley and stir gently until coated.

Cover and refrigerate for at least 2 hours or overnight. Stir well before serving.

70. Garlic Toast

Preparation time: 5 minutes
Cooking time: 5 minutes
Servings: 1 slice

Ingredients

1 teaspoon coconut oil, or olive oil

Pinch sea salt

1 to 2 teaspoons Nutritional yeast

1 small garlic clove, pressed, or ¼ teaspoon garlic powder

1 slice whole-grain bread

Directions:

In a small bowl, mix together the oil, salt, Nutritional yeast, and garlic.

You can either toast the bread and then spread it with the seasoned oil, or brush the oil on the bread and put it in a toaster oven to bake for 5 minutes.

If you're using fresh garlic, it's best to spread it onto the bread and then bake it.

Nutrition (1 slice) calories: 138; total fat: 6g; carbs: 16g; fiber: 4g; protein: 7g

71.Vietnamese-Style Lettuce Rolls

Preparation time: 15 minutes
Cooking time: 0 minutes
Servings: 4 servings

Ingredients

2 green onions

2 tablespoons soy sauce

2 tablespoons rice vinegar

1 teaspoon sugar

1/8 teaspoon crushed red pepper

3 tablespoons water

3 ounces rice vermicelli

4 to 6 soft green leaf lettuce leaves

1 medium carrot, shredded

1/2 medium english cucumber, peeled, seeded, and cut lengthwise into 1/4-inch strips

1/2 medium red bell pepper, cut into 1/4-inch strips

1 cup loosely packed fresh cilantro or basil leaves

Directions

Cut the green part off the green onions and cut them lengthwise into thin slices and set aside. Mince the white part of the green onions and transfer to a small bowl. Add the soy sauce, rice vinegar, sugar, crushed red pepper, and water. Stir to blend and set aside.

Soak the vermicelli in medium bowl of hot water until softened, about 1 minute. Drain the noodles well and cut them into 3-inch lengths. Set aside.

Place a lettuce leaf on a work surface and arrange a row of noodles in the center of the leaf, followed by a few strips of scallion greens, carrot, cucumber, bell pepper, and cilantro. Bring the bottom edge of the leaf over the filling and fold in the two short sides. Roll up gently but tightly. Place the roll seam side down on a serving platter. Repeat with

Remaining Ingredients. Serve with the dipping sauce.

72.   Apple Crumble

Preparation time: 20 minutes
Cooking time: 25 minutes

Servings: 6

Ingredients

FOR THE FILLING

4 to 5 apples, cored and chopped (about 6 cups)

½ Cup unsweetened applesauce, or ¼ cup water

2 to 3 tablespoons unrefined sugar (coconut, date, sucanat, maple syrup)

1 teaspoon ground cinnamon

Pinch sea salt

FOR THE CRUMBLE

2 tablespoons almond butter, or cashew or sunflower seed butter

2 tablespoons maple syrup

1½ cups rolled oats

½ Cup walnuts, finely chopped

½ Teaspoon ground cinnamon

2 to 3 tablespoons unrefined granular sugar (coconut, date, sucanat)

Directions:

Preheat the oven to 350°f. Put the apples and applesauce in an 8-inch-square baking dish, and sprinkle with the sugar, cinnamon, and salt. Toss to combine.

In a medium bowl, mix together the nut butter and maple syrup until smooth and creamy. Add the oats, walnuts, cinnamon, and sugar and stir to coat, using your hands if necessary. (if you have a small food processor, pulse the oats and walnuts together before adding them to the mix.)

Sprinkle the topping over the apples, and put the dish in the oven.

Bake for 20 to 25 minutes, or until the fruit is soft and the topping is lightly browned.

Nutrition calories: 356; total fat: 17g; carbs: 49g; fiber: 7g; protein: 7g

73. Cashew-Chocolate Truffles

Preparation time: 15 minutes
Cooking time: 0 minutes • plus 1 hour to set
Servings: 12 truffles

Ingredients

1 cup raw cashews, soaked in water overnight

¾ Cup pitted dates

2 tablespoons coconut oil

1 cup unsweetened shredded coconut, divided

1 to 2 tablespoons cocoa powder, to taste

Directions:

In a food processor, combine the cashews, dates, coconut oil, ½ cup of shredded coconut, and cocoa powder. Pulse until fully incorporated; it will resemble chunky cookie dough. Spread the remaining ½ cup of shredded coconut on a plate.

Form the mixture into tablespoon-size balls and roll on the plate to cover with the shredded coconut. Transfer to a parchment paper–lined plate or baking sheet. Repeat to make 12 truffles.

Place the truffles in the refrigerator for 1 hour to set. Transfer the truffles to a storage container or freezer-safe bag and seal.

Nutrition (1 truffle): calories 238: fat: 18g; protein: 3g; carbohydrates: 16g; fiber: 4g; sugar: 9g; sodium: 9mg

74.   Banana Chocolate Cupcakes

Preparation time: 20 minutes
Cooking time: 20 minutes
Servings: 12 cupcakes
Ingredients

3 medium bananas

1 cup non-dairy milk

2 tablespoons almond butter

1 teaspoon apple cider vinegar

1 teaspoon pure vanilla extract

1¼ cups whole-grain flour

½ Cup rolled oats

¼ Cup coconut sugar (optional)

1 teaspoon baking powder

½ Teaspoon baking soda

½ Cup unsweetened cocoa powder

¼ Cup chia seeds, or sesame seeds

Pinch sea salt

¼ Cup dark chocolate chips, dried cranberries, or raisins (optional)

Directions:

Preheat the oven to 350°f. Lightly grease the cups of two 6-cup muffin tins or line with paper muffin cups.

Put the bananas, milk, almond butter, vinegar, and vanilla in a blender and purée until smooth. Or stir together in a large bowl until smooth and creamy.

Put the flour, oats, sugar (if using), baking powder, baking soda, cocoa powder, chia seeds, salt, and chocolate chips in another large bowl, and stir to combine. Mix together the wet and dry Ingredients, stirring as little as possible. Spoon into muffin cups, and bake for 20 to 25 minutes. Take the cupcakes out of the oven and let them cool fully before taking out of the muffin tins, since they'll be very moist.

Nutrition (1 cupcake) calories: 215; total fat: 6g; carbs: 39g; fiber: 9g; protein: 6g

75.   Minty Fruit Salad

Preparation time: 15 minutes
Cooking time: 5 minutes

Servings: 4

Ingredients

¼ Cup lemon juice (about 2 small lemons)

4 teaspoons maple syrup or agave syrup

2 cups chopped pineapple

2 cups chopped strawberries

2 cups raspberries

1 cup blueberries

8 fresh mint leaves

Directions:

Beginning with 1 mason jar, add the Ingredients in this order:

1 tablespoon of lemon juice, 1 teaspoon of maple syrup, ½ cup of pineapple, ½ cup of strawberries, ½ cup of raspberries, ¼ cup of blueberries, and 2 mint leaves.

Repeat to fill 3 more jars. Close the jars tightly with lids.

Place the airtight jars in the refrigerator for up to 3 days.

Nutrition: calories: 138; fat: 1g; protein: 2g; carbohydrates: 34g; fiber: 8g; sugar: 22g; sodium: 6mg

76. Mango Coconut Cream Pie

Preparation time: 20 minutes • chill time: 30 minutes

Servings: 8

Ingredients

FOR THE CRUST

½ Cup rolled oats

1 cup cashews

1 cup soft pitted dates

FOR THE FILLING

1 cup canned coconut milk

½ Cup water

2 large mangos, peeled and chopped, or about 2 cups frozen chunks

½ Cup unsweetened shredded coconut

Directions:

Put all the crust Ingredients in a food processor and pulse until it holds together. If you don't have a food processor, chop everything as finely as possible and use ½ cup cashew or almond butter in place of half the cashews. Press the mixture down firmly into an 8-inch pie or springform pan.

Put the all filling Ingredients in a blender and purée until smooth (about 1 minute). It should be very thick, so you may have to stop and stir until it's smooth.

Pour the filling into the crust, use a rubber spatula to smooth the top, and put the pie in the freezer until set, about 30 minutes. Once frozen, it should be set out for about 15 minutes to soften before serving.

Top with a batch of coconut whipped cream scooped on top of the pie once it's set. Finish it off with a sprinkling of toasted shredded coconut.

Nutrition (1 slice) calories: 427; total fat: 28g; carbs: 45g; fiber: 6g; protein: 8g

77.   Cherry-Vanilla Rice Pudding (pressure cooker)

Preparation time: 5 minutes

Serves 4-6

Ingredients

1 cup short-grain brown rice

1¾ cups nondairy milk, plus more as needed

1½ cups water

4 tablespoons unrefined sugar or pure maple syrup (use 2 tablespoons if you use a sweetened milk), plus more as needed

1 teaspoon vanilla extract (use ½ teaspoon if you use vanilla milk)

Pinch salt

¼ Cup dried cherries **or** ½ cup fresh or frozen pitted cherries

Directions

In your electric pressure cooker's cooking pot, combine the rice, milk, water, sugar, vanilla, and salt.

High pressure for 30 minutes. Close and lock the lid, and select high pressure for 30 minutes.

Pressure release. Once the cook time is complete, let the pressure release naturally, about 20 minutes. Unlock and remove the lid. Stir in the cherries and put the lid back on loosely for about 10 minutes. Serve, adding more milk or sugar, as desired.

Nutrition calories: 177; total fat: 1g; protein: 3g; sodium: 27mg; fiber: 2g

78.   Mint Chocolate Chip Sorbet

Preparation time: 5 minutes
Cooking time: 0 minutes
Servings: 1
Ingredients

1 frozen banana

1 tablespoon almond butter, or peanut butter, or other nut or seed butter

2 tablespoons fresh mint, minced

¼ Cup or less non-dairy milk (only if needed)

2 to 3 tablespoons non-dairy chocolate chips, or cocoa nibs

2 to 3 tablespoons goji berries (optional)

Directions:

Put the banana, almond butter, and mint in a food processor or blender and purée until smooth.

Add the non-dairy milk if needed to keep blending (but only if needed, as this will make the texture less solid). Pulse the chocolate chips and goji berries (if using) into the mix so they're roughly chopped up.

Nutrition calories: 212; total fat: 10g; carbs: 31g; fiber: 4g; protein: 3g

79.   Peach-Mango Crumble (pressure cooker)

Preparation time: 10 minutes

Serves 4-6

Ingredients

3 cups chopped fresh or frozen peaches

3 cups chopped fresh or frozen mangos

4 tablespoons unrefined sugar or pure maple syrup, divided

1 cup gluten-free rolled oats

½ Cup shredded coconut, sweetened or unsweetened

2 tablespoons coconut oil or vegan margarine

Directions

In a 6- to 7-inch round baking dish, toss together the peaches, mangos, and 2 tablespoons of sugar. In a food processor, combine the oats, coconut, coconut oil, and remaining 2 tablespoons of sugar. Pulse until combined. (if you use maple syrup, you'll need less coconut oil. Start with just the syrup and add oil if the mixture isn't sticking together.) Sprinkle the oat mixture over the fruit mixture.

Cover the dish with aluminum foil. Put a trivet in the bottom of your electric pressure cooker's cooking pot and pour in a cup or two of water. Using a foil sling or silicone helper handles, lower the pan onto the trivet.

High pressure for 6 minutes. Close and lock the lid, and select high pressure for 6 minutes.

Pressure release. Once the cook time is complete, quick release the pressure. Unlock and remove the lid.

Let cool for a few minutes before carefully lifting out the dish with oven mitts or tongs. Scoop out portions to serve.

Nutrition calories: 321; total fat: 18g; protein: 4g; sodium: 2mg; fiber: 7g

80. Zesty Orange-Cranberry Energy Bites

Preparation time: 10 minutes • chill time: 15 minutes
Servings: 12 bites

Ingredients

2 tablespoons almond butter, or cashew or sunflower seed butter

2 tablespoons maple syrup, or brown rice syrup

¾ Cup cooked quinoa

¼ Cup sesame seeds, toasted

1 tablespoon chia seeds

½ Teaspoon almond extract, or vanilla extract

Zest of 1 orange

1 tablespoon dried cranberries

¼ Cup ground almonds

Directions:

In a medium bowl, mix together the nut or seed butter and syrup until smooth and creamy. Stir in the rest of the Ingredients, and mix to make sure the consistency is holding together in a ball. Form the mix into 12 balls.

Place them on a baking sheet lined with parchment or waxed paper and put in the fridge to set for about 15 minutes.

If your balls aren't holding together, it's likely because of the moisture content of your cooked quinoa. Add more nut or seed butter mixed with syrup until it all sticks together.

Nutrition (1 bite) calories: 109; total fat: 7g; carbs: 11g; fiber: 3g; protein: 3g

81. Almond-Date Energy Bites

Preparation time: 5 minutes • chill time: 15 minutes

Servings: 24 bites

Ingredients

1 cup dates, pitted

1 cup unsweetened shredded coconut

¼ Cup chia seeds

¾ Cup ground almonds

¼ Cup cocoa nibs, or non-dairy chocolate chips

Directions:

Purée everything in a food processor until crumbly and sticking together, pushing down the sides whenever necessary to keep it blending. If you don't have a food processor, you can mash soft medjool dates. But if you're using harder baking dates, you'll have to soak them and then try to purée them in a blender.

Form the mix into 24 balls and place them on a baking sheet lined with parchment or waxed paper. Put in the fridge to set for about 15 minutes. Use the softest dates you can find. Medjool dates are the best for this purpose. The hard dates you see in the baking aisle of your supermarket are going to take a long time to blend up. If you use those, try soaking them in water for at least an hour before you start, and then draining.

Nutrition (1 bite) calories: 152; total fat: 11g; carbs: 13g; fiber: 5g; protein: 3g

Pumpkin pie cups (pressure cooker)

Preparation time: 5 minutes

Serves 4-6

Ingredients

1 cup canned pumpkin purée

1 cup nondairy milk

6 tablespoons unrefined sugar or pure maple syrup (less if using sweetened milk), plus more for sprinkling

¼ Cup spelt flour or all-purpose flour

½ Teaspoon pumpkin pie spice

Pinch salt

Directions

In a medium bowl, stir together the pumpkin, milk, sugar, flour, pumpkin pie spice, and salt. Pour the mixture into 4 heat-proof ramekins. Sprinkle a bit more sugar on the top of each, if you like. Put a trivet in the bottom of your electric pressure cooker's cooking pot and pour in a cup or two of water. Place the ramekins onto the trivet, stacking them if needed (3 on the bottom, 1 on top).

High pressure for 6 minutes. Close and lock the lid, and select high pressure for 6 minutes.

Pressure release. Once the cook time is complete, quick release the pressure. Unlock and remove the lid. Let cool for a few minutes before carefully lifting out the ramekins with oven mitts or tongs. Let cool for at least 10 minutes before serving.

Nutrition calories: 129; total fat: 1g; protein: 3g; sodium: 39mg; fiber: 3g

Coconut and almond truffles

Preparation time: 15 minutes
Cooking time: 0 minutes

Servings: 8 truffles

Ingredients

1 cup pitted dates

1 cup almonds

½ Cup sweetened cocoa powder, plus extra for coating

½ Cup unsweetened shredded coconut

¼ Cup pure maple syrup

1 teaspoon vanilla extract

1 teaspoon almond extract

¼ Teaspoon sea salt

Directions:

In the bowl of a food processor, combine all the **Ingredients** and process until smooth. Chill the mixture for about 1 hour.

Roll the mixture into balls and then roll the balls in cocoa powder to coat.

Serve immediately or keep chilled until ready to serve.

Fudgy Brownies(Pressure cooker)

Preparation time: 10 minutes

Serves 4-6

Ingredients

3 ounces dairy-free dark chocolate

1 tablespoon coconut oil or vegan margarine

½ Cup applesauce

2 tablespoons unrefined sugar

⅓ Cup all-purpose flour

½ Teaspoon baking powder

Pinch salt

Directions

Put a trivet in your electric pressure cooker's cooking pot and pour in a cup or two of two of water. Select sauté or simmer. In a large heat-proof glass or ceramic bowl, combine the chocolate and coconut oil. Place the bowl over the top of your pressure cooker, as you would a double boiler. Stir occasionally until the chocolate is melted, then turn off the pressure cooker. Stir the applesauce and sugar into the chocolate mixture. Add the flour, baking powder, and salt and stir just until combined. Pour the batter into 3 heat-proof ramekins. Put them in a heat-proof dish and cover with aluminum foil. Using a foil sling or silicone helper handles, lower the dish onto the trivet. (alternately, cover each ramekin with foil and place them directly on the trivet, without the dish.)

High pressure for 6 minutes. Close and lock the lid, and select high pressure for 5 minutes.

Pressure release. Once the cook time is complete, quick release the pressure. Unlock and remove the lid.

Let cool for a few minutes before carefully lifting out the dish, or ramekins, with oven mitts or tongs. Let cool for a few minutes more before serving.

Top with fresh raspberries and an extra drizzle of melted chocolate.

Nutrition calories: 316; total fat: 14g; protein: 5g; sodium: 68mg; fiber: 5g

Chocolate macaroons

Preparation time: 10 minutes

Cooking time: 15 minutes

Servings: 8 macaroons

Ingredients

1 cup unsweetened shredded coconut

2 tablespoons cocoa powder

⅔ Cup coconut milk

¼ Cup agave

Pinch of sea salt

Directions:

Preheat the oven to 350°f. Line a baking sheet with parchment paper. In a medium saucepan, cook all the Ingredients over -medium-high heat until a firm dough is formed. Scoop the dough into balls and place on the baking sheet.

Bake for 15 minutes, remove from the oven, and let cool on the baking sheet.

Serve cooled macaroons or store in a tightly sealed container for up to

82.   Chocolate Pudding

Preparation time: 5 minutes
Cooking time: 0 minutes
Servings: 1
Ingredients

1 banana

2 to 4 tablespoons nondairy milk

2 tablespoons unsweetened cocoa powder

2 tablespoons sugar (optional)

½ Ripe avocado or 1 cup silken tofu (optional)

Directions:

In a small blender, combine the banana, milk, cocoa powder, sugar (if using), and avocado (if using). Purée until smooth. Alternatively, in a small bowl, mash the banana very well, and stir in the remaining Ingredients.

Nutrition calories: 244; protein: 4g; total fat: 3g; saturated fat: 1g; carbohydrates: 59g; fiber: 8g

Lime and watermelon granita

Preparation time: 15 minutes • chilling time: 6 hours •
Servings: 4

Ingredients

8 cups seedless -watermelon chunks

Juice of 2 limes, or 2 tablespoons prepared lime juice

½ Cup sugar

Strips of lime zest, for garnish

Directions:

In a blender or food processor, combine the watermelon, lime juice, and sugar and process until smooth. You may have to do this in two batches. After processing, stir well to combine both batches.

Pour the mixture into a 9-by-13-inch glass dish. Freeze for 2 to 3 hours. Remove from the freezer and use a fork to scrape the top layer of ice. Leave the shaved ice on top and return to the freezer.

In another hour, remove from the freezer and repeat. Do this a few more times until all the ice is scraped up. Serve frozen, garnished with strips of lime zest.

83. Coconut-Banana Pudding

Preparation time: 4 minutes
Cooking time: 5 minutes • overnight to set
Servings: 4

Ingredients

3 bananas, divided

1 (13.5-ounce) can full-fat coconut milk

¼ Cup organic cane sugar

1 tablespoon cornstarch

1 teaspoon vanilla extract

2 pinches sea salt

6 drops natural yellow food coloring (optional)

Ground cinnamon, for garnish

Directions:

Combine 1 banana, the coconut milk, sugar, cornstarch, vanilla, and salt in a blender. Blend until smooth and creamy. If you're using the food coloring, add it to the blender now and blend until the color is evenly dispersed.

Transfer to a saucepot and bring to a boil over medium-high heat. Immediately reduce to a simmer and whisk for 3 minutes, or until the mixture thickens to a thin pudding and sticks to a spoon.

Transfer the mixture to a container and allow to cool for 1 hour. Cover and refrigerate overnight to set. When you're ready to serve, slice the remaining 2 bananas and build individual servings as follows: pudding, banana slices, pudding, and so on until a single-serving dish is filled to the desired level. Sprinkle with ground cinnamon.

84. Spiced Apple Chia Pudding

Preparation time: 5 minutes • chill time: 30 minutes

Servings: 1

Ingredients

½ Cup unsweetened applesauce

¼ Cup nondairy milk or canned coconut milk

1 tablespoon chia seeds

1½ teaspoons sugar

Pinch ground cinnamon or pumpkin pie spice

Directions:

In a small bowl, stir together the applesauce, milk, chia seeds, sugar, and cinnamon. Enjoy as is, or let sit for 30 minutes so the chia seeds soften and expand.

Nutrition calories: 153; protein: 3g; total fat: 5g; saturated fat: 1g; carbohydrates: 26g; fiber: 10g

Caramelized pears with balsamic glaze

Preparation time: 5 minutes
Cooking time: 15 minutes

Servings: 4

Ingredients

1 cup balsamic vinegar

¼ Cup plus 3 tablespoons brown sugar

¼ Teaspoon grated nutmeg

Pinch of sea salt

¼ Cup coconut oil

4 pears, cored and cut into slices

Directions:

In a medium saucepan, heat the balsamic vinegar, ¼ cup of the brown sugar, the nutmeg, and salt over medium-high heat, stirring to thoroughly incorporate the sugar. Allow to simmer, stirring occasionally, until the glaze reduces by half, 10 to 15 minutes.

Meanwhile, heat the coconut oil in a large sauté pan over medium-high heat until it shimmers. Add the pears to the pan in a single layer. Cook until they turn golden, about 5 minutes. Add the remaining 3 tablespoons brown sugar and continue to cook, stirring occasionally, until the pears caramelize, about 5 minutes more.

Place the pears on a plate. Drizzle with balsamic glaze and serve.

85.   Salted Coconut-Almond Fudge

Preparation time: 5 minutes • set time: 1 hour •
Servings: 12

Ingredients

¾ Cup creamy almond butter

½ Cup maple syrup

⅓ Cup coconut oil, softened or melted

6 tablespoons fair-trade unsweetened cocoa powder

1 teaspoon coarse or flaked sea salt

Directions:

Line a loaf pan with a double layer of plastic wrap. Place one layer horizontally in the pan with a generous amount of overhang, and the second layer vertically with a generous amount of overhang.

In a medium bowl, gently mix together the almond butter, maple syrup, and coconut oil until well combined and smooth. Add the cocoa powder and gently stir it into the mixture until well combined and creamy.

Pour the mixture into the prepared pan and sprinkle with the sea salt. Bring the overflowing edges of the plastic wrap over the top of the fudge to completely cover it. Place the pan in the freezer for at least 1 hour or overnight, until the fudge is firm.

Remove the pan from the freezer and lift the fudge out of the pan using the plastic-wrap overhangs to pull it out. Transfer to a cutting board and cut into 1-inch pieces.

86. Caramelized Bananas

Preparation time: 5 minutes
Cooking time: 10 minutes

Servings: 2

Ingredients

2 tablespoons vegan margarine or coconut oil

2 bananas, peeled, halved crosswise and then lengthwise

2 tablespoons dark brown sugar, demerara sugar, or coconut sugar

2 tablespoons spiced apple cider

Chopped walnuts, for topping

Directions:

Melt the margarine in a nonstick skillet over medium heat. Add the bananas, and cook for 2 minutes. Flip, and cook for 2 minutes more.

Sprinkle the sugar and cider into the oil around the bananas, and cook for 2 to 3 minutes, until the sauce thickens and caramelizes around the bananas. Carefully scoop the bananas into small bowls, and drizzle with any remaining liquid in the skillet. Sprinkle with walnuts.

Nutrition calories: 384; protein: 4g; total fat: 24g; saturated fat: 13g; carbohydrates: 46g; fiber: 5g

Mixed berries and cream

Preparation time: 10 minutes

Cooking time: 0 minutes

Servings: 4

Ingredients

Two 15-ounce cans full-fat coconut milk

3 tablespoons agave

½ Teaspoon vanilla extract

1 pint fresh blueberries

1 pint fresh raspberries

1 pint fresh strawberries, sliced

Directions:

Refrigerate the coconut milk overnight. When you open the can, the liquid will have separated from the solids. Spoon out the solids and reserve the liquid for another purpose.

In a medium bowl, whisk the agave and vanilla extract into the coconut solids. Divide the berries among four bowls. Top with the coconut cream. Serve immediately.

87. Peanut Butter Cups

Preparation time: 20 minutes
Cooking time: 0 minutes
Servings: 12 cups

Ingredients

1½ cups vegan chocolate chips, divided

½ Cup peanut butter, almond or cashew butter, or sunflower seed butter

¼ Cup packed brown sugar

2 tablespoons nondairy milk

Directions:

Line the cups of a muffin tin with paper liners or reusable silicone cups.

In a small microwave-safe bowl, heat ¾ cup of the chocolate chips on high power for 1 minute. Stir. Continue heating in 30-second increments, stirring after each, until the chocolate is melted.

Pour about 1½ teaspoons of melted chocolate into each prepared muffin cup. Set aside, and allow them to harden.

In a small bowl, stir together the peanut butter, brown sugar, and milk until smooth. Scoop about 1½ teaspoons of the mixture on top of the chocolate base in each cup. It's okay if the chocolate is not yet hardened.

Melt the remaining ¾ cup of chocolate chips using the **Directions** in step 1;pour another 1½ teaspoons of chocolate on top of the peanut butter in each cup, softly spreading it to cover. Let the cups sit until the chocolate hardens, about 15 minutes in the refrigerator or several hours on the counter. Leftovers will keep in the refrigerator for up to 2 weeks.

Nutrition (1 cup) calories: 227; protein: 4g; total fat: 14g; saturated fat: 6g; carbohydrates: 22g; fiber: 3g

Spiced rhubarb sauce

Preparation time: 10 minutes
Cooking time: 15 minutes

Servings: 4

Ingredients

½ Cup water

½ Cup sugar

¼ Teaspoon grated nutmeg

¼ Teaspoon ground ginger

¼ Teaspoon ground cinnamon

1 pound rhubarb, cut into ½- to 1-inch pieces

Directions

In a large saucepan, bring the water, sugar, nutmeg, ginger, and cinnamon to a boil. Add the rhubarb and cook over medium-high heat, stirring frequently, until the rhubarb is soft and saucy, about 10 minutes. Chill for at least 30 minutes before serving.

88.   Chocolate-Coconut Bars

Preparation time: 20 minutes • chill time: 20 minutes

Servings: 16 bars

Ingredients

¼ Cup coconut oil or unsalted vegan margarine, plus more for preparing the baking dish (optional)

2 cups unsweetened shredded coconut

¼ Cup sugar

2 tablespoons maple syrup or *simple syrup*

1 cup vegan chocolate chips

Directions:

Coat the bottom and sides of an 8-9 inch-square baking-dish with coconut oil or line it with parchment paper, set aside.

In a bowl, stir the coconut, sugar, maple syrup, and coconut oil. Transfer the mixture to the prepared baking dish, and press it down firmly with the back of a spoon.

Heat the chocolate chips on high power for 1 minute, (in a microwave-safe bowl). Stir. Continue heating in 30-second increments, stir, until the chocolate is melted. Pour the melted chocolate over the coconut base, and let it sit until the chocolate hardens, about 20 minutes. Cut into 16 bars. Keep covered and refrigerated for up to 1 week.

Nutrition (1 bar) calories: 305; protein: 3g; total fat: 26g; saturated fat: 22g; carbohydrates: 19g; fiber: 6g

SAUCES AND DIPS
89.   Cucumber Bites

Preparation time: 10 minutes (excluding soaking time)
Soaking time: 1-3 hours
Servings: 14 bites
Ingredients:
1 cup almonds – soaked 1-3 hours
¼ Cup cashew nuts – soaked 1-3 hours
Juice of 1 lemon
1 clove garlic –minced
Salt & pepper
1 tsp. Olive oil
1 large cucumber – sliced into approximately 1 inch pieces
1 tomato – diced
½ Cup fresh parsley – roughly chopped

Preparation:
Soak almonds and cashew nuts in warm water for 1-3 hours. The longer you soak them, the softer and creamier they will be.

Put all Ingredients (except cucumber, parsley and tomato) into a blender or food processor.

Blend or process until you get a creamy paste.

If the mix is too thick for your likings you can add a little bit of water.

Remove the mixture from the blender.

Add the diced tomato and fresh parsley and gently mix with a spoon.

Scoop one spoonful of mixture onto each cucumber slice.

8. Sprinkle with black pepper and serve.

90.　Broccoli Crispy Bread

Preparation time: 5 minutes

Cooking time: 30 minutes

Servings: 3-4

Ingredients:

4 cups of broccoli florets – cut into chunks

3 tbsp. Nutritional yeast

1 tbsp. Extra virgin olive oil

2 tbsp. Chia seeds

1 tsp. Baking powder

Salt & pepper

½ Cup fresh basil

Preparation:

Preheat oven to 375f.

Soak the chia seeds with 6 tablespoons of water for about 5 minutes.

Put broccoli into a food processor and pulse until you get a texture similar to rice.

Add Nutritional yeast, basil, salt and pepper, and pulse until Ingredients are well combined.

Transfer the mix into a bowl, add olive oil, baking powder, chia seeds and stir well.

Line a baking tray with a sheet of baking paper.

Pour the dough onto the baking paper and spread evenly. The thinner you make it, the crispier it will be.

Bake in the oven for approximately 30 minute until golden and crispy. Make sure it is cooked in the middle.

Remove from the oven and cut into bars.

Enjoy while still warm or cold.

91. Roasted Pumpkin Seeds

Preparation time: 5 minutes

Cooking time: 25 minutes

Servings: as many as you'd like

Ingredients:

Pumpkin seeds

Extra virgin olive oil

Salt & pepper

Preparation:

Preheat oven to 350f.

Line a baking tray with baking paper or aluminium foil. Either will do.

Place the seeds into a bowl, drizzle with not too much oil but enough to evenly coat them.

Sprinkle with salt and pepper and toss well together.

Pour the seeds onto the baking tray and roast in the oven for approximately 20 minutes or until they become very lightly brown. Keep an eye on them not to burn them.

During cooking remove the tray a few times to stir the seeds.

When completely roasted, remove from oven and let them cool.

Enjoy as nibbles or sprinkle on your salad or soup.

92.   Multi Seeds Crackers

Preparation time: 10 minutes

Cooking time: 1 hour

Servings: 20-30 crackers (depending on your cuts)

Ingredients:

½ Cup chia seeds

½ Cup sunflower seeds

½ Cup pumpkin seeds

½ Cup sesame seeds

1 cup water

1 large clove garlic or 2 small – minced

Salt & pepper

Preparation:

Preheat oven to 300f.

Put all seeds into a large bowl and add water. Stir well until combined.

Let the seeds rest for 3-5 minutes until the chia seeds absorb the water.

Stir again. There should be no more water on the bottom of the bowl.

Use a spatula to spread the mixture onto the baking paper. Spread into two rectangles approximately 12"x 7" in size and approximately 1/8 to ¼ inch thick.

Sprinkle with salt and pepper.

Bake in the oven for 35 minutes.

Remove from oven and turn the rectangles around very carefully with a spatula.

Put back in the oven and back for another 25-35 minutes.

Keep an eye on them to make sure they don't burn.

Remove from oven when the edges are lightly golden.

Set aside to cool down for approximately 10 minutes.

Break the rectangles into crackers and let to cool completely.

You can store these crackers in an airtight container for up to 1 month, but we honestly think they will not last you that long as they are too moreish!

93. Almond Cauliflower

Preparation time: 5 minutes

Cooking time: 30 minutes

Servings: 4

Ingredients:

4 cups cauliflower florets – chopped into bite size chunks

1 tbsp. Extra virgin olive oil

2 tbsp. Almonds – chopped in very small pieces

Preparation:

Preheat oven to 425f.

Line a baking tray with baking paper.

Place cauliflower into a bowl, add olive oil, salt and pepper, almonds and toss everything well together.

Pour the cauliflower onto the baking paper.

Bake in oven for approximately 30 minutes or until golden brown and soft. Stir occasionally.

Remove from oven, sprinkle with ground black pepper and serve.

94. Tahini Dressing

Preparation time: 5 minutes

Servings: 4-5

Ingredients:

¼ Cup tahini paste

Juice of 1 lemon

1 tbsp. Apple cider vinegar

2 tbsp. Extra virgin olive oil

2 clove of garlic – minced

Salt & pepper

Preparation:

Place all Ingredients into a blender (except for water).

Blend until creamy.

If the dressing is too thick, add a little bit of water until it reaches the desired consistency.

95.   Lemon & Mustard Vinaigrette

Preparation time: 5 minutes

Servings: 6 tablespoons

Ingredients:

Juice of 1 lemon

½ Tsp. Dijon mustard

4 tbsp. Extra virgin olive oil

Salt & pepper

Preparation:

Put lemon juice, mustard, salt and pepper into a bowl.

Whisk well until combined.

While whisking, drizzle in the extra virgin olive oil.

Keep whisking vigorously until all Ingredients are combined and you have a medium creamy dressing.

The dressing should be ready at this point. You can taste and adjust any of the Ingredients to taste.

96.   Cheesy Sauce

Preparation time: 5 minutes

Servings: 4

Ingredients:

2 tbsp. Extra virgin olive oil

2 tbsp. Nutritional yeast

Juice of 1 lemon

Salt & pepper

Preparation:

Combine all Ingredients together into a bowl and whisk vigorously.

Serve as an accompaniment to your dishes.

97. Chimichurri Style Sauce

Preparation time: 1-2 minutes

Cooking time: 5 minutes

Servings: 2/3 cup

Ingredients:

½ Cup extra virgin olive oil

1 tsp. Fresh rosemary

1 tsp. Fresh oregano

2 medium cloves garlic – crushed

2 tsp. Smoked paprika

1 bay leaf

¼ Tsp. Sea salt

1 tbsp. Lemon juice

Pinch of black pepper flakes

Preparation:

Put the herbs into a mortar and pestle and lightly pound them. If you do not have a mortar and pestle you can chop them very finely.

Pour olive oil into a pan and warm over medium-low heat.

When oil is hot, remove from heat.

Stir paprika, black pepper flakes, bay leaf and a pinch of salt into the oil.

Add herbs and lemon juice.

Put the sauce into a jar in the fridge and leave it to infuse for a couple of days before using.

98. Peanut Sauce

Preparation time: 10 minutes

Cooking time: 5 minutes

Servings: 1 cup

Ingredients:

½ Cup creamy peanut butter

2 tbsp. Thai red curry paste

¾ Cup coconut milk

2tbsp. Apple cider vinegar

1/2 tbsp. Coconut palm sugar

2 tbsp. Ground peanuts

Salt

Preparation:

Add all Ingredients together into a saucepan and whisk well.

Transfer the pan to the stove and heat up the mix over a low heat while continuing whisking.

Keep a constant eye on the sauce and as soon as it starts bubbling remove from heat. If you like the sauce more liquid, add a little bit of water and whisk. Keep adding water bit by bit until it reaches your desired consistency.

Move the sauce into a bowl and top with ground peanuts.

99. Spicy Almond & Garlic Dip

Preparation time: 5 minutes

Soaking time: overnight

Servings: 1 large cup

Ingredients:

1 cup raw almonds

1 cup almond milk

2 cloves garlic

½ Tsp. Chili powder

¼ Tsp. Smoked paprika

Pinch of salt

Pinch of cayenne pepper

Preparation:

Soak almonds overnight.

Put all **Ingredients** into a blender.

Blend until smooth and creamy.

You can use immediately or refrigerate covered.

100. Cauliflower Hummus

Preparation time: 5 minutes

Cooking time: 5 minutes

Servings: 2 cups

Ingredients:

4 cups cauliflower stems and florets – chopped

2 tbsp. Tahini paste

5 tbsp. Extra virgin olive oil

Juice of 2 lemons

Salt & pepper

Pinch of cumin

Preparation:

Steam or lightly boil cauliflower for approximately 5 minutes or until soft.

Drain and let it cool down completely.

Combine cauliflower, tahini paste, extra virgin olive oil, lemon juice and cumin into a food processor. Process until creamy. Alternatively, you can use a blender.

Add salt and pepper to taste.

You might want to taste it and add more lemon juice or olive oil according to taste.

Serve with raw vegetables.

101. Eggplant & Walnut Spread

Preparation time: 10-15 minutes
Cooking time: 45 minutes
Servings: 1 large cup
Ingredients:
2 x medium round eggplants
1 tbsp. Extra virgin olive oil
1 cup walnuts – chopped
2 cloves garlic
Juice of 1 large lemon
Salt & pepper
1 tsp. Cumin
1/3 cup tahini paste
½ Cup fresh parsley leaves
Preparation:
Preheat oven to 375f.

Place eggplants on a baking tray and rub them with the olive oil.

Stab them with a knife a couple times.

Roast for 45 minutes until they look deflated and wrinkled.

In the meantime, toast the walnuts in a pan over medium-high heat for 3-4 minutes. Leave to cool.

When eggplant is cooked, remove from oven and let it cool down.

Cut the eggplants in half and scoop the flesh out into a food processor.

Add walnuts and all other Ingredients. Process until obtaining a paste.

Serve into a bowl with a drizzle of extra virgin olive oil accompanied by crackers or raw vegetables.

102. Coconut Yogurt Dip

Preparation time: 10 minutes

Servings: 2 cups

Ingredients:

1 ½ cup coconut yogurt

1 large cucumber – peeled and cut into chunks

3 cloves garlic

Juice of 1 lemon

2 tbsp. Extra virgin olive oil

½ Cup fresh coriander – finely chopped

Salt & pepper

Preparation:

Place all Ingredients (except coriander) into a blender and blend until smooth.

Add salt and pepper to taste and the coriander.

Mix well with a spoon.

Refrigerate for about 1 hour to let the flavors infuse.

Stir the dip well before serving.

103. Olive Tapenade

Preparation time: 5 minutes

Servings: 1 cup

Ingredients:

½ Cup black olives

½ Cup green olives

2 cloves garlic

1tsp. Lemon juice

Ground black pepper

Preparation:

Put all Ingredients together into a food processor and process for few seconds. You basically want all Ingredients finely chopped and well mixed together. Be careful not processes for too long otherwise you will have a paste.

Serve to spread onto your favorite crackers.

104. Chunky Rocket Spread

Preparation time: 15 minutes

Servings: 1 cup

Ingredients:

1 ½ cup roasted cashew nuts

1 clove garlic

3 cups rocket leaves

¼ Cup Nutritional yeast

¼ Cup extra virgin olive oil

Juice of ½ lemon

Salt & pepper

Preparation:

Place the cashew nuts, garlic and Nutritional yeast into a food processor.

Pulse gently until the nuts are still chunky and mixed well together with the other Ingredients.

Transfer the mix into a bowl.

Place olive oil and lemon juice into the food processor, then add rocket leaves and pulse to blend.

Transfer the rocket mixture into the bowl with the cashews, season with salt and pepper and mix together with a spoon.

Serve with crackers or other low carb breads.

CONCLUSION

There you have it. You are now well on your way to weight the Vegan way!

Be prepared to feel great, have energy you never had before and achieve the weight loss results you always desired! Thank you for taking the time to read my book and stay tuned for more books on Veganism in the future.

Thanks again for your support!

Plant-based high protein cookbook.

Nutrition guide for athletic performance and muscle growth for a strong body while maintaining.

INTRODUCTION.

Maybe you got a smart pet and decided you had to go vegan. Maybe you're cutting back on eating beef to lighten your environmental footprint. Whatever the reason, when you reduce meat in your diet, getting enough plant-based protein becomes important.

Why? Every meal should include protein since it contributes to satiety (AKA prevents overeating), provides energy, and helps maintain and build muscle (especially if you're a gym junkie).

The good news; Our food supply is now filled with plant-based protein sources. Hemp and chia seeds weren't sitting on grocery store shelves five years ago; neither were high-quality vegan protein powders. We can now meet our needs without burgers or wings. How to do that in the healthiest way possible? Here's everything you need to know about plant-based protein.

What is Plant-based Diet?

Plant-based or plant-forward eating patterns focus on foods primarily from plants. This includes not only fruits and vegetables, but also nuts, seeds, oils, whole grains, legumes, and beans. It doesn't mean that you are vegetarian or vegan and never eat meat or dairy. Rather, you are proportionately choosing more of your foods from plant sources.

Mediterranean and vegetarian diets

What is the evidence that plant-based eating patterns are healthy? Much nutrition research has examined plant-based eating patterns such as the Mediterranean diet and a vegetarian diet. The Mediterranean diet has a foundation of plant-based foods; it also includes fish, poultry, eggs, cheese, and yogurt a few times a week, with meats and sweets less often. The Mediterranean diet has been shown in both large population studies and randomized clinical trials to reduce risk of heart disease, metabolic syndrome, diabetes, certain cancers (specifically colon, breast, and prostate cancer), depression, and in older adults, a decreased risk of frailty, along with better mental and physical function.

Vegetarian diets have also been shown to support health, including a lower risk of developing coronary heart disease, high blood pressure, diabetes, and increased longevity. Plant-based diets offer all the necessary protein, fats, carbohydrates, vitamins, and minerals for optimal health, and are often higher in fibre and phytonutrients. However, some vegans may need to add a supplement (specifically vitamin B12) to ensure they receive all the nutrients required.

Vegetarian diet variety.

Vegetarian diets come in lots of shapes and sizes, and you should choose the version that works best for you.

- Semi-vegetarian or flexitarian includes eggs, dairy foods, and occasionally meat, poultry, fish, and seafood.
- Pescatarian includes eggs, dairy foods, fish, and seafood, but no meat or poultry.
- Vegetarian (sometimes referred to as lacto-ovo vegetarian) includes eggs and dairy foods, but no meat, poultry, fish, or seafood.
- Vegan includes no animal foods.

8 WAYS TO GET STARTED WITH A PLANT-BASED DIET

Here are some tips to help you get started on a plant-based diet.

- **Eat lots of vegetables**: Fill half your plate with vegetables at lunch and dinner. Make sure you include plenty of colours in choosing your vegetables. Enjoy vegetables as a snack with hummus, salsa, or guacamole.
- **Change the way you think about meat**: Have smaller amounts. Use it as a garnish instead of a centrepiece.
- **Choose good fats**: Fats in olive oil, olives, nuts and nut butters, seeds, and avocados are particularly healthy choices.
- **Cook a vegetarian meal at least one night a week**: Build these meals around beans, whole grains, and vegetables.
- **Include whole grains for breakfast**: Start with oatmeal, quinoa, buckwheat, or barley. Then add some nuts or seeds along with fresh fruit.
- **Go for greens**: Try a variety of green leafy vegetables such as kale, collards, Swiss chard, spinach, and other greens each day. Steam, grill, braise, or stir-fry to preserve their flavor and nutrients.
- **Build a meal around a salad**: Fill a bowl with salad greens such as romaine, spinach, Bibb, or red leafy greens. Add an assortment of other vegetables along with fresh herbs, beans, peas, or tofu.
- **Eat fruit for dessert**: A ripe, juicy peach, a refreshing slice of watermelon, or a crisp apple will satisfy your craving for a sweet bite after a meal.

INSPIRATION FOR PLANT-BASED EATING THROUGHOUT THE DAY.

Over time, eating a plant-based diet will become second nature. Here are some ideas to get you started.

Breakfast:

- ✓ Rolled oats with walnuts, banana, and a sprinkle of cinnamon.
- ✓ Breakfast wrap: Fill a whole-wheat tortilla with scrambled egg, black beans, peppers, onions, Monterey jack cheese, and a splash of hot sauce or salsa.
- ✓ Whole-wheat English muffin topped with fresh tomato and avocado slices, and blueberries.

Lunch:

- ✓ Greek salad: Chopped mixed greens with fresh tomato, Kalamata olives, fresh parsley, crumbled feta cheese, extra virgin olive oil, and balsamic vinegar. Whole-wheat pita on the side, fresh melon for dessert.
- ✓ Tomato basil soup, whole-grain crackers with tabbouleh, and an apple.
- ✓ Vegetarian pizza topped with mozzarella cheese, tomatoes, broccoli, onions, peppers, and mushroom. Fresh strawberries for dessert.

Dinner:

- ✓ Grilled vegetable kabobs with grilled tofu, and a quinoa and spinach salad.
- ✓ Whole-wheat pasta with cannellini beans and peas, and a romaine salad with cherry tomatoes, dressed with extra virgin olive oil and balsamic vinegar.
- ✓ Vegetarian chili with a spinach-orzo salad.

These ideas are a great way to begin the plant-based dieting, but surely, we have more for you as we go on.

We're increasingly being told about the benefits of including more plant foods in our diets – both for health and sustainability purposes. In this material, we just want to help you all eat a little more goodness every day.

This means eating healthy staples such as vegetables, fruits, starchy carbohydrates, and unless you're following a vegetarian or vegan diet, fish and lean meat. Eating healthily also means taking in a wide variety of plant-based proteins – but what are these, and how can you incorporate them while retaining protein quality?

WHAT PLANTS ARE HIGH IN PROTEIN?

Plant protein is simply a meaningful food source of protein which is from plants. This group can include pulses, tofu, soya, tempeh, seitan, nuts, seeds, certain grains and even peas. Pulses are a large group of plants, which include chickpeas, lentils, beans (such as black, kidney and adzuki beans) and split peas.

Plant proteins are highly nutritious – not only as good sources of protein, but also because they provide other nutrients such as fibre, vitamins and minerals. Our intake of fibre tends to be too low, however by incorporating certain plant proteins into your diet, such as pulses, peas and nuts, you can easily boost your fibre intake. Did you know that our peas, soya beans and green beans are all a great source of plant fibre?

WHY PROTEIN IS IMPORTANT.

Protein is a vital nutrient responsible for the growth, maintenance and repair of our bodies. So, we must ensure we eat enough high-quality protein every day to keep our bodies healthy. Essentially, protein is fundamental to the basic structure of our body.

There are 9 essential amino acids, and when you eat a protein source containing all of these it is called a 'complete' protein. Animal protein sources are complete, and they include fish, poultry such as chicken and red meat.

Plant sources of protein, with the exception of soya and quinoa, are 'incomplete'. This is because plant protein sources tend to lack at least 1 of the 9 essential amino acids. So how can you ensure that you consume all of the essential amino acids when eating plant proteins? The answer is protein combining.

What is protein combining?

Put simply, protein combining means eating a selection of incomplete plant protein sources, to ensure you consume all of the essential amino acids. As a general rule of thumb, pulses and grains lack different essential amino acids. So, eating a pulse and a grain provides an overall complete protein source.

With this in mind, it's easy to get all the essential amino acids your body needs. For example, a serving of rice and peas or bread and hummus would give you a complete protein source. And remember, you needn't eat your combined proteins in just one meal – they can be eaten at different points during the day or even the week!

Starting a plant-based diet for your optimum health.

Diets centred on a wide variety of plant foods offer affordable, tasty and nutritious options. Plant-based diets which are rich in beans, nuts, seeds, fruit and vegetables, whole grains such as oats, rice, and cereal based foods such as breads, and pasta can provide all the nutrients needed for good health. This includes essential fats, protein, vitamins, minerals and plenty of fibre too.

Well balanced plant-based diets that are also low in saturated fat, can help you manage your weight and may reduce your risk of type 2 diabetes, cardiovascular disease and some cancers. However, as with any diet, plant-based nutrition needs to be planned.

Most nutrients are abundantly available in plant-based diets, but if you are avoiding all or minimising your consumption of animal-derived foods there are a few nutrients that you need to pay attention to.

Calcium: Calcium is essential for bone health, along with weight bearing exercise and a healthy diet. An adult requires approximately 700mg per day. Dairy foods are rich in calcium but if you are not eating these make sure you obtain calcium from other sources like fortified plant based dairy alternatives, dried fruit e.g. figs, nuts such as almonds, leafy green vegetables, red kidney beans, sesame seeds, tahini and tofu to lower your risk of bone fractures.

Omega 3 fatty acids: These fats have been shown to be important for health and are commonly found in oily fish. However, if you are not eating fish, plant sources of omega 3 include walnuts, flax (linseed), hemp seeds, chia seeds and soya beans. Oils such as hemp, rapeseed and flaxseed oil provide essential omega 3 fats and are preferable to corn/sunflower oils.

Vitamin D: Vitamin D is needed to keep bones, teeth and muscles healthy and is made in our bodies when our skin is exposed to appropriate sunlight. In the UK this is usually between April and September. During the winter months, we need to get vitamin D from our diet because the sun isn't strong enough for the body to make it.

Plant-based sources of vitamin D include sun-exposed mushrooms and fortified foods such as vegetable spreads, breakfast cereals and plant based dairy alternatives. Since it's difficult to get enough vitamin D from food alone, everyone should consider taking a daily supplement of 10mcg/ day during the autumn and winter months. Some vitamin D supplements are not suitable for vegans. Vitamin D2 and lichen-derived vitamin D3 are suitable.

Iodine: The major sources of iodine in our diet are dairy products and fish. The iodine content of plant foods depends on the iodine content of the soil which is variable. Foods grown closer to the ocean tend to be higher in iodine. Where soils are iodine deficient, iodised salt and seaweed provide iodine which is needed in moderation. As the iodine content of seaweed is variable, and sometimes too high, guidance is not to consume sea vegetables more than once a week. An excess of iodine is also unhealthy so if you are taking a supplement, discuss this with your dietician.

Vitamin B12: We need vitamin B12 for many reasons. Too little can result in fatigue, anaemia and nerve damage and increase homo-cysteine levels leading to cardiovascular disease. Most people get vitamin B12 by eating animal products. If you are eliminating all animal derived foods, the only reliable sources of vitamin B12 are fortified foods and supplements. Suitable B12-fortified foods include some breakfast cereals, yeast extracts, soya yoghurts and non-dairy milks. To make sure you get enough vitamin B12, either eat fortified foods at least twice a day, aiming for 3mcg of vitamin B12 a day, or take a supplement, 10mcg daily or at least 2000mcg weekly. If you are worried whether you are obtaining sufficient vitamin B12, a dietician can calculate your intake from food/supplements or a doctor can check your blood homo-cysteine levels.

Iron: Plant sources of iron include dried fruits, whole grains, nuts, green leafy vegetables, seeds and pulses. The form of iron in plant foods is absorbed far less efficiently compared to iron from animal derived sources such as meat and eggs. Eat plenty of fruits and vegetables rich in vitamin C to help the iron to be absorbed e.g. citrus fruits, strawberries, green leafy vegetables and peppers.

Zinc: Phytates found in plant foods such as whole grains and beans reduce zinc absorption, so it's important to eat good sources of zinc-containing foods. Eat fermented soya such as tempeh and miso; beans (soak dried beans then rinse before cooking to increase zinc absorption); whole grains; nuts; seeds and some fortified breakfast cereals.

Selenium: Plant sources of this mineral include grains, seeds and nuts. Just two Brazil nuts daily will provide you with your daily requirement of selenium.

Protein: Plant-based sources of protein include lentils, beans, chickpeas, seeds, nuts and nut butters (e.g. peanut butter), and tofu. Eggs, and dairy are also good sources if you are eating these. Meat substitutes like vegetarian burgers, soya sausages, and other meat alternatives can be useful for those adapting to a plant-based diet and can provide a source of protein. However, as with any processed foods, these can often be high in salt and fat so should be used in moderation.

These products may contain animal ingredients such as eggs, milk derivatives and honey so careful label reading is necessary if you wish to follow a vegan diet.

It's a warm reminder that, well-planned plant-based diets can support healthy living at every age and life-stage. Include a wide variety of healthy whole foods to ensure your diet is balanced and sustainable. Eat your veggies! Compared to the average Western diet, plant-based diets are rich in everything you've been told to eat more of: fibre from fruits and vegetables, and fats from nuts and seeds—while generally low in the saturated fat that animal-based foods can be rich in.

SOAKING METHODS AND COOKING.

Whenever "soaking" is mentioned, we "think" beans and that's correct. We know that beans is one of the most potent source of protein and contains fractions of other nutrients too as recently confirmed by health experts.

Beans are the musical fruit, the more you eat the more you...well, toot. Let's face it, beans are yummy. But the gas sucks. So to keep your beans more tasty and less musical it's always a good idea to learn about the best methods for soaking beans. Soaking beans is not hard. Sure, it may take a few hours but it's not like you have to stand there watching them get submerged. Just be sure to plan a little ahead of time when making recipes calling for dried beans or legumes.

Soaking your beans helps them cook faster and more evenly, and it can also make them easier to digest. If you add salt to the soaking water (in other words, make a brine), your beans will cook even faster; the salt helps break down their skins. Here are a few methods; choose the one that best fits your schedule. And keep in mind that you never need to soak legumes like lentils or split peas.

To help make the most of your frugal and yummy bean meals I've summarized three easy methods for soaking beans, they are: the long soak method (where you soak beans overnight), the quick soak method, and the quick cook method.

The Long Soak
The "Long Soak" method is the most common way to soak your beans. Just put your beans in a large bowl or pot of water and let them sit submerged for 8-12

hours overnight. Soaking beans overnight actually begins bean germination and promotes enzyme release. The germination process is what breaks down all the complex bean sugars. Breaking down the complex sugar is a good thing as this is what gives us gas. Apparently, soaking beans overnight using the "Long Soak" method can reduce complex sugars by up to 60 percent. I usually use this method of soaking dried beans with exceptional results – no gastrointestinal gusts.

Quick Soaking Beans (The Power Soak).

I have tried the "Quick Soaking Beans or Power Soak" method a few times. But basically, just bring a pot of water to boil, add your beans, and then let them boil for about three minutes. After boiling, remove the beans from the stove and let them sit in the hot water for 2-6 hours. This method apparently removes 80 percent of complex bean sugars. How does that toot your horn?

Quick Cook

While bigger beans like red beans, chick peas, and navy beans do require soaking – some smaller beans and legumes require little to no soaking. Legumes like lentils, mung beans, or split peas can be added to soup (like lentil soup) without ever needing time soaked in water before cooking. If you're using smaller beans and legumes, then use the "Quick Cook" or "no soak method" where you just throw your dried beans into a pot and cook it till you're satisfied with its degree of softness. I wouldn't recommend the "Quick Cook" method for tougher beans like kidney or chick peas cause you'll have a lot of gas and may not feel your stomach normally for a couple of days.

More on beans soaking and cooking.

Easy, forgiving, healthy and economical, beans are a home cook's secret weapon. Yes, canned beans are convenient, but knowing how to cook dried beans gives you flexibility, and makes for a far more delicious meal.

A few handy tips:

- Check for a date on the beans; freshness matters. Dried beans last up to two years, but are best cooked within a year of harvest. Always rinse beans before cooking, and check for stray rocks, twigs and leaves.
- Leave substantial time for bean soaking (either overnight or using our shortcut method) and cooking. If you are short on time, choose lentils or adzuki beans, which cook quickly and don't need soaking.
- To add more flavour, consider cooking your beans in stock or broth instead of water.

Choosing Your Bean

There are dozens of varieties of beans, but these are the ones you're most likely to encounter. Use this list to figure out what to buy when you want them to fall apart into a soup or dal (lentils, flageolet and split peas), or hold their shape for salads (adzuki, black-eyed peas, chickpeas, cranberry and kidney). As a general rule, 1 cup dried beans make about 3 cups cooked.

Above, from left: cranberry beans, lentils, black beans, chickpeas, red kidney beans, split peas, pinto beans and cannellini beans.

Adzuki: These small, scarlet beans cook quickly, with a sweet flavour. They're often used in Japanese bean paste desserts, but are versatile enough for salads, soups and stews.

Black: Also known as turtle beans, these full-flavored beans are classic in Latin American cooking, usually for soups and stews.

Black-eyed peas: These small earthy-flavoured beans, also known as Crowder peas and cowpeas, are particularly cherished in Southern cooking.

Cannellini: These mild, starchy white beans are often used in soups and stews, particularly in Italian cooking.

Chickpeas: These nutty-tasting legumes, also known as garbanzo beans, are used all the globe in many guises: soups, stews, dips and even fried or roasted as a snack.

Cranberry: These red-and-brown speckled beans have a rich, toasty flavour. They hold their shape well for salads, soups and stews.

Fava: Dried favas, also known as broad beans, have a very strong, meaty flavour and a somewhat thick skin. Beloved in Middle Eastern cuisine, they are made into soups, stews and salads.

Flageolet: These are a creamy, smooth, pale green-to-white-hued bean from France with a thin skin. They work well for soups and purées.

Great Northern: These large white beans with a firm texture and gentle, nutty flavour are great for stews and soups.

Kidney: These large red beans are often used in salads and chili. Some people find them particularly hard to digest, but soaking and rinsing before cooking can help, as does using a pressure cooker.

Lentils: There are several varieties of these tiny legumes, ranging from shiny black beluga lentils, which remain nicely intact for salads, to orange-hued "red" lentils, which collapse into a thick purée when simmered. In between, there are brown lentils (good all-purpose lentils) and more expensive French green lentils, also called Puy lentils, which take a bit longer to cook and have a nice sweet flavour. All lentils are relatively quick-cooking and don't need any pre-soaking.

Lima: Large white dried lima beans take on a velvety, creamy texture after simmering, and hold their shape well.

Navy: These small white beans have a nutty flavour, and cook more quickly than other white beans. They are the traditional choice for Boston baked beans. Like red kidney beans, they can be easier to digest if you soak and rinse before cooking.

Pinto: These are small brownish-pink beans frequently used in Mexican and other Latin American cooking, particularly for refried beans, stews and chili.

Split peas: Green or yellow split peas are small legumes often used in soups, and in the case of the yellow ones, Indian dals. They do not need to be soaked before cooking.

Seasoning

You can simmer beans and other legumes in nothing but plain water with salt and get great results. But before you start cooking, take a minute to add the herbs, spices, stock and aromatics that make beans even better. Even a humble onion and a bay leaf works wonders.

There's a myth out regarding beans and salt — specifically, that you should never salt your beans before cooking because the salt keeps them from cooking through.

That's just not true. You can add salt to your bean pot at the beginning of cooking, and your beans will be better seasoned for it.

If you've ever cooked beans for hours without them softening, it's probably because you're using old beans, or you've got hard (mineral-rich) water, or there's an acidic ingredient in the pot, which can slow down cooking. Using distilled water solves the hard water problem. (And soaking your beans in salt water before cooking not only adds flavour, it can also help them cook more quickly.)

Don't stop at salt and black pepper. Spices like cumin, cinnamon, coriander, ground chilies and allspice add depth and complexity to your bean pot and are traditional additions in many cultures. To give spices a richer character, toast them in the pot for a few minutes until you can smell them, then add beans and liquid.

Cooking

You've soaked your beans (or maybe not) and they're ready for some heat. Simmering them on the stove is the time-honoured method, and I'll tell you how to do it. But you can also cook them in a slow cooker or a pressure cooker — whatever you prefer.

STOVETOP METHOD

Place your beans in your pot and cover them with at least 2 inches of water, and turn the heat to low. Stir them gently and occasionally, never letting them hit a strong boil; this can burst their skins and make them mushy or unevenly cooked. Depending upon the variety, dried beans will cook quickly (about 15 minutes for red lentils) or slowly (up to 3 to 4 hours for un-soaked chickpeas or lima beans).

SLOW-COOKER METHOD

To use a slow cooker, cover your beans with 2 inches of water or broth and salt to taste, and toss any aromatics you like into the pot. Set your machine to the low setting and cook until the beans are done, usually 3 to 6 hours. If you are cooking kidney beans, you need to boil them on the stove for 10 minutes first before adding them to the slow cooker. This makes them much more digestible.

PRESSURE-COOKER METHOD

To cook beans in a pressure cooker, place your soaked or un-soaked beans with enough water to cover by 2 inches into the pressure cooker. Add salt, any aromatics you like, and a tablespoon of neutral oil to help keep the foam from clogging the vent. Make sure not to exceed the maximum fill line for your brand of pressure cooker. This is usually around the halfway mark for beans. Cook at high pressure for anywhere from 5 to 10 minutes for small beans such as black-eyed peas, lentils and split peas, to up to 35 to 40 minutes for larger beans such as chickpeas. Soaked beans will cook more quickly than un-soaked beans.

TESTING FOR DONENESS

How do you know when your beans are ready to eat? Read on for the signs that it's time to taste — and don't toss that cooking liquid.

To make sure your beans are cooked thoroughly, scoop up a couple of beans and blow on them. The skin should curl and wrinkle. Then taste. They are done when they're tender and cooked through to the centre (but not mushy). Let them cool in their cooking liquid.

A tip: Don't throw out your bean cooking liquid, that tasty pot liquor. Salt it if need be, and save it. It's basically a rich vegetarian stock that freezes well for up to six months; use it as you would any other chicken or vegetable stock.

Would you like one of my favourite recipes? I bet you would! Here you go:

SIMPLE PINTO BEANS.

Pinto beans are emblematic of the Old West — good cheap hearty fare. These plain ones are good with just about anything or as a meal in a tin plate, cowboy-style, with a chunk of cornbread. For the best tasting beans, cook at a bare simmer, and keep the liquid level just 1 inch above the beans' surface as they cook.

Ingredient: 1-pound pinto beans, 1 small onion, halved, 1 bay leaf, ¾ pound slab bacon, 1 tablespoon kosher salt, 1 tablespoon paprika, ¼ teaspoon cayenne.

Preparation: Pick over the beans for small rocks or debris. Rinse well, then cover with cold water and soak for 6 hours or overnight. Transfer beans to a soup pot and add water to cover by 1 inch. Add onion, bay leaf and bacon and bring to a boil. Reduce heat to a bare simmer, partly cover pot with lid, and cook for 1 hour, stirring occasionally.

Stir in salt, paprika and cayenne, then continue simmering until beans are soft and creamy and the broth is well seasoned and lightly thickened, about 1 hour more. Remove bacon and chop roughly, then return to pot. (Dish may be prepared up to 2 days ahead.)

Enjoy the treat!

STORAGE

How and where you store your beans, lentils and more, both before and after cooking, can dramatically affect flavour and texture. Store uncooked dried beans in a dark, cool cabinet for up to a year. They really go downhill after two years, so throw out all your old beans, especially if you can't remember when you bought them. If you can find a harvest date on your package of beans, all the better. Some beans may have been stored in a warehouse for months or even a year before they arrive at your market.

Cooked beans are best stored in their cooking liquid in the refrigerator for up to 5 days. Or drain the beans and toss them with a little oil, salt and pepper (or a vinaigrette) before chilling. This both preserves them and flavours them. Beans can turn mushy in the freezer, but if you do want to try to freeze them, do so in their cooking liquid.

THE PLANT-BASE ATHLETE.

Have you ever wondered if athletes can succeed eating plant-based or if your physical performance will plummet if you eat fewer animal foods? I myself am by no means an athlete but I am well-versed in plant-based nutrition and know that athletes can thrive on a plant food if they wish. It does take a little extra planning (and as most athletes know, no matter your dietary preferences, you need to be mindful about how you feed your body before, during and after an event or tough training session).

So, whether you're decreasing or ditching animal foods for ethical, environmental or health reasons, or just want to see what all the fuss is about with plant-based eating, I hope you learn some valuable strategies as we go on!

To provide top-notch information I interviewed my friend, long-time vegan and plant-based nutrition expert Matt Ruscigno, MPH, RD. Matt co-authored the books No Meat Athlete and Plant-Based Sports Nutrition and founded Vegan Nutrition Consulting, a network of nutrition experts to provide science-based vegan nutrition education for both individuals and corporate wellness. He's also done some extreme endurance events and knows first-hand what it's like to fuel for intense activity. I also chatted with a female plant-based athlete who's experienced some cool changes in her performance since tweaking her eating pattern. Now let's get into it!

Can Athletes Succeed While Eating Plant-Based?

Whether you're simply eating more plant foods or going vegan, there is lots of evidence to support plant-based eating for optimal athletic performance. According to the Vegetarian Nutrition Dietetic Practice Group of the Academy of Nutrition and Dietetics, *"Vegetarian diets are linked to decreased risk for chronic diseases including cardiovascular disease, type 2 diabetes, and certain cancers, while their naturally high carbohydrate and phytochemical content may help athletes optimize their training, performance and recovery."*

In other words, you're more likely to experience benefits from this style of eating than disadvantages. As long as you're meeting your fuelling needs and eating satisfying foods, a plant-based eating style can support your sports performance and your overall health!

Amanda Wagner, who is a plant-based athlete and nutrition student, said that her performance and recovery has improved since switching to a plant-based eating style. She even qualified for the Boston Marathon while eating vegan! Now if that's not a successful athlete, I don't know what is. *"I'm training for my second marathon now on a vegan diet and feeling the best I've felt in years and running personal bests in all my races so far this summer. I am confident my vegan diet has played a key role in my strong athletic performances this year,"* she says.

How do Athletes Get the Nutrients They Need from Plant-Based Foods?

No matter your eating style, carbohydrates are key for fuelling workouts. You're probably familiar with carb-rich plant-based foods including grains, potatoes and fruit. It's not tough to get enough carbs while eating plant-based! Sometimes all the fibre in plant foods can fill you up too fast and it's OK to eat some refined grains such as white pasta and white rice.

Many of us have been trained to believe that we need protein from meat, dairy and eggs to maintain strong muscles and bones. In actuality, plant foods can provide all the amino acids and protein we need! Protein-rich plant foods include beans, lentils, nuts and soy foods such as tofu and tempeh. Bonus: these foods tend to be way more affordable than animal-based protein foods!

Another concern about plant-based eating as an athlete may be getting enough calories. While it's true that vegetables are low in calories, there are calorie-dense foods in the plant kingdom including nuts, seeds, avocados and olives. "*Nuts and seeds and nut and seed butters are crucial for athletes. And there's no shame in so-called 'processed foods' like veggie burgers and vegan meats*," Matt says.

"*Try to cook whenever possible, but do not shy away from packaged vegan foods, frozen dinners, or restaurant meals as they can help you fill your daily vegan athlete plate*," Amanda says. She echoes Matt's sentiments about processed foods and incorporates protein bars and powders into her day for an extra boost, especially during heavy training periods.

Beyond the macronutrients (carbs, protein, fat), athletes also need to be mindful of certain micronutrients (vitamins and minerals). According to Matt, "Iron should be on the mind of all athletes, especially plant-based and vegan ones. Fortunately, plenty of plant foods have iron and absorption is increased by combining them with vitamin-C containing foods. This pairing happens naturally — salsa in burritos, tomatoes in falafel sandwiches and bell peppers in tofu scrambles."

Keep in mind that women need more iron than men so this is a nutrient that females of child-bearing age (or anyone who menstruates) need to be mindful of. I recommend asking your health care provider to check your iron status when you go in for your yearly check-up (yes, you should be going in for those yearly visits, and not just for your lady bits!). It involves a simple blood draw and an inexpensive lab test. This is for all females, not just those who are eating plant-based or who are active (but especially if you fall into these categories).

How Can Athletes Get Started with Plant-Based Eating?

Think substitution rather than elimination. Substitute meat with tofu, tempeh, beans and lentils. Substitute dairy-based milk, cheese and yogurt with fortified plant-based versions of these foods. Hopefully you're already eating a wide variety of colourful vegetables and fruits, but if you're not, make it a goal to add at least two different colours of produce to every meal! Colours in vegetables and fruits represent different nutrients which are crucial for fuelling and recovery.

You'll also need to do some additions along with your substitutions. I love adding baked tofu to pasta for a protein boost of an otherwise carb-centric meal. And trying some legume-based pastas for even more of a boost. Adding peanut butter to smoothies is great for adding protein, fat and calories. Avocado in salads and wraps is another great way to add fat, calories and deliciousness to plant-based meals. And remember that it's OK to cook with oils such as olive oil. Just because you're eating plant-based doesn't mean you need to start overly restricting certain foods.

Looking for specific ideas for plant-based meals and snacks? "*Bean dips are so good! In taste and for easy, quick calories and protein. You can eat them with fresh veggies, on sandwiches, with a spoon, in sauces — the application is unlimited. And there's more than hummus! I make white bean and black bean dips regularly*," Matt says.

Some of Amanda's favourite meals are pasta with kidney beans and vegetables; black beans, rice, and vegetables; and tofu and vegetable stir-fry. "You do have to eat a greater volume of food as a vegan athlete, but it does not have to be annoying. Make it fun by trying as many new meals and snacks as your time and budget will allow," she says.

Have fun with it, experiment with different recipes and enjoy the taste and benefits of plant-based eating! For personalized guidance on food, nutrition and dietary supplements, consider working with a registered dietician nutritionist who specializes in plant-based nutrition.

HANDY TIPS AS A PLANT-BASED ATHLETE.

If you have been inspired by the knowledge here so far, and adopted a whole-food, plant-based diet as your foundation for health, perhaps you are ready to pursue meaningful fitness goals but don't know where to start. Or perhaps you have been working out for a long time and are concerned that your new diet will affect your performance. With the knowledge and relationship, I've gathered from as many plant-based athlete, I've sorted through all of the issues unique to vegan athletes and guided thousands to successfully incorporate physical activity into their vegan lifestyle routine. Here are some of my top tips:

- ✓ ***Unlearn the Most Common Nutrition Myth***— a common question that comes up among many people new to a plant-based diet is, "what do I eat?" What to avoid on a plant-based it quite clear: all animal products. If we want that plant-based diet to be a healthy one, we take things a step farther, also eliminating processed foods, including oils and refined carbohydrates. But knowing only what not to eat leaves many wondering how to get adequate nutrition, especially protein. The human requirement for protein is so low (5 to 10 percent of our total caloric intake) that as long as you consume adequate calories to maintain your weight, it is virtually impossible to have a protein deficiency. Further, if you are eating nothing but a variety of whole, natural plants, you will get enough of every single essential amino acid, regardless of which foods you choose (the complete protein myth has long been debunked). You would experience a calorie deficiency before a protein deficiency, and both are virtually non-existent in first-world societies.

✓ ***Know Which Foods Best Fuel Your Fitness*—** Nobody is fuelled by kale, so don't fool yourself into thinking you will get sufficient energy to perform athletic activities from leafy greens and other non-starchy vegetables (which average about 100 and 150 calories per pound, respectively). For long-lasting fuel, vegan athletes and non-athletes alike need to centre their diets around the more calorically dense whole plant foods that are rich in complex carbohydrates such as potatoes, beans, lentils, squash, brown rice, oats, quinoa, and other starchy vegetables, legumes, and grains (which range from about 350 to 600 calories per pound). Fruits (which average about 250 calories per pound) are also an excellent source of fuel. This is especially true right before exercise, because they digest quickly and will not weigh heavily in your stomach during cardiovascular exercise. When you consume an abundance of whole, unprocessed plant foods, you get not only get the fuel, but also the full range of macronutrients (protein, fat, carbohydrates, water, and fibre) and micronutrients (vitamins, minerals, enzymes, antioxidants, and other important phytochemicals). Since most whole plant foods contain 600 or fewer calories per pound (with the exception of nuts and seeds, which range from 2,500 to 3,000 calories per pound, on average), you can eat a lot of food, experiencing many flavours and textures, and the volume will fill you up before you overdose on calories. Overeating is easy to do when consuming refined and processed foods. By consuming foods high in nutrients and low in calorie density, you can support energy production and muscle recovery without excess fat gain, while avoiding the energy-sucking process of digesting refined foods.

✓ ***Eat Many Small Meals per Day***— when it comes to what to eat, know that your options are boundless, with ample varieties of fruits, vegetables, legumes, grains, nuts, and seeds. Because whole plant foods are lower in calorie density (see #2), you may find that you need to eat more volume than you did before. Simply choose the foods you like the most and eat 5 or 6 small meals throughout the day until you are comfortably full. This way, you'll find it easier not to under- or overeat. You will have sufficient fuel to work out any time, rather than finding yourself too hungry, too full, or too tired to exercise, as is common when we eat three more substantial meals each day. The two biggest obstacles that keep people from exercising regularly are shortages of time and energy. You can now put the energy issue to rest and work on time management to ensure that regular exercise is part of your routine. If you aren't losing or gaining weight as you'd like, then it's a good idea to get a general sense of how many calories you need to eat in a day. To determine your own personal caloric needs, simply use an online Harris-Benedict calculator, and enter five simple bits of data. This will reveal two numbers: (1) your estimated BMR (basal metabolic rate), the average number of calories you would burn if you slept all day and (2) your daily calorie needs, taking into account your activity level.

✓ ***Get Moving ... and Have Fun***! — Over the years, one thing I have discovered to be profoundly true is that if it isn't fun, I am unlikely to do it regularly. This clearly applies to fitness. If your current exercise routine is not enjoyable, you will find yourself consciously or unconsciously avoiding exercise by finding other ways to occupy your time, such as putting in extra hours at work or distracting yourself with entertainment or hobbies. This approach will not lead to fitness success. To succeed, you will need to find genuine enjoyment in whatever activity you choose. Exercise is not just putting on spandex and grunting while lifting weights. Exercise is hiking, swimming, jogging, playing team sports, and anything else that increases your heart rate, gets your body moving vigorously, and puts stress on your muscles. Find a physical activity you enjoy, and do it regularly. I suggest exercising for 30 to 90 minutes a day, three to five days per week, which allows at least a couple of days off for recovery.

ENERGY AND PERFORMANCE.

Whether training for a local 10 km run or the Euro 2020 Championship, athletes of all shapes, sizes and levels share a common goal: to perform to the best of their ability. Technical expertise and training are the cornerstones of improving athletic performance, but good nutrition is equally crucial for success. Over the last two decades, our understanding of the important role that dietary protein plays in muscle building and recovery has grown vastly. We now know that it is not simply the quantity of protein consumed, but also the quality of that protein and when we consume it that dictates muscle health and function.

- o ***Adequate does not mean optimal*** — the daily recommended allowance (RDA) for protein is 0.8

grams per kilogram of body weight per day, which translates to 56 g for a 70 kg/178-pound man. The vast majority of people consuming a typical western style diet easily achieve this level. But at Kerry's recent Scientific Advisory Council Meeting, Professor Stuart Phillips, Director of the Centre for Nutrition, Exercise, and Health Research at McMaster University, warned that RDAs are minimum levels set to prevent deficiency rather than levels that will optimise health. Protein has countless functions in the human body; however, it is especially important for the maintenance and recovery of muscle. Muscle health is a critical determinant of athletic performance, so, for athletes, achieving optimal rather than merely adequate protein intake is key. Intense exercise causes the proteins that make up muscle to be broken down. This damage is responsible for muscle soreness and can ultimately reduce strength and function if the proteins are not replenished. Consuming protein in the diet can offset this effect. Eating a high protein meal decreases muscle breakdown and increases muscle repair and synthesis (Moore D et al., 2015). As a result, the American College of Sports Medicine advocates protein intakes higher than the RDA. Individuals who take part in endurance sports (runners, cyclists, swimmers) are advised to consume between 1.2 – 1.4 g per kg body weight per day (84-98 g per day for a 70 kg/178 pound man) while for power disciplines (strength or speed) intakes of up to 1.7g per kg body weight per day (119 g/d) are recommended.

DAILY PROTEIN NEEDS For a 70kg (178lb) man
Types of Training

56 grams (Sedenatary)

119 grams (Strength or Speed)

84 - 98 grams (Endurance)

- o **Quality Matters**— it's not just the amount of protein, but also the type of protein in the diet that athletes need to take note of. Scientific research shows that simply consuming enough protein will not optimise muscle repair and synthesis because not all types of protein are equally beneficial. In order to utilise the protein, we eat, the body breaks it down into basic building blocks, called amino acids. The source of the protein influences our ability to digest it properly and, therefore, the availability of these crucial building blocks. Protein from plants such as vegetables, nuts, seeds, grains, and legumes are not as well digested as protein from animal sources or soy protein. In addition, not all proteins contain all of the amino acids the human body needs. Some amino acids, called essential amino acids, cannot be produced by the human body and must be consumed in the diet. Most plant proteins lack one or more of these essential amino acids, meaning plant sources must be combined in the diet to provide for the body's needs. Egg, milk and soy proteins are highly digestible and contain all of the essential amino acids, meaning they are considered the highest quality proteins for humans. Recent scientific research has allowed us to refine this list even further for athletes because when it comes to building muscle, one specific amino acid, leucine, plays a critical role (Layman D et al., 2015). Leucine acts like a molecular switch that turns on the body's machinery for manufacturing muscle. Whey protein contains more leucine than any other source of protein and clinical studies have shown that whey stimulates muscle synthesis more effectively than other high-quality proteins, especially when consumed after exercise. As a result, whey protein recovery supplements have become extremely popular.

- ○ ***Timing is of the essence*—** Focusing on post-exercise whey supplementation is only part of a bigger picture. Optimal muscle repair and synthesis will not be achieved simply by drinking a protein shake after a workout. Frequent training is required to improve performance. As a result, muscle breakdown, repair and synthesis become an ongoing process and regular intake of high-quality protein is needed. We now know that consuming around 20-30g of protein can "switch on" muscle protein synthesis, but this effect plateaus when more protein is consumed (Moore D et al., 2015). This means that consuming larger amounts of protein at that same meal offers no additional benefit. For this reason, spreading protein intake throughout the day, such that 20-30g of high-quality protein is consumed at breakfast, lunch and dinner, is more beneficial. This type of meal pattern will lead to more muscle synthesis and less muscle breakdown throughout the day. A recent study carried out by researchers at Maastricht University in the Netherlands suggests that one additional snack before sleeping may further optimise muscle synthesis (Snijders T et al., 2015). Sleep is crucial, not only for athletic performance but also for general health and wellness. The hours we spend sleeping, however, constitute a period of fasting and this leaves the body vulnerable to muscle breakdown. The researchers found that consuming 20-30g of high quality protein before bed minimised muscle break down and promoted muscle synthesis during sleep, meaning that a protein packed bedtime snack could be beneficial.

What does all of this mean in terms of diet?

Thanks to our improved understanding of the way in which dietary protein affects muscle health, we can now define not just the quantity of protein, but also the quality and timing of intake needed to optimise muscle recovery and function, and ultimately, performance.

1. **Quantity**: RDAs for protein are minimum rather than optimum levels. To maximize muscle health target 1.2-1.7g per kg of body weight per day
2. **Quality**: As you are a vegetarian, combine plant sources of protein to ensure your body gets all of the essential amino acids.
3. **Timing**: It is important to consume protein regularly throughout the day. Aim to include 20-30g of high-quality protein at breakfast, lunch, dinner and as a bedtime snack.

Six reasons you'd want to embrace the plant-based diet as an athlete.

- Even athletes are at risk for heart disease: In one study, 44 percent of endurance cyclists and runners had coronary plaques. A plant-based diet keeps athletes' hearts strong by reversing plaque, bringing down blood pressure and cholesterol, and reducing weight.

- Meat consumption and high cholesterol levels exacerbate inflammation, which can result in pain and impair athletic performance and recovery. Studies show that a plant-based diet may have an anti-inflammatory effect.
- A plant-based diet, which is low in saturated fat and free of cholesterol, helps improve blood viscosity, or thickness. That helps more oxygen reach the muscles, which improves athletic performance.
- Plant-based diets improve arterial flexibility and diameter, leading to better blood flow. One study found that even a single high-fat meal, including sausage and egg McMuffins, impaired arterial function for several hours.
- Compared with meat-eaters, people eating a plant-based diet get more antioxidants, which help neutralize free radicals. Free radicals lead to muscle fatigue, reduced athletic performance, and impaired recovery.
- Plant-based diets, which are typically low in fat and high in fibre, can reduce body fat. Reduced body fat is associated with increased aerobic capacity—or the ability to use oxygen to fuel exercise. Studies show that athletes on a plant-based diet increase their VO2 max—the maximum amount of oxygen they can use during intense exercise—leading to better endurance.

Let's Put the Protein Myth to Rest

The idea that plant sources are insufficient to meet protein requirements is an outdated myth. The Academy of Nutrition and Dietetics supports the notion that an appropriately planned vegan or vegetarian diet can meet the energy and macronutrient needs (including protein) of athletes.

But the key words here are appropriately planned. Meeting your protein needs as a vegan athlete isn't rocket science, but it may take a little effort or at least forethought.

- Eat a variety of foods throughout the day.
- Include high-lysine foods when possible.
- Know roughly how many grams you need and plan accordingly.

While the protein question may never go away completely, at least you know you can be healthy and reach your goals.

And now you know the science to prove it.

PROTEIN AND RECOVERY.

Recovery after exercise is just as important (if not more) than the exercises you do while you're working out. The body can only run off what we give it, and what we give it determines our health in more ways than one. After exercise, the body needs to be refuelled with a delicate mix of protein and carbohydrates from quality foods. Not cheap protein shakes, fast food, processed bars, or junk food. Good, clean food is what it needs. Muscles can utilize these foods better than anything else, and these foods are better for our blood sugar which should be considered post-workout too.

What Happens in the Body Post-Workout?

After we workout, our cortisol levels are normally high while insulin is usually low. This happens because we've put stress on the body which then causes stress hormones to pump out more abundantly in the body (namely cortisol) and insulin levels drop because glucose has been depleted which lowers blood sugar levels. This might be one reason you feel so hungry after you work out and are more likely to just grab something to help yourself feel better. Blood sugar should be managed by eating something that will provide quality carbohydrates to the body, but also to allow those carbs to enter in rapidly into the bloodstream so they can help reach muscle cells and replenish muscle glycogen stores. The key is not to choose refined carbs, but whole food-based carbs.

We all know eating well is essential for a healthy lifestyle. Getting the right nutrients affects everything from your mood and risk of injury and illness, to your weight and even how you look.

A good diet for any regular exerciser should be made up of a good balance of macronutrients: healthy carbohydrates to provide energy and fuel your training; fats to provide energy and support cell growth; and lean protein to help rebuild and recover. When you're asking your body to do things like 4-hour bike rides or 26.2-mile runs, getting enough protein becomes a key focus, to help your body's cells and tissues – such as muscle – recover, repair and grow.

Protein is made up of 20 different organic compounds known as amino acids. While some of these amino acids are made by our bodies, there are nine – known as essential amino acids – the body doesn't create. These have to be provided through diet.

Studies have shown that leucine – a branch chain amino acid (BCAA) found in protein-rich foods and not created by the body – is particularly important as it's one of the key drivers of muscle protein synthesis. To put that in simpler terms, it helps you build muscle mass. Leucine is used by muscles as fuel and so is depleted after exercise.

While leucine is found in many animal-based proteins such as chicken, eggs, beef and whey it's also found in a number of plant-based foods. Vegan foods high in leucine include soybeans, hemp seeds, peanuts, almonds, oats and soy and pea protein powders. Vegan or non-vegan, to supercharge your recovery you should be aiming to eat some form of protein and carbohydrate – to replace the energy used by your body – within two hours of exercising and ideally within the first 45 minutes.

How does your body get protein from vegan diets?

The body gets protein from a vegan diet in the same way it does from a diet that includes animal products, by eating protein-rich foods. You may have heard a theory that you need to combine plant-based protein types to ensure you're getting a 'complete' protein but luckily, that complicated concept has been disproved.

Complete vs. incomplete proteins: the latest thinking

All animal proteins contain each of the nine essential amino acids and are termed 'complete protein', some plant-based proteins are deficient in certain amino acids, leading these to be termed 'incomplete'.

This labelling promotes the thinking that you'd need to combine different plant-based proteins in one sitting to ensure you got enough of each amino acid, but the reality is that as long as you're eating a variety of different proteins on a regular basis, your body will be able to pull from this pool of amino acids as it needs.

There are also a number of plant-based proteins including quinoa, hemp seeds, soy, and chia seeds which contain all nine essential amino acids in roughly equal amounts.

How much protein do I actually need to consume?

According to the British Nutrition Foundation, the protein requirements of a normal adult are 0.75g per kilogram of body weight per day. If you're regularly cycling, running, hitting the gym or working out, your protein needs go up to help promote muscle tissue growth and repair.

The general advice is that strength and endurance athletes should aim for 1.2-1.7g of protein per kilogram of bodyweight daily. So, if you weigh in at around 11 stone or 70 kg, you should be eating 84-119g of protein a day.

Protein should also be restored, which is best utilized by muscle cells when carbs are eaten with them. Quality carbs help drive amino acids from protein into the muscle cells where they are needed most. While refined sugars will do that just fine too, they will also disrupt insulin levels and are more likely to leave you fatigued not long after. Not to mention they can lead to weight gain and inflammation, which is most definitely not what you want post-workout, right?

So, now that you know what your body needs post-workout, here are 10 great plant-based options to give a try:

- ***Fruit***— Fruit is a high in natural sugars, which makes it best to consume either before or right after your workout. This will allow your muscles to use the sugars from the fruit either for energy, or for restoring glycogen back in the muscle cells to aid in repair and blood sugar regulation. Their fibres will help prevent nasty drops in blood sugar later as well. Just keep in mind, you don't need a lot of fruit to get the benefits — just a piece or one serving. Fruit is healthy for us, but too much isn't necessarily more effective. Choose some berries, an apple, a banana, or perhaps some anti-inflammatory cherries, pineapple, or mango. Whatever you like!
- ***Hemp protein***: Hemp protein powder is a great post-workout meal idea because though it does contain healthy fats, it's lower in fat than whole hemp seeds and higher in protein per serving. Hemp protein is generally anywhere from 4-5 grams of fat per serving and 15-16 grams of protein. It's also an anti-inflammatory protein that's great at reducing muscle

aches and fatigue thanks to the natural magnesium and iron found in hemp. Choose natural, plain hemp protein instead of sweetened options. If you don't like hemp protein, there are other comparable options like brown rice or pea protein you can try, however, no other single plant-based protein offers the complete full spectrum of nutrition benefits that hemp does. You can also find a blend of hemp, pea, and rice protein, along with some others like flax, hemp and pea, etc. Use hemp protein in a post-workout smoothie to get the best benefits, preferably with a piece of fruit to assist with complete nutrition and taste.

- **Sweet potato**: If you're up to sitting down for a meal right after you eat, choose sweet potatoes for a healthy carb source. They're rich in natural sugars but won't spike your blood sugar like refined carbs or even regular potatoes do. They also offer up trytophan, an amino acid that relaxes the body and reduces stress hormones like cortisol. Sweet potatoes are also a good source of potassium, which also helps lower stress hormones and high blood pressure. Not to mention that potassium-rich foods also restore electrolytes in the body that are often depleted right after a workout.

•

- ***Chia seeds*** — Chia seeds make a great post-workout addition to a smoothie because they're full of amino acids, even though not very high in protein or carbs. They're also a good source of fibre, potassium, magnesium, and iron to restore balance to the body after a workout. They can also slow down the insulin spike that might happen when you eat natural sugars such as fruit, but still allow your body to absorb them for optimal repair. Chia seeds are also great options when you're looking to lower inflammation thanks to their omega-3 fatty acids.

- ***Lentils*** — Lentils are a good source of both protein and carbs, which makes them a great post-workout meal choice. They're also fairly easy to digest for most people, which is important right after a workout for optimal absorption. (Just don't eat them before your workout — they're very high in fibre!) Try topping your sweet potato with lentils, adding them to a salad, or even adding some lentils and sweet potatoes to some broth to make a quick soup. You can also make lentil sweet potato veggie burgers as another option.

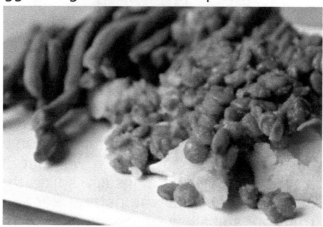

- **_Green smoothie_** — a green smoothie is probably one of the most popular post-workout options we have available to us today. They're amazing sources of antioxidants, fibre, anti-inflammatory chlorophyll, iron, B vitamins, magnesium, and are so easy to add protein to! Use greens like spinach, berries, chia seeds, some plant-based protein powder, and either a small piece of banana or some stevia to sweeten. Green smoothies are also easy to make in a flash when you need some quick replenishment.

- ***Almonds and figs or dates***— if you like quick bites or bars after a workout, make some or buy some with a base of almonds and figs or almonds and dates. These two combinations are a wonderful blend of fibre, natural sugars, and plant-based protein. They also offer up amino acids, B vitamins, and magnesium. Add some hemp seeds to the mix, and you're really in for a delicious, nutritious (and filling) snack!
- ***Spinach***— Spinach is a remarkable source of plant-based protein, iron, magnesium, and B vitamins. It makes a great green to include post-workout either in a smoothie, or with some plant-based protein and another healthy carb (like lentils and sweet potatoes) because it's filling, anti-inflammatory, and delicious! Keeping some organic spinach on hand is a great practice since you'll always have it for meals of all kinds, and to use in your post-workout regimen.

- **Oats**—if you love oats, good news — they love you right back! This is especially true after a workout when your body needs carbs and protein all at once. Oats contain not just fibre, but also other quality carbs your muscles can immediately put to use to restore energy and aid in muscle repair. If you don't eat oats, you can also try quinoa as another option. Oats and quinoa both provide quality sources of protein, with around 4-5 grams per serving, though quinoa is a complete source of protein while oats are not.
- **Pumpkin seeds**— Snacking on a few pumpkin seeds or adding them to your smoothie is a fantastic way to get in some plant-based protein, iron, and magnesium. All of these aid in repairing your muscle cells, but their high alkaline feature and high amino acid profile are what really makes pumpkin seeds so awesome. These tiny seeds reduce inflammation, keep your blood sugar stable, promote a more positive mood, and yes, keep you lean and fit too! They're also a great source of zinc to improve your immune health, which can be depleted without proper post-workout nutrition.

These are what I call "My ten green monsters" for post-workout and recovery. You can invent yours with any healthy combination of plant protein.

PROTEIN MUSCLE SYNTHESIS.

Manufacturers of sports supplements and protein powders often claim that their products can increase muscle protein synthesis (MPS). While this suggests that sports supplements somehow facilitate changes in muscle mass, the process is actually more complicated than that. Muscle growth is ultimately achieved with the combination of resistance training and protein intake. What MPS provides us is the means to gauge how effectively those interventions work. MPS is ultimately a physiological process by which increases are linked to improved muscle growth, although the actual gains can vary from one person to the next.

Muscle protein synthesis is the process of building muscle mass. Muscle protein synthesis is essential for exercise recovery and adaptation. As such, it's a really popular topic in the fitness community. But the methods used to measure muscle protein synthesis in studies are very complicated. Some basic knowledge of the various methods is essential to draw proper conclusions from the research as you'll read.

Protein is the main building block of your muscle. Protein synthesis is the process of building new proteins. This process happens in all organs. Muscle protein synthesis is the process of building specifically muscle protein. Think of a muscle as a wall. Each brick is a protein. Muscle protein synthesis is the addition of new bricks to the wall. Now, this would mean the wall would become larger and larger. However, there is an opposing process. On the other side of the wall, a process is removing bricks. This process is called muscle protein breakdown, sometimes referred to as muscle proteolysis or muscle degradation. The speed of these two opposing processes determines the net change of the wall.

If muscle protein synthesis exceeds muscle protein breakdown, the wall will become larger (your muscles are growing). If muscle protein breakdown exceeds muscle protein synthesis, the wall is shrinking (you're losing muscle mass). The sum of these two processes determines your net balance:

Net muscle protein balance = muscle protein synthesis – muscle protein breakdown.

You can also compare it to your bank account.

balance = income – expenses

Muscle protein synthesis is the process of building muscle mass. Muscle protein breakdown is the opposing process of breaking down muscle tissue. If muscle protein synthesis exceeds muscle protein breakdown, your muscles will grow.

How Muscle Protein Synthesis Works

Protein is the building block of muscles. Muscle protein synthesis is a naturally occurring process in which protein is produced to repair muscle damage caused by intense exercise. It is an opposing force to muscle protein breakdown (MPB) in which protein is lost as a result of exercise. The ratio of MPS to MPB determines whether muscle tissues are built or lost. If MPS outpaces MPB, muscle growth is achieved. If MPB outpaces MPS, the opposite occurs.

MPS can be enhanced by increasing your protein intake immediately following exercise. The amino acids derived from protein will then be shuttled to your muscles, replacing any lost to exercise. Learning how to stimulate MPS through exercise and diet can help accelerate muscle growth, improve recovery and athletic performance, and increase overall endurance.

Effects of Exercise

Protein balance is used to describe the relationship between muscle protein breakdown and muscle protein synthesis. When your body is in protein balance, no muscle growth or wasting is occurring, and you're considered to be in a healthy state of biological equilibrium (homeostasis). To stimulate muscle growth, you essentially need to unsettle the protein balance. While it may seem counterintuitive, exercise can break down muscle protein but rarely in excess of protein synthesis. In fact, the greater the intensity of a workout, the greater the MPS.

Scientists measure intensity by something called the one-repetition maximum (1-RM), meaning the maximum weight you can lift for one repetition. According to research from the University of Nottingham, workout intensities of under 40 percent of the 1-RM will not affect MPS, whereas intensities greater than 60 percent will double or triple the MPS. Even if exercising to failure, low-intensity exercise will do little to increase MPS and, as such, will not increase muscle mass.

Effects of Diet

The relationship between diet and protein balance is less straightforward. Even with increased protein intake, MPS is triggered for only a finite period of time. This is because the body can only utilize so much of the essential amino acids (EAAs) it receives; anything more will be broken down and excreted by the liver. To stimulate MPS, it is important to consume the appropriate amount of protein following exercise. Eating too much will not improve muscle growth but may increase the accumulation of potentially harmful by-products such as urea. A study from the University of Birmingham looked into MPS response rates in men prescribed 10, 20, or 40 grams of whey protein immediately following resistance training. According to the researchers:

- A 10-gram dose of whey protein had no effect on MPS.

- A 20-gram dose increased the MPS by 49 percent.
- A 40-gram dose increased the MPS by 56 percent but also caused the excessive accumulation of urea.

Consuming 20 grams to 40 grams of whey protein after resistance training also increased concentrations of phenylalanine, leucine, and threonine, EAAs associated with lean muscle growth.

Why muscle protein breakdown is of less importance

We'll almost exclusively talk about muscle protein synthesis, and not focus much on muscle protein breakdown. That might sound like you're missing out on a whole lot, but you're not. Changes in muscle protein synthesis are much greater in response to exercise and feeding than changes in muscle protein breakdown in healthy humans.

While feeding can reduce muscle protein breakdown by approximately 50%, very little is needed to reach this maximal inhibition. This is best illustrated by a study which clamped (maintained) insulin at different concentrations and also clamped amino acids at a high concentration.

There were five conditions:

- Fasted state
- high amino acids + low insulin
- high amino acids + medium insulin
- high amino acids + high insulin
- high amino acids + very high insulin

In the illustration below, you see the effects on muscle protein breakdown.

Muscle protein breakdown

Fasted
AA + low insulin
AA + medium insulin
AA + high insulin
AA + very high insulin

Greenhaff, 2008

In a fasted state, muscle protein breakdown rates were relatively high (condition 1). Amino acid infusion did not reduce muscle protein breakdown when in ¨ kept low (condition 2). But when insulin was ii reach a moderate concentration, muscle protein breakdown rates went down (condition 3). Further increasing insulin did not have an additional effect on muscle protein breakdown (conditions 4 and 5).

This study shows us a couple of things.

Firstly, insulin inhibits muscle protein breakdown, but you only need a moderate insulin concentration to reach the maximal effect. In this study the medium insulin concentration already resulted in the maximal 50% muscle protein breakdown, but other research has shown that even half the insulin concentration of the medium group is already enough for the maximal effect.

Secondly, protein ingestion does not directly inhibit muscle protein breakdown. While protein intake can decrease muscle protein breakdown, this is because it increases the insulin concentration.

You only need a minimal amount of food to reach insulin concentrations that maximally inhibit muscle protein breakdown. In agreement, adding carbohydrates to 30 g of protein does not further decrease muscle protein breakdown rates.

Therefore, it often doesn't make much sense to measure muscle protein breakdown in nutrition studies. All study groups that got at least some amount of food will have the 50% inhibition of fasted muscle protein breakdown rates. If the effect on muscle protein breakdown is the same between groups, then changes in muscle protein net balance would be entirely be explained by differences in muscle protein synthesis.

It should be noted that HMB decreases muscle protein breakdown in an insulin independent way. It is not known of the effects of HMB and insulin on muscle protein breakdown are synergistic. However, HMB supplementation appears to have minimal effects of muscle mass gains in long-term studies.

Of course, you can speculate that muscle protein breakdown becomes more relevant during catabolic conditions during which there is significant muscle loss, such as dieting or muscle disuse (e.g. bed rest or immobilization). However, it cannot be simply assumed that the observed muscle loss in such condition is the result of increased muscle protein breakdown. After just 3 days of dieting, there is already a large decrease in muscle protein synthesis. In agreement, there is a large decrease in muscle protein synthesis during muscle disuse. Therefore, muscle loss may be largely (or even entirely) caused by a reduction in muscle protein synthesis, and not by an increase in muscle protein breakdown.

But let's say that muscle protein breakdown does go up a bit during catabolic conditions. Then the first question would be, could nutrition prevent this? If the answer is no, muscle protein breakdown is still not that relevant to measure. If nutrition does have an effect, how much would it take? Let's say you need double the amount of insulin you normally need to maximally inhibit muscle protein breakdown. That would still be a small amount of insulin that any small meal would release and all nutritional interventions have the same effect. So even during catabolic conditions, muscle protein synthesis rates are likely much more relevant than muscle protein breakdown.

While it sounds that muscle protein breakdown is a bad thing and we should try to completely prevent it, that is not necessarily true. Muscle proteins get damaged from exercise, physical activity, and metabolism (e.g. oxidative stress, inflammation etc). Muscle protein breakdown allows you to break down those damaged muscle proteins into amino acids and recycle most of them into new functional muscle proteins again.

In fact, muscle protein breakdown has beneficial roles in muscle growth and adaptation! If mice are genetically engineered so that they can't properly break down muscle protein, they are actually weaker and smaller than normal mousses. This highlights that at least some amount of muscle protein breakdown is necessary to optimally adapt to training and maximize muscle growth. So anytime you eat just about anything, you'll reduce muscle protein breakdown by 50%. We don't know how to reduce muscle protein breakdown even further, but it's not clear if we would even want that, as at least some muscle protein breakdown seems necessary for optimal muscle growth.

While muscle protein breakdown is an important process, it doesn't fluctuate much, which makes

it far less important for muscle gains than muscle protein synthesis.

ENERGIZING BREAKFAST.

Vegan diets always get so much praise due to their benefits towards our health and the environment. Regardless of that, you will always run into people that are still concerned if such diets can provide all necessary nutrients. Thankfully, with the abundance of resources out there it's that much easier to find dishes suitable for all dietary needs. Look no further than these high-protein vegan breakfasts with enough plant power that will kickstart the day for you and even your non-veggie mates.

Tip: Protein content is an approximation calculated by adding the grams in the ingredients that are considered a source of protein. It is subject to change depending on optional toppings.

ORANGE FRENCH TOAST: Aquafaba is the not-so-secret ingredient that make this vegan French toast recipe soft, thick, and eggy—without the eggs. Use your favourite bread or berries to create your own signature version.

Ingredient:

1 ½ cup unsweetened, unflavoured plant milk, ½ cup almond flour, 1 cup aquafaba, 2 tablespoons pure maple syrup, ¼ teaspoon ground cinnamon, 2 pinches of salt (optional), ½ tablespoon orange zest (from half an orange), 8 whole-grain bread slices (about ¾ inches thick). 4.5 ounces (about 1 cup) blueberries or raspberries (fresh, or frozen and thawed), ½ cup applesauce, 1 teaspoon pure maple syrup.

Preparation:

Preheat the oven to 400°F. Place a wire rack over a baking sheet. Combine the plant milk, flour, aquafaba, maple syrup, cinnamon, and salt (if using) in a bowl and stir until the mixture is smooth. Transfer to a shallow pan. Stir in the orange zest and mix well. Warm a non-stick skillet over medium heat. Dip each bread slice into the mixture and let soak for a few seconds. Turnover and soak for a few seconds more. Place in the skillet and cook over medium-low heat for 2 to 3 minutes. Turn over gently, then cook the other side for 2 to 3 minutes, until golden brown. Place the toast on the wire rack and bake in the oven for 10 to 15 minutes, until crisp. Combine berries, applesauce, and maple syrup in a blender and pulse until sauce reaches a chunky consistency. Serve the French toast warm with the berry compote.

CHOCOLATE CHIP BANANA PANCAKES: These pancakes are so simple and delicious, and they're just as good for dessert as they are for breakfast! Plus, they freeze really well, so you can make an extra batch and freeze them. Use a large griddle so that you can cook three or four at a time.

Ingredient:

1 tablespoon flaxseeds

1¼ cups buckwheat flour

¼ cup old-fashioned rolled oats

2 tablespoons unsweetened coconut flakes

1 tablespoon baking powder

Pinch of sea salt

1 cup unsweetened, unflavoured plant milk

½ cup unsweetened applesauce

¼ cup pure maple syrup

1 teaspoon pure vanilla extract

⅓ cup grain-sweetened, vegan mini chocolate chips

Sliced bananas, for serving.

Preparation: Place the flaxseeds in a small saucepan with ½ cup water. Cook over medium heat until the mixture gets a little sticky and appears stringy when it drips off a spoon, 3 to 4 minutes. Immediately strain the mixture into a glass measuring cup and set aside. Discard the seeds. In a large bowl, whisk together the buckwheat flour, oats, coconut flakes, baking powder, and salt. In a medium bowl, whisk together the milk, applesauce, maple syrup, vanilla, and 2 tablespoons of the reserved flax water. Add the liquid mixture to the dry mix and stir together to blend; the batter will be thick. Stir in the chocolate chips.

Heat a non-stick griddle over medium-low heat. Pour ⅓ cup batter for each pancake onto the griddle and spread gently. Cook for 6 to 8 minutes, until the pancakes look slightly dry on top, are lightly browned on the bottom, and release easily from the pan. Flip and cook for about 5 minutes on the other side. Repeat for the remaining batter, wiping off the griddle between batches. Serve hot with sliced bananas.

BANANA ALMOND GRANOLA: This recipe was inspired by my favourite banana almond muffins. Whether in muffins or in cereal, bananas and almonds pair perfectly.

Ingredient:

8 cups rolled oats

2 cups pitted and chopped dates

2 ripe bananas, peeled and chopped

1 teaspoon almond extract

1 teaspoon salt

1 cup slivered almonds, toasted (optional).

Preparation: Preheat the oven to 275°F. Add the oats to a large bowl and set aside. Line two 13 × 18-inch baking sheets with parchment paper. Place the dates in a medium saucepan with 1 cup of water and bring to a boil. Cook over medium heat for 10 minutes. Add more water if needed to keep the dates from sticking to the pan. Remove from the heat and add the mixture to a blender with the bananas, almond extract, and salt. Process until smooth and creamy. Add the date mixture to the oats and mix well. Divide the granola between the two prepared baking sheets and spread out evenly. Bake for 40 to 50 minutes, stirring every 10 minutes, until the granola is crispy. Remove from the oven and let cool before adding the slivered almonds (if using). (The cereal will get even crispier as it cools.) Store the granola in an airtight container.

CHICKPEA OMELETTE: This wonderful egg-free omelette is easy to make and is good for breakfast, lunch, or dinner.

Ingredient: 1 cup chickpea flour

½ teaspoon onion powder

½ teaspoon garlic powder

¼ teaspoon white pepper

¼ teaspoon black pepper

1/3 cup nutritional yeast

½ teaspoon baking soda

3 green onions (white and green parts), chopped

4 ounces sautéed mushrooms (optional).

Preparation: Combine the chickpea flour, onion powder, garlic powder, white pepper, black pepper, nutritional yeast, and baking soda in a small bowl. Add 1 cup water and stir until the batter is smooth. Heat a frying pan over medium heat. Pour the batter into the pan, as if making pancakes. Sprinkle 1 to 2 tablespoons of the green onions and mushrooms into the batter for each omelette as it cooks. Flip the omelette. When the underside is browned, flip the omelette again, and cook the other side for a minute. Serve your amazing Chickpea Omelette topped with tomatoes, spinach, salsa, hot sauce, or whatever heart-safe, plant-perfect fixings you like.

POLENTA WITH PEARS AND CRANBERRIES: This polenta recipe is one of my favourites! For this recipe use the ripest pears you can find on the market—Bosc, Asian, or D'anjou—and fresh cranberries when they are in season (usually from October through December).

Ingredient:

1/4 cup brown rice syrup

2 pears, peeled, cored, and diced

1 cup fresh or dried cranberries

1 teaspoon ground cinnamon

1 batch Basic Polenta, kept warm

Preparation: Heat the brown rice syrup in a medium saucepan. Add the pears, cranberries, and cinnamon and cook, stirring occasionally, until the pears are tender, about 10 minutes. To serve, divide the polenta among 4 individual bowls and top with the pear compote.

FRUIT AND NUT OATMEAL: Oatmeal is one of my favourite breakfast foods. It is quick to prepare and easily adaptable to my ever-changing moods—some days I want it with fruit, some days I want it plain, and sometimes I want a little bit of everything in it (that's when I include all of the optional ingredients listed here!). This basic recipe is all you need to get started ... add as much or as little of the extras as you like.

Ingredient:

¾ cup rolled oats

¼ teaspoon ground cinnamon

Pinch of sea salt

¼ cup fresh berries (optional)

½ ripe banana, sliced (optional)

2 tablespoons chopped nuts, such as walnuts, pecans, or cashews (optional)

2 tablespoons dried fruit, such as raisins, cranberries, chopped apples, chopped

Apricots (optional)

Maple syrup (optional).

Preparation: Combine the oats and 1½ cups water in a small saucepan. Bring to a boil over high heat. Reduce the heat to medium-low and cook until the water has been absorbed, about 5 minutes. Stir in the cinnamon and salt. Top with the berries, banana, nuts, and/or dried fruit, as you like. If desired, pour a little maple syrup on top. Serve hot.

EGYPTIAN BREAKFAST BEANS: This traditional Egyptian breakfast (pronounced fool mudammis) is almost always made with dried fava beans. They need to soak at least 8 hours before cooking, so start this dish the day before you want to serve it, to let the beans soak overnight. Full Medames is usually served with pita bread and a fried egg, but take some liberty and serve it over brown rice with fresh lemon instead.

Ingredient:

1½ pounds dried fava beans, soaked for 8 to 10 hours

1 medium yellow onion, peeled and diced small

4 cloves garlic, peeled and minced

1 teaspoon ground cumin

Zest and juice of 1 lemon

Sea salt

1 lemon, quartered.

Preparation: Drain and rinse the beans and add them to a large pot. Cover with 4 inches of water and bring to a boil over high heat. Reduce the heat to medium, cover, and cook until the beans are tender, 1½ to 2 hours. While the beans are cooking, sauté the onion in a medium skillet or saucepan over medium heat for 8 to 10 minutes, or until it is tender and starting to brown. Add the garlic, cumin, and lemon zest and juice and cook for 5 minutes longer. Set aside. When the beans are fully cooked, drain all but ½ cup of the liquid from the pot and add the onion mixture to the beans. Mix well and season with salt to taste. Serve garnished with the lemon quarters.

APPLE LEMON BREAKFAST: Fresh and deliciously filling, this apple-lemon breakfast bowl is beautifully flavoured with dates, cinnamon, and walnuts.

Ingredient:

4 to 5 medium apples, any variety

5 to 6 dates, pitted

Juice of 1 lemon (about 3 tablespoons)

2 tablespoons walnuts (about 6 walnut halves)

¼ teaspoon ground cinnamon.

Preparation: Core the apples and cut into large pieces. Place dates, half of the lemon juice, walnuts, cinnamon, and three quarters of the apple in the bowl of a food processor. Puree until finely ground, scraping down the sides of the bowl as needed. Add the remainder of the apples and lemon juice and pulse until the apples are shredded and the date mixture is evenly distributed.

BREAKFAST SCRAMBLE: There are many very good recipes for scrambles, but most call for tofu. In this recipe, cauliflower takes the place of the tofu—with delicious results.

Ingredient:

1 red onion, peeled and cut into ½-inch dice

1 red bell pepper, seeded and cut into ½-inch dice

1 green bell pepper, seeded and cut into ½-inch dice

2 cups sliced mushrooms (from about 8 ounces whole mushrooms)

1 large head cauliflower, cut into florets, or 2 (19-ounce) cans ackee, drained and gently rinsed

Sea salt

½ teaspoon freshly ground black pepper

1½ teaspoons turmeric

¼ teaspoon cayenne pepper, or to taste

3 cloves garlic, peeled and minced

1 to 2 tablespoons low-sodium soy sauce

¼ cup nutritional yeast (optional).

Preparation: Place the onion, red and green peppers, and mushrooms in a medium skillet or saucepan and sauté over medium-high heat for 7 to 8 minutes, or until the onion is translucent. Add water 1 to 2 tablespoons at a time to keep the vegetables from sticking to the pan. Add the cauliflower and cook for 5 to 6 minutes, or until the florets are tender. Add the salt to taste, pepper, turmeric, cayenne, garlic, soy sauce, and nutritional yeast (if using) to the pan, and cook for 5 minutes more, or until hot and fragrant.

BROWN RICE BREAKFAST PUDDING: My mom used to serve a version of this for breakfast—cooked with milk, sugar, and a hint of cinnamon. It is still one of my favourite breakfasts, although now I make a more wholesome version with almond milk and chopped dates.

Ingredient:

3 cups cooked brown rice

2 cups unsweetened almond milk

1 cinnamon stick

⅛ to ¼ teaspoon ground cloves, to taste

1 cup dates, pitted and chopped

1 tart apple (such as Granny Smith), cored and chopped

¼ cup raisins

Salt to taste

¼ cup slivered almonds, toasted.

Preparation: Combine the rice, almond milk, cinnamon stick, cloves, and dates in a medium saucepan and cook, stirring occasionally, over medium-low heat for 12 minutes, or until the mixture thickens. Remove the cinnamon stick. Add the apple, raisins, and salt and mix. Serve garnished with the toasted almonds.

CHOCOLATE BUTTERMILK PANCAKES: Everybody deserves to have a little chocolate for breakfast once in a while. These pancakes got five-star reviews from all of my testers. This recipe requires a non-stick skillet to keep the pancakes from sticking. Serve with whatever fresh fruit you like—we enjoy them with strawberries, raspberries, bananas, or a combination of all three.

Ingredient:

1¼ cups whole-grain gluten-free flour (see Notes)

2 tablespoons unsweetened cocoa powder

1 tablespoon baking powder

1 tablespoon ground flaxseed

1 tablespoon vegan mini chocolate chips (optional; see Notes)

¼ teaspoon sea salt

1 cup unsweetened, unflavoured almond milk

1 tablespoon pure maple syrup or ¼ teaspoon stevia powder

1 teaspoon vanilla extract

1 tablespoon apple cider vinegar

¼ cup unsweetened applesauce.

Preparation: Combine the dry ingredients (flour, cocoa powder, baking powder, flax, chocolate chips, and salt) in a medium bowl. Whisk until fully combined. Combine the wet ingredients (almond milk, maple syrup, vanilla, and vinegar) in a small bowl, and whisk well. This will create a vegan buttermilk for your pancakes. Add the vegan buttermilk and the applesauce to the flour mixture, and stir until the batter is just combined. Let the batter stand for 10 minutes while it rises and thickens as the flaxseeds soak; it may nearly double in size.

Heat a non-stick skillet or electric skillet griddle over medium heat and mist with a tiny bit of non-stick spray, if desired. (If you have a large skillet, you can cook multiple pancakes at once.) Scoop the batter into 3-inch rounds. Cook for 2 to 3 minutes or until the bubbles have burst in each of the pancakes and the tops start to appear dry. Flip the pancakes and cook for 1 to 2 minutes more. You should get 12 pancakes total.

BLACK BEAN AND SWEET POTATO HASH: This black bean and sweet potato hash can be an ideal breakfast, a lunch, or a light dinner. It can be served simply as a side dish, spooned over brown rice or quinoa, wrapped in a whole-wheat tortilla, or made into soft tacos garnished with avocado, cilantro, and other favourite toppings. Make it in your Instant Pot or other pressure cooker, or do it the old-fashioned way, on the stovetop.

Ingredient:

1 cup chopped onion

1 to 2 cloves garlic, minced

2 cups chopped peeled sweet potatoes (about 2 small or medium)

2 teaspoons mild or hot chili powder

⅓ cup low-sodium vegetable broth

1 cup cooked black beans

¼ cup chopped scallions

Splash of hot sauce (optional)

Chopped cilantro, for garnish.

Preparation:

Stovetop Method— Place the onions in a non-stick skillet and sauté over medium- heat, stirring occasionally, for 2 to 3 minutes. Add the garlic and stir. Add the sweet potatoes and chili powder, and stir to coat the vegetables with the chili powder. Add broth and stir. Cook for about 12 minutes more, stirring occasionally, until the potatoes are cooked through. Add more liquid 1 to 2 tablespoons at a time as needed, to keep the vegetables from sticking to the pan. Add the black beans, scallions, and salt. Cook for

1 or 2 minutes more, until the beans are heated through. Add the hot sauce (if using), and stir. Taste and adjust the seasonings. Top with chopped cilantro and serve.

Pressure Cooker Method — Heat a stovetop pressure cooker over medium heat or set an electric cooker to sauté. Add the onion and cook, stirring occasionally, for 2 to 3 minutes. Add the garlic and stir. Add the sweet potatoes and chili powder. Stir to coat the sweet potatoes with the chili powder. Add the broth and stir. Lock the lid on the pressure cooker. Bring to high pressure for 3 minutes. Quick release the pressure. Remove the lid, tilting it away from you. Add the black beans, scallions, and salt. Cook for 1 or 2 minutes more over medium heat, or lock on the lid for 3 minutes, until the beans are heated through. Add the hot sauce (if using), and stir. Taste and adjust the seasonings. Top with chopped cilantro and serve.

EASY OVERNIGHT OATS WITH CHIA: To get through those busy weeks, try this easy and healthy breakfast that you can make the night before.

Ingredient:

¾ cup gluten-free rolled oats

¼ cup plant milk

½ cup water

1 heaping tablespoon chia seeds

½-1 tablespoon maple syrup

¼ teaspoon cinnamon

Dash of vanilla bean powder or extract

Fruit of choice.

Preparation: Place oats, liquid, chia seeds, maple syrup, cinnamon, and vanilla into a 16-ounce mason jar or container of choice. Mix well. Seal shut and place jar in refrigerator overnight. In the morning, mix again and top with anything you'd like, such as fresh fruit, more chia seeds, or cacao nibs.

WHOLE-WHEAT BLUEBERRY MUFFINS: These are a perfectly delicious breakfast muffin with loads of berry goodness and a tasty, wheat backdrop. If you can find wild blueberries, use them—they are perfect for muffins because they're tiny and distribute beautifully without making the muffin soggy. If you use larger berries, like blackberries, slice them in half; otherwise they'll be too large. If you use frozen berries, bake the muffins for 26 minutes. If you use fresh, then 22 minutes should do it. Either way, check after 22 minutes to make sure you don't overbake.

Ingredient:

⅔ cup unsweetened plant-based milk

1 tablespoon ground flaxseeds

1 teaspoon apple cider vinegar

2 cups whole-wheat pastry flour

2 teaspoons baking powder

¼ teaspoon baking soda

¾ teaspoon salt

½ cup unsweetened applesauce

½ cup pure maple syrup

1½ teaspoons pure vanilla extract

1 cup berries.

Preparation: Preheat the oven to 350°F. Line a 12-cup muffin pan with silicone liners or use a non-stick or silicone muffin pan. In a large measuring cup, use a fork to vigorously mix together the plant-based milk, flaxseeds, and vinegar. Mix for about a minute, until it appears foamy. Set aside. In a medium mixing bowl, sift together the flour, baking powder, baking soda, and salt. Make a well in the centre and pour in the milk mixture. Add the applesauce, maple syrup, and vanilla to the well and stir together. Incorporate the dry ingredients into the wet ingredients until the dry ingredients are moistened (do not overmix). Fold in the berries. Fill each muffin cup three-quarters full and bake for 22 to 26 minutes, or until a knife inserted through the centre of a muffin comes out clean. Let the muffins cool completely, about 20 minutes, then carefully run a knife around the edges of each muffin to remove them from the pan.

APPLE-WALNUT BREAKFAST BREAD: Slightly sweet, oil-free, and totally satisfying, this makes a great breakfast on the run. I know you want to eat it all in one sitting (I do, too), so to avoid that calorie splurge, cut it into single servings, wrap each in plastic wrap, and put them in the freezer until needed. This also makes a great baked gift. Wrap it up, tie it with a bow—now you're everyone's favourite breakfast baker!

Ingredient:

1½ cups unsweetened applesauce

¾ cup packed light brown sugar

⅓ cup plain unsweetened almond milk or plant milk

1 tablespoon ground flax seeds mixed with 2 tablespoons warm water

2 cups all-purpose or whole wheat flour

1 teaspoon baking soda

½ teaspoon baking powder

1 teaspoon salt

1 teaspoon ground cinnamon

½ cup chopped walnuts.

Preparation: Preheat the oven to 375°F. In a large bowl, combine the applesauce, brown sugar, almond milk, and flax mixture and stir until smooth and well mixed. Set aside. In a separate bowl, combine the flour, baking soda, baking powder, salt, and cinnamon. Mix the dry ingredients into the wet ingredients just until blended. Stir in the walnuts, then transfer the batter to a 9x5-inch loaf pan, spreading evenly and smoothing the top. Bake until golden brown and a toothpick inserted in the centre comes out clean, 25 to 30 minutes. Cool in the pan for about 20 minutes, then remove from the pan and cool completely on a wire rack.

HIGH PROTEIN SALADS.

GRILLED HALLOUMI BROCCOLI SALAD: Here is a grilled halloumi salad with grilled baby broccoli, avocado and quinoa.

Ingredient: Fresh Salad

Halloumi Cheese (about 2/3 of a packet)

Half an Avocado

Baby Broccoli

Quinoa (half a cup)

Olive Oil (dressing).

Preparation: The first thing to do is to prepare your salad. Wash and dry it well. Once the halloumi is ready, you're going to want to eat it straight away as it tends to get very rubbery as it cools off so preparing everything else beforehand makes everything easier. Prepare half an avocado by slicing it into small cubes (it'll add creaminess to your salad which is why I tend to only use olive oil as my dressing).

In a pot, add some water to boil (with a pinch of salt) for the baby broccoli. I like mine fairly crunchy so 2-3 minutes was enough. Once your salad and avocado are done and your broccoli is cooking, start with your quinoa. Put half a cup of quinoa into a small pot, add about one cup of water and leave to boil (salt isn't necessary here because of the saltiness of the halloumi cheese) on a medium flame.

As your broccoli is cooking, prepare your grill pan for the halloumi cheese. On a medium flame, add a few drops of olive oil and leave it to heat up. Slice the halloumi into about centimetre thick pieces, then add to the grill pan. Your broccoli should be ready by now so add those too. For a golden-brown colour, I grilled my halloumi and broccoli for about 6 minutes, making sure to flip the cheese over to cook it evenly.

Don't forget to check on the quinoa. It should be ready once the water is gone (about 7-8 minutes), but taste to be sure (it should have a somewhat crunchy texture). Once the halloumi, broccoli, and quinoa are ready, throw everything into your salad bowl and mix well. Season with some olive oil and serve while the halloumi is hot.

BLACK BEAN LENTIL SALAD WITH LIME DRESSING: Healthy black bean lentil salad with cumin-lime dressing! Perfect for lunches, snacks, potlucks, picnics, etc.! (Vegan, gluten-free)

Ingredient: 1 cup green/brown lentils (uncooked)

15 oz. can black beans

1 red bell pepper

1/2 small red onion

1-2 roma tomatoes

2/3 cup cilantro (stems removed)

Optional: green onion.

Juice of 1 lime

2 Tbsp. olive oil (omit for oil-free)

1 tsp. Dijon mustard

1-2 cloves garlic (minced)

1 tsp. cumin

1/2 tsp. oregano

1/8 tsp. salt

Optional: chipotle powder, chili powder, pepper, hot sauce, other seasonings, etc.

Preparation: Cook lentils according to package directions, leaving firm not mushy. Drain.

While lentils are cooking, make the dressing: place all ingredients in a small bowl and whisk to combine. Set aside. Finely dice the bell pepper, onion, and tomatoes. Roughly chop the cilantro. In a large bowl, place the black beans (rinsed and drained), bell pepper, onion, tomatoes, and lentils. Add the dressing and toss to combine. Add cilantro, and lightly toss. Serve immediately or chill covered in the fridge for at least an hour to let the flavours combine.

ARUGULA LENTIL SALAD: Arugula Lentil Salad with easy to find ingredients. It's simple, tasty, vegan and really healthy!

Ingredient: ¾ cups cashews (¾ cups = 100 g)

1 onion

3 tbsp olive oil

1 chilli / jalapeño

5-6 sun-dried tomatoes in oil

3 slices bread (whole wheat)

1 cup brown lentils, cooked (1 cup = 1 / 15oz / 400 g)

1 handful arugula/rocket (1 handful = 100 g)

1-2 tbsp balsamic vinegar

salt and pepper to taste.

Preparation: Roast the cashews on a low heat for about three minutes in a pan to maximize aroma. Then throw them into the salad bowl. Dice up and fry the onion in one third of the olive oil for about 3 minutes on a low heat. Meanwhile chop the chilli/jalapeño and dried tomatoes. Add them to the pan and fry for another 1-2 minutes. Cut the bread into big croutons. Move the onion mix into a big bowl. Now add the rest of the oil to the pan and fry the chopped-up bread until crunchy. Season with salt and pepper. Wash the arugula and add it to the bowl. Put the lentils in too, and mix them all around. Season with salt, pepper and balsamic vinegar. Serve with the croutons. Super tasty!

RED CABBAGE SALAD WITH CURRIED SEITAN: If you cook vegetarian dishes long enough, eventually you'll wind up cooking seitan. It's a "high-protein wheat gluten product" that's a staple of meatless meals.

Ingredient:

1 Tbs. olive oil

1 8-oz. pkg. seitan, cut into bite-size strips

3 cloves garlic, minced (1 Tbs.)

¾ tsp. mild curry powder

6 cups shredded red cabbage (½ small head)

1 small cucumber, sliced into thin half-moons (¾ cup)

3 green onions, thinly sliced (½ cup)

⅓ cup prepared mango chutney

⅓ cup creamy natural peanut butter.

Preparation: To make Dressing: Blend chutney, peanut butter, and 1/3 cup water in blender until smooth. Set aside. To make Salad: Heat 2 tsp. oil in large skillet over medium heat. Add seitan, and season with salt, if desired. Sauté 5 to 7 minutes, or until browned. Add garlic and remaining 1 tsp. oil, and sauté 30 seconds. Sprinkle with curry powder, and sauté 2 minutes more. Remove from heat, and keep warm. Toss cabbage and cucumber with Dressing in large bowl. Top with warm seitan and green onions.

CHICKPEA, RED KIDNEY BEAN AND FETA SALAD: rich in Protein, Fibre, anti-oxidants, and other minerals.

Ingredient:

1 can chickpeas

1 can red kidney beans

1 piece small of ginger grated or shredded

1 medium onion diced

2- 3 cloves garlic

1   tbsp olive oil

A pinch of red chili flakes

3-4 spring onions green part only, chopped, scallions

1 cup chopped parsley OR coriander I used cilantro

Juice of one lemon

150 g feta cheese – almost half cup size

Salt and Black pepper.

Preparation: Heat 1 tablespoon of olive oil and cook the onion till lightly golden. Do not overdo it and the onions should still be crunchy. Add garlic, ginger and chili and cook till the garlic is fragrant. Set aside to cool so it doesn't melt the feta when you mix it in. Drain the chickpeas and red kidney beans, rinse and place in the salad bowl. Add crumbled feta, spring onion, parsley (or coriander) and lemon juice, season with salt and pepper. Add the cooled onion and garlic mixture and remaining oil and mix well.

THE AMAZING CHICKPEA SPINACH SALAD: These bad boy legumes are high in both fibre and protein, essential for good health and a strong digestive system.

Ingredient: 1 can chickpeas (drained and rinsed)

1 handful spinach

3.5 oz feta cheese (or similar cheese)

1 small handful raisins

½ tbsp lemon juice (white or malt vinegar is also good)

3 tsp honey

4 tbsp olive oil

0.5 - 1 tsp cumin

1 pinch salt

½ tsp chili flakes (or dried cayenne pepper will do the trick nicely).

Preparation: Chop the cheese and add with the spinach and chickpeas to a large bowl

Mix the honey, oil, lemon juice and raisins in a small bowl. Add the cumin, salt and pepper to the dressing bowl and mix well. Drizzle devilishly delicious dressing over the salad.

CURRIED CARROT SLAW WITH TEMPEH: Bold in flavour and dense in nutrition, this crunchy-nutty-sassy-savoury-sweet meal is a golden delight you will make again and again.

Ingredient: 8 ounces tempeh, sliced into triangles

1/4 tsp liquid smoke (optional)

1 1/2 Tbsp maple syrup, grade B

1 tsp extra virgin olive oil or virgin coconut oil

2-3 tsp tamari or 2 tsp soy sauce

1 Tbsp crushed raw walnuts

4 cups shredded carrots

1 small onion, diced

1 Tbsp curry powder

1/4 tsp turmeric powder (for added turmeric power, optional)

1/8 tsp black pepper

2 Tbsp tahini

1/4 cup fresh lemon juice

sweet stuff: 1 – 1 1/2 Tbsp maple syrup + an optional handful or raisins

1/2 cup flat leaf parsley, finely chopped + some for garnish

a few pinches of cayenne for heat (optional)

salt and pepper for carrot salad – to taste.

Preparation: Warm a skillet up over high heat and add in the coconut or olive oil. When oil is hot, add the tempeh triangles, tamari, maple and liquid smoke. Flip the tempeh around a bit to allow it to absorb the liquid. Cook for about 5 minutes, flipping the tempeh a few times throughout the cooking process. When tempeh is browned and edges blackened a bit, and all liquid absorbed, turn off heat. Sprinkle the walnut pieces and some black pepper over top the tempeh and set pan aside to keep triangles warm in skillet. In a large mixing bowl, add the carrots, tahini, lemon juice, spices, parsley, maple syrup, optional raisins and onion. Toss very well for a few minutes to marinate the carrots with the dressing. For a creamier salad, add another spoonful of tahini. To thin things out and make the salad zestier, add another splash of lemon juice or a teaspoon of apple cider vinegar. Finally, add salt and pepper to the carrot salad to taste. Pour the carrot salad in a large serving bowl and top with the tempeh. Serve right away or place in the fridge to serve in a few hours or up to a day later. The carrots will soften the longer they set in the fridge.

BLACK & WHITE BEAN QUINOA SALAD: This salad packs not only a protein punch but also good amounts of fibre and iron.

Ingredient:

⅓ cup (75 mL) quinoa

1 can (19 oz/540 mL) black beans, drained and rinsed

1 can (19 oz/540 mL) navy beans, drained and rinsed

1 cup (250 mL) diced cucumbers

¼ cup (50 mL) diced red onion

1 jalapeno pepper, seeded and minced (I've never used it and find the dish spicy enough for me, but feel free to add it if you like things hot!)

¼ cup (50 mL) chopped fresh coriander (cilantro)

¼ cup (50 mL) vegetable oil (I use cold pressed extra-virgin olive oil)

2 tbsp (25 mL) lime juice

1 tbsp (15 mL) cider vinegar

1 clove garlic, minced

½ tsp (2 mL) chili powder

1 tsp (5 mL) ground coriander

½ tsp (2 mL) dried oregano

¼ tsp (1 mL) salt

¼ tsp (1 mL) pepper.

Preparation: In saucepan of boiling salted ⅔ C water, cook quinoa until tender, about 12 minutes. Drain and rinse. Dressing: In large bowl, whisk together oil, lime juice, vinegar, garlic, chili powder, coriander, oregano, salt and pepper. Add quinoa, black beans, navy beans, cucumber, onion, jalapeño pepper and coriander; toss to combine.

GREEK SALAD WITH SEITAN GYROS STRIPS: You can't really mess with this classic so I have just veganised it and added some Greek style 'meat' strips and a bad ass dressing!

Ingredient: 4 tomatoes

1 punnet cherry tomatoes

1 1/2 crunchy cucumbers

1 big handful kalamata olives

1/2 Spanish onion finely sliced

1/4 stick of Cheesy mozzarella style cheese.

Fresh oregano and mint

1/4 cup good quality extra virgin olive oil

2 Tablespoons vinegar (red wine or balsamic)

1 teaspoon castor sugar

2 teaspoons mixed dried Italian herbs

1 clove finely chopped garlic

1 teaspoon soy sauce

salt

pepper.

Preparation: In a small frying pan, place gyros strips and fry until slightly blackened on the edges. Leave to cool. Cut up all your veggies roughly and place in a large bowl. Add olives, oregano, mint and chopped cheese. In a jar add all dressing ingredients. Shake well and taste. Combine the cooled gyros strips, salad and dressing and coat well.

CHICKPEA AND EDAMAME SALAD: The best part about this salad is it's so simple to whip up. It's perfect for a summer picnic with some fresh fruit, sparkling water and a warm baguette.

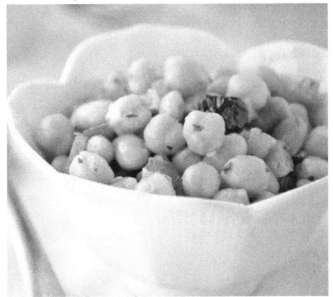

Ingredient: 2 15.5oz each cans chickpea (garbanzo beans) rinsed and drained

3/4 cup edamame soy beans

1/3 cup chopped red pepper

1/3 cup chopped green pepper

1/4 cup diced carrots

3 tablespoons dried cranberries

1 garlic clove minced

Dressing

2 tablespoons grapeseed oil

2 tablespoons olive oil

1 teaspoon white distilled vinegar

1 teaspoon sugar

1/4 teaspoon dried oregano

1/4 teaspoon dried basil

1/4 teaspoon dried rosemary

Salt and pepper

Preparation: In a large bowl combine chickpeas, edamame, red pepper, green pepper, carrots, dried cranberries, minced garlic and set aside. In a small bowl combine grapeseed oil, olive oil, vinegar, sugar, oregano, basil and rosemary. Whisk until blended. Pour dressing over chick peas and gently toss. Season with salt and pepper to taste. Chill for at least 30 minutes for flavours to blend. Serve chilled.

WHOLE FOOD DINNERS.

COCONUT CAULIFLOWER CURRY: Everybody loves this cauliflower curry! This easy dinner recipe is warm-spiced, nutrient packed, and ready in just over 30 minutes. Dinnertime win.

Ingredient: 1 yellow onion

1-pound sweet potato (4 cups chopped)

1 head cauliflower (5 cups chopped)

2 tablespoons olive oil

1 teaspoon kosher salt, divided

2 tablespoons curry powder*

1 tablespoon garam masala

1 teaspoon cumin

¼ teaspoon cayenne

28-ounce can dice tomatoes, San Marzano if possible

15-ounce can full-fat coconut milk

15-ounce can chickpeas

4 cups spinach leaves

Cilantro, for garnish

Brown or white rice, for serving

Preparation: Make the rice according to How to Cook White Rice, How to Cook Brown Rice, or Instant Pot Rice. Dice the onion. Chop the sweet potato into bite-sized chunks (do not peel). Chop the cauliflower into florets. Heat 2 tablespoons olive oil in a large non-stick skillet over medium-high heat. Add onion and sauté 2 minutes, then add the sweet potato and sauté 3 minutes. Add cauliflower and ½ teaspoon kosher salt and sauté another 5 minutes. Stir in 2 tablespoons curry powder, 1 tablespoon garam masala, 1 teaspoon cumin, and ¼ teaspoon cayenne. Add the Muir Glen tomatoes and coconut milk. Bring to a boil, then cover, reduce heat and simmer for about 10 minutes until the cauliflower and sweet potato are tender. Drain and rinse the chickpeas. When the vegetables are tender, add the chickpeas and 4 cups spinach and stir for 2 minutes until the spinach is wilted. Add another ½ teaspoon kosher salt to taste, adding additional salt if necessary. Garnish with chopped cilantro, and serve with brown rice.

3-Bean Healthy Chili Recipe: This healthy chili recipe is full of good-for-you ingredients and big flavour, featuring a trio of beans, quinoa, and lots of hearty spices.

Ingredient: 3/4 cup Simply Nature Organic Quinoa

2 small or 1 medium yellow onion

3 cloves garlic

2 tablespoons olive oil

1/2 cup Simply Nature Organic Ketchup

1/4 cup chili powder

2 tablespoons dried oregano

1 tablespoon garlic powder

1 teaspoon cumin

1 cup water

3 15-ounce cans Simply Nature Organic Beans (we did 1 can each black, pinto and kidney), drained.

2 28-ounce cans Simply Nature Organic Diced Tomatoes

1 cup frozen corn

1 tablespoon yellow mustard

1 tablespoon Worcestershire sauce, vegan if desired

2 tablespoons ground Simply Nature Flax Seed (optional)

1 1/2 teaspoons kosher salt

Optional: 1 tablespoon adobo sauce (from a can of chipotle chilis).

To garnish: Sour cream or Greek yogurt (or Vegan Sour Cream or Cashew Cream for vegan), Mexican blend shredded cheese, and Southern Grove Pepitas.

Preparation: Cook the quinoa: Place the quinoa in a saucepan with 1 1/2 cups water. Bring to a boil, then reduce the heat to very low. Cover the pot, and simmer where the water is just bubbling for about 15 to 20 minutes, until the water has been completely absorbed. (Check by pulling back the quinoa with a fork to see if water remains.) Turn off the heat and let sit covered to steam for 5 minutes. Dice the onions. Mince the garlic. In a large pot or Dutch oven, heat the olive oil over medium heat. Add the onions and sauté for 5 to 7 minutes, until tender. Add the garlic and cook for 2 minutes until lightly browned. Add the ketchup and spices and cook for 1 minute until fragrant. Add all other ingredients, and throw in the quinoa whenever it is cooked. Simmer for 25 minutes. Serve immediately with toppings. Store leftovers refrigerated for up to 3 days, or frozen for 3 months.

BBQ Bean Tacos with Pineapple Salsa: These plant-based BBQ bean tacos with pineapple salsa are a delicious fast and easy dinner recipe! They're on the table in less than 30 minutes.

Ingredient: 2 15-ounce cans pinto beans

2 tablespoons Dijon mustard

1 tablespoon maple syrup

3/4 cup organic ketchup (or with natural sugars)

1/2 teaspoon garlic powder

1/2 teaspoon chili powder

3/4 teaspoon kosher salt, divided

20-ounce can (11/2 cups) pineapple chunks packed in juice* (or substitute Mango Salsa)

1/4 cup minced red onion

1/4 cup finely chopped cilantro, plus additional for garnish

1 small green cabbage

3 radishes

1 lime (wedges for squeezing)

Tortillas, for serving.

Preparation: Drain both cans of beans (no need to rinse). In a large skillet, place the beans, mustard, maple syrup, ketchup, garlic powder, chili powder, and 1/2 teaspoon kosher salt. Heat on low until thickened and warm, while making the remainder of the recipe. Drain the pineapple and finely chop it. Mince the red onion, and chop the cilantro. Mix the pineapple, red onion and cilantro together with 1/4 teaspoon kosher salt. Thinly slice the green cabbage and radishes. Slice the lime into wedges. If desired, char the tortillas by placing them on an open gas flame on medium for a few seconds per side, flipping with tongs, until they are slightly blackened and warm. To serve, place the beans in a tortilla, then add cabbage, radishes and a squeeze of lime (important, do not omit!). Top with pineapple salsa and additional cilantro if desired.

BEST WILD RICE SOUP: This wild rice soup recipe is impossibly creamy, packed with flavour and full of tender veggies and hearty rice. Everyone asks for the recipe—it's that good.

Ingredient: 1/2 cup cashews*

1 medium yellow onion

2 celery stalks

3 medium carrots

8 ounces baby Bella mushrooms

6 cloves garlic

2 tablespoons olive oil

1 tablespoon dried thyme

1 tablespoon dried oregano

8 cups vegetable broth

1 cup wild rice (not a wild rice blend)

2 teaspoons kosher salt, divided

2 15-ounce cans white beans, drained and rinsed

1/2 teaspoon black pepper

2 teaspoons dried sage

1 tablespoon soy sauce, tamari, or liquid amino.

Preparation: Place the cashews in a bowl and cover them with water. Leave them to soak while you make the recipe. Dice the onion. Thinly slice the celery. Cut the carrot into rounds. Slice the mushrooms. Mince the garlic. Add the olive oil to a Dutch oven. Add the onion, celery and carrot and cook, stirring occasionally for 5 minutes until lightly browned. Add mushrooms and sauté for 2 minutes. Add garlic, thyme and oregano and stir for 2 minutes. Add the broth, wild rice, 1 1/2 teaspoon kosher salt, and black pepper. Bring to a simmer. Simmer uncovered for 20 minutes. Then add the beans (drained and rinsed), and continue to simmer uncovered for 30 to 35 minutes more, or until rice breaks open. Using a liquid cup measure, carefully remove 2 cups of the hot soup (including broth, veggies and rice) to a blender. Add 1 cup water. Drain the cashews and add them to the blender, along with the dried sage. Blend on high for about 1 minute until creamy. Then pour the creamy mixture back into the soup. Add the soy sauce and the remaining 1/2 teaspoon kosher salt. Taste, and adjust seasonings as desired. Garnish with fresh ground pepper.

Thai Salad with Peanut Sauce Dressing: A fast and easy dinner recipe, this colourful Thai salad recipe features a flavourful peanut sauce dressing. It's vegan, gluten-free, and delicious!

Ingredient: 14-ounce package extra firm tofu

   2 tablespoons olive oil

   1/2 cup coconut milk

   1/4 cup peanut butter

   2 tablespoons soy

   1 tablespoon lime juice

   2 teaspoons honey

   ¼ teaspoon kosher salt

   1 red pepper

   1 yellow pepper

   2 green onions

¼ red cabbage

4 carrots

10 ounces Earthbound Farm Organic Half & Half Baby Spinach and Spring Mix

1/4 cup crushed peanuts

Cilantro, to garnish

Lime wedges, to garnish.

Preparation: Remove the tofu from the package and blot it dry with a clean dish towel. With tofu block flat, slice it into 3 long strips, and cut the strips in half crosswise. Slice each piece into thirds. On a non-stick griddle or large skillet over low heat, warm 2 tablespoons olive oil. Place the tofu on the griddle, sprinkle with kosher salt and fresh ground pepper, and cook for 10 to 15 minutes, flipping every few minutes, until light brown and crisp on both sides. Remove from the heat and allow to cool for a few minutes, and then cut into smaller bite-sized pieces if desired. In a small bowl, whisk together coconut milk, peanut butter, soy, lime, honey, and kosher salt. Taste, and add additional peanut butter if desired (we added 1 additional tablespoon). Thinly slice the peppers, green onions and cabbage. Shred the carrots (using a julienne peeler, or us a vegetable peeler to make ribbons). To serve, place greens in a bowl. Top with vegetables and tofu and drizzle with dressing, then garnish with crushed peanuts, cilantro leaves, and a squeeze of lime.

PERFECT VEGAN BLACK BEAN BURGER: This easy vegan black bean burger is bursting with flavour: the patties are also gluten free and topped with spicy mayo & sprouts.

Ingredient: 1 small sweet potato (½ pound)

3/4 cup Bob's Red Mill gluten-free old-fashioned rolled oats

2 green onions

15-ounce can black beans

½ cup sunflower seeds (shelled)

1/2 teaspoon kosher salt

1/2 teaspoon garlic powder

2 teaspoons smoked paprika

1 ½ tablespoons soy sauce

1 ½ tablespoons mirin

4 shiitake mushrooms

1 splash each olive oil, mirin, and soy sauce

¼ cup vegan mayonnaise

2 teaspoons Sriracha hot sauce (or less to taste)

4 English muffins (gluten-free if desired, or omit)

Alfalfa sprouts, for serving.

Preparation: Preheat oven to 375°F. Wash the sweet potato and prick it with a fork. Microwave until cooked through, about 8 minutes, turning halfway through. Slice open and allow to cool until the steam dissipates and it is cool to the touch.

Place oats on cutting board and roughly chop with a knife to obtain a mixed texture. Thinly slice green onions. Drain and rinse the beans. In a bowl, combine onions, oats, beans, sunflower seeds, kosher salt, garlic powder, smoked paprika, soy sauce and mirin. Mix with your hands and lightly mash the beans with your fingers. Add ½ cup sweet potato and mix to combine. Line a baking sheet with parchment paper. Form into 4 patties and place on the baking sheet. Bake 20 minutes on one side, then flip and bake 20 minutes on the other side. Cool slightly before serving. Remove the stems and slice the shiitake mushroom caps. In a small skillet, add a splash of olive oil, mirin, and soy sauce, then sauté the mushrooms until soft, about 1 minute. Mix the mayonnaise with Sriracha. To serve, place the burgers on toasted English muffins and top with mushrooms, spicy mayo, and alfalfa sprouts.

"GET YOUR GREENS" NAAN PIZZA: This naan pizza is a quick and easy vegetarian dinner recipe, topped with hummus, kale, broccoli, and a tahini miso drizzle!

Ingredient: 1 tablespoon miso

2 tablespoons fresh orange juice

1/4 cup tahini

1/4 teaspoon ground ginger

1/4 teaspoon maple syrup or honey

1 large head broccoli, chopped into small florets (5 cups chopped)

1 bunch chard, kale, or spinach (4 cups chopped)

2 green onions

2 tablespoons olive oil

2 tablespoons soy sauce

1/2 teaspoon kosher salt

Fresh ground black pepper

7 ounces canned artichokes (1/2 14-ounce can)

2 radishes

4 naan breads (or vegan pita or flatbread)

1 cup hummus (purchased or homemade).

Preparation: Preheat the oven to 450°F. In a medium bowl, whisk the miso into the orange juice. Whisk in the tahini, ginger, and maple syrup, and 1 tablespoon water. Stir until a drizzle-able consistency is reached, adding additional water if necessary.

Chop the broccoli into small florets. Destem and chop the greens. Thinly slice the green onion. In a large skillet, heat the olive oil over medium high heat. Add the broccoli and sauté for 2 minutes. Add the chard and green onion, and cook until the chard is wilted, about 2 minutes. Add the soy sauce and 1/4 teaspoon kosher salt and sauté for another minute, until the broccoli is bright green and crisp tender. Taste, and add another 1/4 teaspoon kosher salt if desired. Roughly chop the artichoke. Slice the radish into matchsticks. Place naan directly on the oven grate and pre-bake 3 to 4 minutes per side. Remove the naan from the oven and allow to cool slightly. To serve, spread each pita with hummus. Top with greens and broccoli, artichokes, and radishes, and drizzle with the tahini miso sauce.

CHICKPEA FATTOUSH SALAD BOWL: This chickpea Fattoush salad bowl is a take on the traditional Lebanese salad; adding chickpeas makes it a filling meatless healthy dinner idea.

Ingredient: 1 garlic clove

1 large lemon (1/4 cup lemon juice plus zest)

11/2 teaspoons kosher salt, divided

1/4 teaspoon cinnamon

1/4 teaspoon allspice

11/2 teaspoons maple or honey

Fresh ground black pepper

1/2 cup plus 2 tablespoons olive oil

2 15-ounce cans chickpeas

2 teaspoons cumin

3 romaine hearts

10 ounces Village Farms heavenly Villaggio Marzano tomatoes

1 small English cucumber

2 scallions (green onions)

3 to 4 radishes

1 handful fresh mint leaves

Sumac (optional).

Preparation: Preheat the oven to 350F. Brush the pita breads on both sides with olive oil and sprinkle with a few pinches kosher salt. Slice each pita into 8 wedges with a pizza cutter. Place the wedges on a baking sheet and bake until golden and crispy, about 20 minutes.

Allow to cool slightly, then break the wedges into irregular pieces. Meanwhile, mince the garlic, then use the flat blade of your knife to scrape it into a paste. In a medium bowl whisk together the garlic, 1/4 cup lemon juice, 1/2 teaspoon kosher salt, cinnamon, allspice, maple, and several grinds of black pepper. Gradually whisk in 1/2 cup olive oil a tablespoon or two at a time until a creamy emulsion form. Drain and rinse the chickpeas, shaking off as much water as possible. In a large skillet, heat 2 tablespoons olive oil over medium heat. Add the chickpeas, cumin, 1 teaspoon kosher salt, and several grinds of black pepper and sauté for 5 minutes until the chickpeas are golden and warmed through. Chop the romaine hearts. Slice the tomatoes in half. Dice the cucumber. Thinly slice the scallions and radishes; slice the radishes in half. Thinly slice the mint leaves. To serve, place the greens in the bowl and arrange the vegetables, chickpeas, and toasted pita on top, adding a few pinches of kosher salt to the tomatoes and cucumber. Drizzle with dressing and garnish with mint and lemon zest (or sumac, if desired).

SWEET POTATOES WITH THAI PEANUT BUTTER SAUCE: These sweet potatoes topped with a zesty slaw and creamy Thai peanut butter sauce are an irresistible plant-based dinner recipe!

Ingredient: 4 medium to large sweet potatoes (10 to 12 ounces each)

   1/4 red cabbage (3 cups shredded)

   1/2 red bell pepper

   1/2 yellow bell pepper

   1 green onion

   1/4 cup chopped cilantro

   2 tablespoons fresh lime juice (1 lime)

   1/4 teaspoon kosher salt

   Crushed peanuts, for the garnish

   1/3 cup peanut butter

   2 tablespoons soy sauce

   2 tablespoons lime juice (1 lime)

   1 teaspoon maple syrup

   2 tablespoons water.

Preparation: Cook the sweet potatoes: Go to Instant Pot Sweet Potatoes or Quick Baked Sweet Potatoes. Make the slaw: Thinly slice the red cabbage, enough for 3 cups. Thinly slice the peppers. Thinly slice the green onion. Chop the cilantro. In a large bowl, mix together the cabbage, peppers, green onion and cilantro with the lime juice and kosher salt. Make the Thai peanut butter sauce: In a small bowl, whisk together the peanut butter, soy sauce, lime juice, maple syrup, and water. Taste and add a bit of kosher salt if desired (this depends on the salt content of the peanut butter). Serve: Slice the sweet potatoes in half and top them with the slaw. Drizzle with the Thai peanut butter sauce and sprinkle with chopped peanuts.

MOROCCAN STEW WITH CHICKPEAS & SWEET POTATOES: This Moroccan stew with chickpeas and sweet potatoes is an easy plant-based dinner recipe: it's incredibly flavourful featuring a blend of Moroccan spices.

Ingredient: 2 cups uncooked quinoa

1 large onion

3 cloves garlic

2 large sweet potatoes (about 1 ¾ pounds)

2 tablespoons olive oil

1 teaspoon paprika

1 teaspoon ground cumin

½ teaspoon ground coriander

½ teaspoon turmeric

½ teaspoon ground ginger

1/4 teaspoon ground cinnamon

½ teaspoon kosher salt

½ teaspoon ground black pepper

2 pinches cayenne pepper

1 15-ounce can diced tomatoes

2 cups vegetable broth

15 ounce can chickpeas, drained (or 1 1/2 cups cooked)

3 cups spinach

2 tablespoons chopped fresh cilantro, for garnish

1 lemon, for garnish

1 cup Greek yogurt, for garnish.

Preparation: Make the quinoa using the stovetop method or Instant Pot method. Dice the onion and mince 3 cloves garlic. Chop the sweet potatoes into bite-sized pieces. In a large pot, heat 2 tablespoons olive oil. Sauté the onion for about 5 minutes. Add minced garlic and sauté about 1 minute. Stir in 1 teaspoon paprika, 1 teaspoon ground cumin, ½ teaspoon ground coriander, ½ teaspoon turmeric, ½ teaspoon ground ginger, 1/4 teaspoon ground cinnamon, ½ teaspoon kosher salt, ½ teaspoon ground black pepper, and 2 pinches cayenne pepper. Stir about 30 seconds, then add diced tomatoes and 2 cups broth. Bring to a boil, then add sweet potatoes and drained and rinsed chickpeas. Simmer 25 to 30 minutes until the potatoes are tender. Stir in 3 cups spinach in the last 2 minutes. Serve garnished with chopped cilantro, fresh squeezed lemon juice, and a dollop of Greek yogurt.

Snack and Energy Recovery.

Chocolate Chia Pudding: This easy and healthy chocolate chia pudding is perfect as a breakfast, snack or dessert. Vegan and naturally sweetened with dates, this is one sweet recipe you will make again and again.

Ingredient: 2 cups water

1/2 cup Brazil nuts unsalted

5 dried dates Medjool

4 mint leaves medium/large

1/2 cup chia seeds

2 tbsp cacao powder pure, unsweetened

1/2 tsp cinnamon powder

1/4 tsp sea salt iodized.

Preparation: Blend Brazil nuts, water, dates, mint and cacao in a high-speed blender until you get smooth, creamy milk.

In two clean and dry mason jars, add 1/4 cup chia seeds.

Pour Brazil nut milk equally among the two jars. Stir well and let them sit several minutes (or overnight) in the fridge, until desired consistency is reached. Serve & enjoy with fresh strawberries!

CHEESY ROASTED CHICKPEAS: Cheesy roasted chickpeas make a delicious snack or savoury topping for soups, salads, and grain bowls. You don't need to be vegan to fall in love with this plant-based recipe!

Ingredient: 1 can chickpeas, drained and rinsed

2 tablespoons grapeseed oil

2 tablespoons nutritional yeast

1 teaspoon crushed rosemary

1 teaspoon dry thyme

1 teaspoon oregano

1/2 teaspoon onion powder

1/2 teaspoon garlic powder

Salt and pepper.

Preparation: Preheat oven to 400º F and prepare a baking pan. Dry chickpeas by rolling them in between paper towel sheets or a clean kitchen towel and transfer to a large mixing bowl. Stir in grapeseed oil, nutritional yeast, crushed rosemary, thyme, oregano, onion powder, garlic powder, and salt and pepper. Spread on baking pan and place on the centre rack of oven. Cook 20 minutes, or until chickpeas are crispy and golden.

VEGAN WILD BLUEBERRY CAULIFLOWER SMOOTHIE:
How about some veggies in your smoothie? Wild blueberries and purple cauliflower add brilliant colour to this breakfast.

Ingredient: ¾ cup unsweetened cashew milk

½ cup plain cashew yogurt

¾ cup frozen wild blueberries

¼ cup frozen strawberries

½ cup cauliflower florets (I used purple cauliflower), coarsely chopped

5 Tablespoons powdered peanut butter

1 teaspoon vanilla extract

2 teaspoons maple syrup.

Preparation: Blend ingredients together, and enjoy! Makes 1 smoothie.

WHITE BEAN MUFFINS (OR BARS!): These White Bean Muffins (or bars!) pack an entire can of great northern beans into a dozen muffins. They're full of protein and fibre and perfect for breakfast or snack time!

Ingredient: 1 (15 oz can) great northern beans, drained and rinsed

2 eggs

1/3 cup maple syrup

3/4 cup rolled oats

1/2 cup peanut butter (or almond butter)

1 tsp baking soda

1 tsp cinnamon

1 tsp vanilla

1/2 tsp salt

chocolate chips, craisins, shredded coconut etc for optional mix-ins.

Preparation: Combine beans, eggs and maple syrup in the food processor and blend until smooth. Add oats, peanut butter, baking soda, cinnamon, vanilla and salt and blend again. Add mix-ins, pulse a few times to mix. Pour into greased or lined muffin tins (or 9×9 pan). Add additional toppings if desired. Bake at 375 degrees for 18-20 minutes.

PANTRY CHIA SEED CRACKERS: These energizing, travel-friendly chia seed crackers are made only with pantry staples, I believe you can whip yourself something nice with what you already have of gather a few more.

Ingredient: 1/2 cup chia seeds

1 cup water

1/2 cup pumpkin seeds

1/2 cup chopped pecans

1/4 cup ground flax

1/4 cup nutritional yeast

1/2 teaspoon cayenne pepper optional

salt and pepper.

Preparation: Preheat oven to 325ºF and line baking sheet with parchment. Mix chia seeds and water together and set aside to thicken. In a separate large mixing bowl, combine remaining ingredients. Stir in chia water mixture and mix until dough forms, using hands as needed. Press dough into baking sheet and roll out to about ¼" thick. Place on centre rack of oven and bake about 30 minutes. Remove baking sheet from the oven, carefully flip the dough, and then cut into squares or desired cracker shape. Spread and place the baking sheet back into the oven and bake for an additional 30 minutes or until browned and crispy. Remove from oven and allow to cool before eating. Store in an airtight container for up to a week.

VEGAN PROTEIN BARS: These Vegan Protein Bars are a wholesome, on-the-go option that provide a filling combination of protein and fibre and is a great allergy free option for those allergic to nuts, gluten or dairy.

Ingredient: 15 oz can chickpeas, drained and rinsed

½ cup oats (use gluten-free if needed)

½ cup sunflower seed butter

1/3 cup coconut sugar

1/2 tsp baking powder

1/4 tsp baking soda

½ tsp salt

1.5 tsp vanilla extract

¼ cup maple syrup (or honey if not vegan)

1/3 cup sunflower seeds

1/3 cup chocolate chips

sea salt, for sprinkling (optional).

Preparation: Preheat oven to 350. Rinse and drain chickpeas and place in ninja or food processor. Add in other ingredients and blend until smooth, adding sunflower seeds and chocolate chips in last. Spoon batter into 8x8 pan and spread evenly, sprinkling with sea salt. Bake for 25-30 minutes, or until lightly browned and set. Let cool for 10-15 minutes before eating. Bars will harden slightly upon cooling. Store cooled bars in refrigerator for up to a week.

SAVOURY HUMMUS NO BAKE ENERGY BITES: A healthy snack recipe that is full of protein and fibre, and perfect for when you are craving something savoury and want to recover some lost energy.

Ingredient:

2 cups old-fashioned oats*

1 cup Sabra Toasted Pine Nut hummus (or flavour of choice)

1 tablespoon olive oil

1/4 cup roasted chickpeas

1/4 cup sunflower seeds

1/4 cup pumpkin seeds

1/4 teaspoon salt

1/4 teaspoon pepper

1/4 teaspoon red pepper flakes

1 tablespoon nutritional yeast (optional)

seasoning blends, (optional).

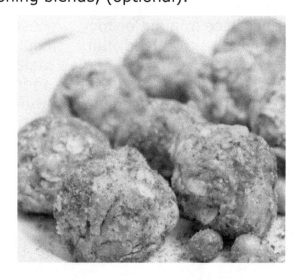

Preparation: In a large bowl, stir together all ingredients until combined. Roll into 12 balls. Sprinkle or roll into seasoning blends if using. Store in an airtight container in the refrigerator for up to 4 days, or freeze for up to 3 weeks.

MAPLE TAHINI CASHEW CLUSTERS: These maple tahini cashew clusters are a delicious snack that's easy to make with just 5 simple ingredients, but hard to stop eating! (gluten-free, vegan, refined sugar free).

Ingredient: 2 cups raw cashews

   2 tbsp tahini

   2 tbsp pure maple syrup

   2 tsp sesame seeds

   Coarse sea salt.

Preparation: Heat oven to 350°F. Line a baking sheet with parchment paper. In a bowl, Stir together cashews, tahini and maple syrup. Spread on baking sheet in close together in one large clump in a single layer. This will help it to stick into clusters instead of just single cashews. Sprinkle with sesame seeds and sea salt. Bake 20-25 min, or until golden but not burned. Remove from oven and let cool completely before breaking into clusters. Store in an airtight container on the counter.

HEALTHY EDIBLE VEGAN COOKIE DOUGH: This flour-less, vegan, low sugar "cookie dough" is full of protein and fibre thanks to the secret ingredient: beans! I assure you it has no hint of legume flavour, just guilt-free chocolatey yumminess.

Ingredient: 1 can chickpeas drained and well rinsed

.25 c sunflower seed butter can sub other nut butter if not allergic

1 tbsp lemon juice

1 tsp salt

2-3 dropper's liquid stevia or 4tbsp maple syrup

5 c allergy friendly chocolate chips.

Preparation: Add all ingredients except the chocolate chips to a food processor. Blend until smooth, stopping to scrape sides as desired. A few tablespoons of water or non-dairy milk of your choice may be needed to achieve cookie dough texture– add a bit at a time if too dry. Once fully blended, taste for desired sweetness and adjust as needed. Transfer to a medium sized bowl, add chocolate chips and mix thoroughly.

CARROT AND WHITE BEAN VEGAN BLONDIES: These healthy, vegan blondies are made with creamy peanut butter, Great Northern beans, and shredded carrots! Sneak in a few extra veggies with these gluten free treats.

Ingredient: 1/2 cup old fashioned oats – ground into a powder; be sure to get gluten free oats if needed

1/4 tsp salt

1/2 tsp baking powder

1 15.5 oz can Great Northern beans – ~1.5 cups, drained and rinsed

1/2 cup maple syrup

1 tsp vanilla extract

1/4 cup creamy peanut butter

1 cup shredded carrots – more for topping

1/4 cup chocolate chips.

Preparation: Preheat oven to 350 degrees F. Grease an 8×8 baking dish and set aside. In a high-powered blender or food processor, process/grind the old-fashioned oats into a flour. Add the salt, baking powder, Great Northern beans, maple syrup, vanilla extract, peanut butter, and shredded carrots. Blend/process at high speed for 1-2 minutes, or until you get a thick, smooth batter. You may need to stop the blender or food processor from time to time and use a rubber spatula to promote blending. Transfer the batter to the baking dish and spread it out evenly with a rubber spatula. Top with more shredded carrots and the chocolate chips. Bake for 21 to 24 minutes or until the edges of the bars get slightly brown. Remove from oven and let them sit for a few minutes before slicing them into 9 squares. Store the squares in an airtight refrigerator in the fridge for up to 5-7 days.

Conclusion.

Protein is an excellent source of fuel, nutrition and replenishment for our muscles and cells in general; whether you be an athlete or just a regular person that wants to maintain a healthy vegan diet whilst improving on every segment of your body, this guide must have helped in a way or two.

It is our sincere hope that you are able to largely benefit from all of there and become your best self; as an athlete or just a regular vegan.

THE HEALTHY MEAL PREP INSTANT POT COOKBOOK

VEGAN MEAL PREP

Delicious Vegan Meal Prep Recipes That Will Have You Covered for Convenient Plant-based Breakfasts, Lunches, Dinners and Snacks!

INTRODUCTION.

Health is a one of the greatest factors of a happy life and that comprises mainly of what we eat. If cutting out meat, dairy and eggs leaves you confused about how to eat a healthy, balanced diet, you're holding in your hands, the best guide for you!

You've probably heard that eating more vegetables and less meat is healthy. Maybe you're even feeling inspired to try eating a vegan diet-which excludes all animal products, including dairy and eggs-to improve your health or lose a little weight. Eating a vegan diet can be a healthy way to eat when your meals are full of vegetables, fruits, legumes and whole grains. You need a well-planned vegan diet to make sure you don't miss out on essential nutrients or end up eating only processed vegan foods.

In this material, we are going to share a lot about the foundational purposes of veganism, the advantages and how it affects vegans positively. We have also made a great blend of vegan foods (to include all; from breakfast to lunch, dinner, great ideas for desserts and sauce) to get you living your best life whilst enjoying the savoury taste of good food.

We hope that this material guides you to that exceptional balance between health and dieting that you've been aiming for as a vegan.

Best.

WHAT IS VEGANISM?

Veganism is a way of living which seeks to exclude, as far as is possible and practicable, all forms of exploitation of, and cruelty to, animals for food, clothing or any other purpose. Veganism is the practice of minimizing harm to all animals, which requires abstention from animal products such as meat, fish, dairy, eggs, honey, gelatine, lanolin, wool, fur, silk, suede, and leather. Some call veganism a moral baseline for animal rights activists. A few notable points:

- Veganism is more than a diet: it's a philosophy that excludes exploitation and cruelty in all forms.

- Veganism is different from vegetarianism; not all vegetarians are vegans, though all vegans are vegetarians.

- A vegan diet excludes all animal-based foods and food products but does not exclude cooked, processed, canned, or frozen foods.

- Vegan diets can help lower cholesterol and control weight but should be carefully managed to include sufficient protein, fat, calcium, and necessary vitamins.

- Vegans ensure that their food, clothing, household products, and energy are ethically and sustainably sourced.

- It's best to go vegan slowly and seek out support and help both locally and online.

VEGAN DEFINITION

Unlike vegetarianism, veganism is not a diet. Instead, it is a moral philosophy which, when strictly followed, according to the Vegan Society, "is a way of living which seeks to exclude, as far as is possible and practicable, all forms of exploitation of, and cruelty to, animals for food, clothing or any other purpose." Thus, a vegan will not only choose plant-based foods but will also avoid the use of animal-derived products (such as animal-tested cosmetics) and will choose not to visit or patronize places that use animals for entertainment or where animals are injured or abused. Many individuals are attracted to the vegan lifestyle because of its many personal, planetary, and ethical benefits.

SO WHAT DO VEGANS EAT?

A great deal - you'll soon find a whole new world of exciting foods and flavours opening up to you. When asking what vegans eat, it would almost be easier to ask what they avoid eating, as a vegan diet is by no means restrictive. A vegan diet is richly diverse and comprises all kinds of fruits, vegetables, nuts, grains, seeds, beans and pulses - all of which can be prepared in endless combinations that will ensure you're never bored. From curry to cake, pasties to pizzas, all your favourite things can be suitable for a vegan diet if they're made with plant-based ingredients.

WHY GO VEGAN?

There's a multitude of reasons to go vegan, the main one being that every vegan saves more than

100 animals a year, and there is simply no easier way to help animals and prevent suffering than by choosing vegan foods. There are also numerous benefits for both your health and the environment, as consuming meat and dairy products is actually one of the worst things that you can do for the Earth. Not only is it wasteful and causes enormous amounts of pollution, and the meat industry is also one of the biggest causes of

climate change. Adopting a vegan diet is more effective than switching to a "greener" car in the fight against climate change.

Let's take a look at some of the major benefits of being a vegan from the many:

- **Health Benefits**. A nutritionally-balanced plant-based diet is, for most people, a very healthy choice. According to a 2013 Nutritional Update for Physicians: "Research shows that plantbased diets are cost-effective, low-risk interventions that may lower body mass index, blood pressure, HbA1C, and cholesterol levels. They may also reduce the number of medications needed to treat chronic diseases and lower ischemic heart disease mortality rates. Physicians should consider recommending a plant-based diet to all their patients, especially those with high blood pressure, diabetes, cardiovascular disease, or obesity.

- **Benefits to Animals**. True vegans are focused on the rights of all animals, including insects. According to the Vegan Society, "many believe that all sentient creatures have a right to life and freedom." Vegans choose cruelty-free products and avoid any clothing, furniture, etc., that is made from an animal product such as leather; many also avoid wool, silk, and other materials made from or by animals.

- **Benefits to the Environment**. Animal husbandry has a significant negative impact on the environment, would be eradicated in a vegan world. Just a few examples include a radical reduction in greenhouse gas emissions, a significant reduction in biodiversity loss, and a major reduction in pollution of waterways.

- **Socio-Economic Benefits**. Animal diets are expensive, both in terms of financial cost and land use. For people in poorer areas of the world, the cost of animal-based products is overwhelmingly high relative to the cost of plant-based foods that offer similar nutrition.

VEGAN VERSUS VEGETARIAN

While vegans neither eat nor use any form of animal-based product, vegetarians vary in their diets, philosophies, and personal choices. In addition, while vegans generally choose veganism for philosophical reasons, vegetarians may choose their diets for a variety of reasons; some, for example, become vegetarians for health or financial reasons.

Some people follow a vegan diet but do not avoid animal products in other parts of their lives. This may be for health, religious, or other reasons. The term "strict vegetarian" is sometimes used in this instance, but it's problematic because it implies that someone who eats eggs or dairy is not a vegetarian or is not a "strict" vegetarian.

There are several types of vegetarianism that actually include animal products of various sorts. For example:

- Lacto-ovo vegetarians eat eggs and dairy products.

- Lacto vegetarians do consume dairy products, though they don't eat eggs.

- Pescatarians do not eat bird or mammal meat but do eat fish and shellfish.

Vegetarians may or may not share vegan views on subjects such as animal welfare or environmentalism. As a result, they may or may not choose to use products such as leather, wool, silk, or honey.

A brief peek into the nutritional contents of vegan meals.

The key is to eat a varied diet full of fruits, vegetables, pulses, legumes and healthy fats, and to make sure you're clued up when it comes to nutrition.

PROTEIN

One thing vegans are often asked, is 'Where do you get your protein from?'. In actual fact there's no shortage of protein in a vegan diet, as many beans, nuts and veggies are packed full of it. The recommendation for protein for adult male vegans is around 63 grams per day, and for adult female vegans it is around 52 grams per day, so if you're consuming plenty of the following it's unlikely you are deficient in protein:

- *Pulses*: peas, beans (aduki beans, blackeye beans, chickpeas (and chickpea flour), kidney beans), lentils, soya foods (tofu, tempeh, soya mince, soya milk)

- **Some nuts**: cashews, almonds, peanuts, pistachios. (Some 'nuts' such as chestnuts and macadamias are poor sources of protein and others such as Brazil nuts, walnuts, pine nuts, pecan nuts and hazel nuts are mediocre sources)

- **Seeds:** pumpkin, sunflower, sesame

- **Grains**: wheat, oats, buckwheat, millet, quinoa, amaranth, pasta, bread, seitan (which contains 75g of protein per 100g). Note that rice is a relatively poor source of protein.

CALCIUM.

Calcium is an essential part of human's diets, and we need it in order to maintain healthy bones and is vital for growth and development. A balanced vegan diet will ensure you receive your recommended daily allowance (700mg for adults, 800-1000mg for adolescents), but it's important to be aware of how much of the calcium you eat is being actively absorbed by your body.

Some foods, such as spinach, contain a high amount of calcium, but unfortunately are bound to a substance called 'oxalate' which means that calcium absorption in hindered. This is why it's important to replace spinach with low-oxalate vegetables such as rocket, cabbage and kale. Interestingly enough, calcium in cow's milk cannot be easily absorbed by the body, which means that vegetables such as kale are actually much better sources of calcium than animal milks or

'dairy'.

IRON

Iron is an essential part of our diets, as we need it in order to make enough healthy oxygencarrying red blood cells. However, research has shown that vegans have an average iron intake that's similar to, and often higher than, non-vegans. Good sources of iron include:

- Dried fruits

- Whole grains (including wholemeal bread)

- Nuts, seeds and pulses

- Other foods rich in iron but which are usually eaten in smaller amounts include soya, some flours, parsley, watercress, black molasses and edible seaweeds.

Note: It's important to remember that you also need plenty of vitamin C to help absorb the iron in your meals.

Good sources of vitamin C include:

- Oranges. ü   Potatoes.

- Cabbage.

- Green leafy vegetables.

- Blackcurrants.

- Broccoli.

- Mango. ü   Kiwis.

- Parsley.

KETO VEGANISM.

A vegan keto diet is a plant based version of the popular ketogenic diet. The ketogenic diet is a high-fat, low-carb, moderate-protein diet promoted for its powerful effects on weight loss and overall health. Though often associated with animal foods, this way of eating can be adapted to fit plant-based meal plans — including vegan diets. Vegan diets exclude all animal products, making it more difficult to eat low-carb. However, with careful planning, vegans can reap the potential benefits of a ketogenic diet.

What is vegan Keto diet?

The vegan keto diet significantly restricts carbohydrate intake and only allows plant based foods. It is high in fats, contains adequate amounts of protein, and does not include any animal products. Carbs are typically reduced to less than 50 grams per day to reach and maintain ketosis — a metabolic process in which your body burns fat for fuel instead of glucose. Since this way of eating is composed mostly of fat — generally around 75% of your intake — keto dieters often turn to high-fat animal products, such as meats, butter and full-fat dairy.

However, those who eat plant-based diets, including vegans, can follow a ketogenic diet as well. People on a vegan diet consume only plant-based foods, such as vegetables, fruits and grains, and avoid animal-based foods like meat, poultry, eggs and dairy. Vegans can reach ketosis by relying on high-fat, plant-based products like coconut oil, avocados, seeds and nuts.

Benefits of keto vegan diet.

The list of benefits from a proper keto vegan diet stretches but mainly, we have a few that really compels many to make the switch to keto vegan dieting especially those who want to do something to their weight loss issues and diabetes. Let's enter into some details.

Point: Choosing a ketogenic diet for diabetes management offers a range of valuable benefits.

Research shows that being in a state of nutritional ketosis notably leads to significant improvement in blood glucose control and weight loss. Other common benefits provided include:

- Reduced dependence on medication

- Improvements in insulin sensitivity

- Lower blood pressure

- Usually improvements in cholesterol levels.

WEIGHT LOSS AND MAINTENANCE

A primary benefit of the ketogenic diet is its ability to achieve rapid weight loss Restricting carbohydrates enough to be in a state of ketosis leads to both a significant reduction in body fat and an increase or retention of muscle mass. Studies show that low-carb, ketogenic diets are able to achieve strong weight loss over an extended period. An Australian study showed that obese people were able to lose, on average, 15 kg over a period of a year. This was 3 kg more than the low-fat diet used in the study achieved.

BLOOD GLUCOSE CONTROL

The other main reason for people with diabetes to follow a ketogenic diet is its ability to lower and stabilise blood sugar levels Carbohydrate is the nutrient (macronutrient) that raises blood sugar the most. Because ketogenic diets are very-low in carbohydrate, they eliminate the larger rises in blood sugar.

Studies into ketogenic diets show them to be very effective at reducing HbA1c – a long-term measure of blood glucose control. A 6-month study ran by Eric Westman and colleagues in 2008 showed an average reduction in HbA1c levels of 17 mmol/mol (1.5%) for people with type 2 diabetes. People with other types of diabetes, such as type 1 diabetes and LADA, should also expect to see a strong reduction in blood sugar levels and an improvement in control.

Note: if an improvement in blood glucose control is maintained over a number of years, this can reduce the risk of complications occurring.

REDUCING RELIANCE ON DIABETES MEDICATION

Because they're so effective at reducing blood sugar levels, ketogenic diets have the additional benefit of helping people with type 2 diabetes to reduce their dependence on diabetes medication In the study by Westman mentioned above, 95% of the people in the study were able to reduce, or come off completely, their diabetes medication.

People on insulin and other hypo-causing medication (such as sulphonylureas and glinides) may need to reduce their doses in advance of starting a ketogenic diet to prevent hypos. Speak to your doctor for advice on this.

INSULIN SENSITIVITY

A ketogenic diet has been shown to help restore insulin sensitivity, as it eliminates the root cause of insulin resistance – which is too high levels of insulin in the body. This diet helps promote sustained periods of low insulin, as low levels of carbohydrate mean lower levels of insulin. A high carbohydrate diet is like putting petrol on the fire of insulin resistance High carbohydrate means a greater need for insulin and this make insulin resistance worse.

By comparison, a ketogenic diet, turns insulin levels down, as fat is the macronutrient that requires the least insulin getting the levels of insulin down also helps with fat burning, because high insulin levels prevent the breakdown of fat. When insulin levels drop for a number of hours, the body is able to break down fat cells.

CHOLESTEROL LEVELS

Overall, ketogenic diets usually result in improvements of cholesterol levels. It is usual for LDL cholesterol levels to go down and HDL cholesterol levels go up, which is healthy. One of the strongest measures of healthy cholesterol is the ratio of total cholesterol to HDL. This can be easily found by taking your total cholesterol result and dividing it by your HDL result. If the number you get is 3.5 or lower, this indicates a healthy cholesterol. Research studies show that ketogenic diets are usually effective at improving this measure of cholesterol health.

Note: some people may show an increase in LDL and total cholesterol after starting a ketogenic. This is usually regarded as a negative sign but if your total cholesterol to HDL ratio is good, this does not necessarily represent a worsening in heart health. Cholesterol is a complicated topic and your doctor is the best source of advice if your cholesterol levels change significantly on a ketogenic diet.

STRONGER MENTAL PERFORMANCE

Mental clarity, an increased ability to focus and a better memory are other commonly reported benefits of eating a ketogenic diet. Increasing intake of healthy fats with omega-3, such as those found in oily fish like salmo, tuna and mackerel, can improve mood and learning ability. This is because omega-3 increases a fatty acid called DHA that makes up between 15 to 30 per cent of our brain. The production of beta-hydroxybutyrate, a form of ketone, helps support long-term memory function.

SATIETY

Ketogenic diets have positive effects on appetite. Once the body adapts to being in a state of ketosis, it gets used to getting energy from breaking down body fat and this can reduce appetite and cravings.

They are effective at:

- Reducing cravings

- Helping you feel full for longer   ▪   Reducing preference for sugary foods.

Weight loss as a result of a ketogenic diet can help lower leptin levels which can improve leptin sensitivity and benefit satiety as a result.

CANDIDA

Ketogenic diets can be good at reducing thrush and yeast infections as they lower blood sugar, which reduces glucose being passed out in the urine. It is glucose in the urine that bacteria feed off that leads to a fertile breeding ground for yeast and bacterial infections.

In addition to that, a higher intake of a saturated fatty acid called lauric acid – found in coconut oil, a staple keto food – has been shown to have anti-microbial properties. It can kill off candida albican and help with yeast infections.

FOODS TO AVOID

When following a vegan keto diet, you must significantly reduce your carb intake and replace carbs with healthy fats and vegan sources of protein. Animal products, including eggs, meat, poultry, dairy and seafood, are excluded on a vegan keto diet.

Here are examples of foods that should be completely avoided:

- *Meat and poultry*: Beef, turkey, chicken, pork.

- *Dairy:* Milk, butter, yogurt.

- Eggs: Egg whites and egg yolks.

- *Seafood*: Fish, shrimp, clams, mussels.

- *Animal-based ingredients*: Whey protein, honey, egg white protein. Here are examples of foods that should be significantly reduced:

- *Grains and starches*: Cereal, bread, baked goods, rice, pasta, grains.

- *Sugary drinks*: Sweet tea, soda, juice, smoothies, sports drinks, chocolate milk.

- *Sweeteners*: Brown sugar, white sugar, agave, maple syrup.

- *Starchy vegetables*: Potatoes, sweet potatoes, winter squash, beets, peas.

- *Beans and legumes*: Black beans, chickpeas, kidney beans.

- *Fruits*: All fruits should be limited. However, small portions of certain fruits like berries are allowed.

- *High-carb alcoholic beverages*: Beer, sweetened cocktails, wine.

- *Low-fat diet foods*: Low-fat foods tend to be high in added sugar.

- *High-carb sauces and condiments*: Barbecue sauce, sweetened salad dressings, marinades. § *Highly processed foods*: Limit packaged foods and increase whole, unprocessed foods.

The level of carbohydrate restriction when following a vegan keto diet varies depending on your health goals and individual needs.

In general, healthy, high-fat vegan foods and vegan protein sources should make up the majority of your diet.

FOODS TO EAT

When following a vegan keto diet, it's important to focus on vegan, healthy foods that are high in fat and low in carbs.

Foods to eat on a vegan keto diet include:

- *Coconut products*: Full-fat coconut milk, coconut cream, unsweetened coconut.

- *Oils*: Olive oil, nut oil, coconut oil, MCT oil, avocado oil.

- *Nuts and seeds*: Almonds, Brazil nuts, walnuts, hemp seeds, chia seeds, macadamia nuts, pumpkin seeds.

- *Nut and seed butter*: Peanut butter, almond butter, sunflower butter, cashew butter.

- *Non-starchy vegetables*: Leafy greens, Brussels sprouts, zucchini, broccoli, cauliflower, peppers, mushrooms.

- Vegan protein sources: Full-fat tofu, tempeh.

- *Vegan full-fat "dairy"*: Coconut yogurt, vegan butter, cashew cheese, vegan cream cheese.

- *Avocados*: Whole avocados, guacamole.

- *Berries*: Blueberries, blackberries, raspberries and strawberries can be enjoyed in moderation.

- *Condiments*: Nutritional yeast, fresh herbs, lemon juice, salt, pepper, spices.

Though the keto diet cuts out many food groups that vegans rely on, such as whole grains and starchy vegetables, a vegan keto diet can be followed with careful planning. Vegan keto dieters should get their calories from whole, unprocessed foods while avoiding highly processed vegan foods.

EATING HEALTHY AND LOSING WEIGHT.

I don't like to put a label on my dietary advice. It is based on scientific research, not ethics, religion or a preconceived notion of what a healthy diet should be like. But if you want to label it, call it a "Low-Carb, Real-Food" based diet (LCRF).

What Does "Low-Carb, Real-Food" Mean?

Let me start by explaining a bit of terminology.

- A low-carbohydrate diet minimizes sugars and starches, replacing them with foods rich in protein and healthy fats.

- "Real food" means choosing foods that humans had access to throughout evolution. Processed, unnatural foods with artificial chemicals are avoided.

LCRF is not a "diet." It is a way of eating, a lifestyle change based on bulletproof scientific evidence. It is a way of eating that emphasizes the foods humans have evolved to eat for hundreds of thousands of years, before the agricultural and industrial revolutions. This type of diet is proven to work better than the low-fat diet still recommended all around the world.

WHAT NOT TO EAT

You should limit the following foods.

- *Sugar:* Added sugar is addictive, fattening and a leading cause of diseases like obesity, diabetes and cardiovascular disease.

- *Grains*: Avoid grains if you need to lose weight, including bread and pasta. Gluten grains (wheat, spelt, barley and rye) are the worst. Healthier grains like rice and oats are fine if you don't need to lose weight.

- *Seed and vegetable oils*: Soybean oil, corn oil and some others. These are processed fats with a high amount of Omega-6 fatty acids, which are harmful in excess.

- *Trans fats*: Chemically modified fats that are extremely bad for health. Found in some processed foods.

- *Artificial sweeteners*: Despite being calorie free, observational studies show a correlation with obesity and related diseases. If you must use sweeteners, choose Stevia.

- *"Diet" and "low-fat" products:* Most of these "health foods" aren't healthy at all. They tend to be highly processed and loaded with sugar or artificial sweeteners. Agave syrup is just as bad as sugar.

- *Highly processed foods*: Foods that are highly processed are usually low in nutrients and high in unhealthy and unnatural chemicals.

You must read ingredient lists. You'll be surprised at the amount of "health foods" that can contain sugar, wheat and other harmful ingredients.

HEALTHY FOODS TO EAT

You should eat natural, unprocessed foods that humans are genetically adapted to eating. Research shows that such foods are great for health. For healthy people who exercise and don't need to lose weight, there is absolutely no proven reason to avoid tubers like potatoes and sweet potatoes, or healthier non-gluten grains like oats and rice. If you are overweight or have metabolic issues (low HDL, high LDL cholesterol, triglycerides, belly fat, etc.) you should restrict all high-carb foods.

- *Meat*: Beef, lamb, pork, chicken, etc. Humans have eaten meat for hundreds of thousands of years. Unprocessed meat is good for you, especially if the animals ate natural foods (like beef from grass-fed cows).

- *Fish:* Fish is great. Very healthy, fulfilling and rich in omega-3 fatty acids and other nutrients. You should eat fish (preferably fatty fish like salmon) every week.

- *Eggs*: Eggs are among the most nutritious foods on the planet. The yolk is the most nutritious and healthiest part. Omega-3 eggs are best.

- *Vegetables*: Contain fibre and many nutrients that are essential for the human body. Eat vegetables every day.

- *Fruit*: Increase variety, taste good, are easy to prepare and rich in fibre and vitamin C. They're still pretty high in sugar, so eat in moderation if you need to lose weight.

- *Nuts and seeds*: Almonds, walnuts, sunflower seeds, etc. Rich in various nutrients, but very high in calories. Eat in moderation if you need to lose weight.

- *Potatoes*: Root vegetables like potatoes and sweet potatoes are healthy, but they're still high in carbs. Eat in moderation if you need to lose weight.

- *High-fat dairy*: Cheese, cream, butter, full-fat yogurt, etc. Rich in healthy fats and calcium.

Dairy from grass-fed cows will be rich in vitamin K2, which is very important for health.

- *Fats and oils*: Olive oil, butter, lard, etc. Choose saturated fats for high-heat cooking like pan frying, they are more stable in the heat.

WHAT TO DRINK?

- *Coffee:* Coffee is healthy and very rich in antioxidants, but people who are sensitive to caffeine should avoid it. Avoid coffee late in the day because it can ruin your sleep.

- *Tea:* Tea is healthy, rich in antioxidants and has a lot less caffeine than coffee.

- *Water:* You should drink water throughout the day and especially around workouts. No reason to drink a whole ton though, thirst is a pretty reliable indicator of your need. § Carbonated soda without artificial sweeteners is fine.

Avoid sodas with sugar and artificial sweeteners, fruit juice, milk and beer.

Simple rule: Don't drink calories.

CONSUME IN MODERATION

These indulgences can be enjoyed from time to time.

- *Dark Chocolate*: Choose organic chocolate with 70% cocoa or more. Dark chocolate is rich in healthy fats and antioxidants.

- *Alcohol*: Choose dry wines and drinks that don't contain added sugar or carbs: vodka, whiskey, etc.

How Many Carbs Per Day?

This varies between individuals. Many people feel best eating very little carbs (under 50 grams) while others eat as much as 150 grams, which is still low-carb.

You can use these numbers as a guideline:

  10-20 grams per day: Very low, can't eat any carbs except low-carb vegetables. Appropriate if you have a lot of weight to lose or if you have diabetes and/or the metabolic syndrome.

- *20-50 grams per day*: If you need to lose weight fast. You can eat quite a bit of vegetables and one piece of fruit per day.

- *50-150 grams per day*: If you want to achieve optimal health and lower your risk of lifestylerelated disease. There is room for several fruit per day and even a little bit of healthy starches like potatoes and rice.

When you lower carbohydrates below 50 grams per day, you can't eat any sugar, bread, pasta, grains, potatoes and a maximum of one fruit per day. I recommend creating a free account on Fitday to log your food intake for a few days. This is great way to get a feel for the amount of carbs you are eating. Warning For Diabetics: Carbs in the diet are broken down into glucose in the digestive tract, then they enter the body as blood sugar. If you eat less carbs, you will need less insulin and glucose-lowering drugs. It is very dangerous if your blood sugar drops below a certain level (hypoglycaemia). If you have diabetes, consult with your doctor before reducing carbohydrate intake.

WHY DOES IT WORK?

Humans evolved as hunter-gatherers for hundreds of thousands of years. Our diet changed drastically in the agricultural revolution, about 10,000 years ago. However, this change is small compared to the massive transformation we've seen in the last few decades with modern food processing. It is quite clear that humans today are eating a diet that is very different from the diet our ancestors thrived on throughout evolution.

There are several "primitive" populations around the world that still live as hunter-gatherers, eating natural foods. These people are lean, in excellent health and most of the diseases that are killing western populations by the millions are rare or non-existent. Studies show that when people eat natural foods that were available to our hunter-gatherer ancestors (also known as the Palaeolithic diet), they lose weight and see massive improvements in health.

THE HORMONE INSULIN

The hormone insulin is well known for its role of moving glucose from the blood and into cells. A deficiency in insulin, or resistance to its effects, causes diabetes. But insulin also has other roles in the body. Insulin tells fat cells to produce fat and to stop breaking down the fat that they carry. When insulin levels are high, the body chooses not to dip in to the fat stores to provide energy.

On a Western, high-carb diet, insulin levels are high all the time, keeping the fat safely locked away in the fat cells. Carbs are the main driver of insulin secretion. A low carb diet lowers and balances blood sugar and therefore lowers insulin levels. When insulin goes down, the body can easily access the calories stored in the fat cells, but it can take a few days to adapt to burning fat instead of carbs.

Low carbohydrate diets are very satiating. Appetite goes down and people start to automatically eat fewer calories than they burn, which causes weight loss. The main advantage of a low-carb diet is that you can eat until fullness and lose weight without counting calories. Eat low-carb and you avoid the worst side effect of calorie restricted diets: hunger.

HEALTH BENEFITS OF A LOW CARB DIET

It is a common misunderstanding, even among health professionals, that low-carb diets are somehow bad for health. People who make such claims obviously haven't bothered to check out the research. Their main argument is that low-carb diets are bad because they're high in saturated fat, which raises cholesterol and causes heart disease.

But recent research suggests that there is nothing to worry about. Saturated fats raise HDL (the good) cholesterol and change the "bad" cholesterol from small, dense LDL (very bad) to large LDL which is benign. The fact is that saturated fat does not cause heart disease. This is simply a myth that has never been proven. Low-carb diets actually lead to more weight loss and further improvements in risk factors compared to a low-fat diet.

- *Body fat*: A low-carb diet, eaten until fullness, usually causes more fat loss than a low-fat diet that is calorie restricted.

  Blood sugar: One of the hallmarks of diabetes and the metabolic syndrome is an elevated blood sugar, which is very harmful over the long term. Low-carb diets lower blood sugar.

- *Blood pressure*: If blood pressure is high, it tends to go down on a low-carb diet.

- *High triglycerides*: These are fats that circulate around in the blood and are a strong risk factor for cardiovascular disease. Low-carb diets lower triglycerides much more than lowfat diets.

- *HDL (the good) cholesterol*: Generally speaking, having more of the "good" cholesterol means you have a lower risk of cardiovascular disease. Low-carb diets raise HDL cholesterol much more than low-fat diets.

- *sdLDL (the bad) cholesterol*: Low-carb diets cause LDL cholesterol to change from small, dense LDL (bad) to large LDL, which is benign.

- Easier: Low-carb diets appear to be easier to stick to than low-fat diets, probably because it isn't necessary to count calories and be hungry, which is arguably the worst side effect of dieting.

The statements above have been shown to be true in randomized controlled trials - scientific studies that are the gold standard of research.

COMMON LOW-CARB SIDE EFFECTS IN THE BEGINNING

When carbs in the diet are replaced with protein and fat, several things need to happen for the body to efficiently use fat as fuel. There will be major changes in hormones and the body needs to ramp up production of enzymes to start burning primarily fat instead of carbs. This can last for a few days and full adaptation may take weeks.

Common side effects in the first few days include:

- Headache

- Feeling Lightheaded

  Tiredness

- Irritability

- Constipation.

Side effects are usually mild and nothing to worry about. Your body has been burning mostly carbs for decades, it takes time to adapt to using fat as the primary fuel source. This is called the "low carb flu" and should be over within 3-4 days. On a low-carb diet, it is very important to eat enough fat. Fat is the new source of fuel for your body. If you eat low-carb and low-fat, then you're going to feel bad and abandon the whole thing.

Another important thing to be aware of is that insulin makes the kidneys hold on to sodium. When you eat less carbs, the kidneys release sodium. This is one of the reasons people lose so much bloat and water weight in the first few days. To counteract this loss of sodium you can add more salt to your food or drink a cup of broth every day. A bouillon cube dissolved in a cup of hot water contains 2 grams of sodium. Many people say they feel better than ever on a low-carb diet, when the initial adaptation period is over. If you don't feel good, adding more fat and sodium should take care of it.

A MEAL PLAN THAT CAN SAVE YOUR LIFE.

This is a sample meal plan for one week that supplies less than 50 grams of carbs per day.

Day 1 — *Monday:*

- Breakfast: Omelet with various vegetables, fried in butter or coconut oil.

- Lunch: Grass-fed yogurt with blueberries and a handful of almonds.

- Dinner: Cheeseburger (no bun), served with vegetables and salsa sauce.

Day 2— *Tuesday:*

- Breakfast: Bacon and eggs.

Lunch: Leftover burgers and veggies from the night before. ▪ Dinner: Boiled Salmon with butter and vegetables.

Day 3— *Wednesday:*

- Breakfast: Eggs and vegetables, fried in butter or coconut oil.

- Lunch: Shrimp salad with some olive oil. ▪ Dinner: Grilled chicken with vegetables.

Day 4— *Thursday:*

- Breakfast: Omelet with various vegetables, fried in butter or coconut oil.

- Lunch: Smoothie with coconut milk, berries, almonds and protein powder.

- Dinner: Steak and veggies.

Day 5— *Friday:*

- Breakfast: Bacon and Eggs.

- Lunch: Chicken salad with some olive oil. ▪ Dinner: Pork chops with vegetables.

Day 6 – *Saturday:*

- Breakfast: Omelet with various veggies.

- Lunch: Grass-fed yogurt with berries, coconut flakes and a handful of walnuts.

- Dinner: Meatballs with vegetables.

Day 7— *Sunday*:

- Breakfast: Bacon and Eggs.

- Lunch: Smoothie with coconut milk, a bit of heavy cream, chocolate-flavoured protein powder and berries.

  Dinner: Grilled chicken wings with some raw spinach on the side.

Do your best to include a variety of vegetables in your diet. If you want to stay below 50g of carbs per day then you can safely have one piece of fruit or some berries every day. Organic and grassfed foods are best, but only if you can easily afford them. Just make an effort to always choose the least processed option within your price range.

WHAT ABOUT SNACKS?

There is no scientific evidence that you should eat more than 3 meals per day. If you do get hungry between meals, here are a few ideas for snacks that are healthy, easily portable and taste good.

- Full-fat yogurt
- A piece of fruit
- Baby carrots
- Hard-boiled eggs
- A handful of nuts
- Leftovers
- Some cheese and meat.

That's about the length you can go with snacks.

NUTRIENT RICH VEGAN FOODS.

As we've already established, that vegan avoid eating animal foods for environmental, ethical or health reasons. Unfortunately, following a diet based exclusively on plants may put some people at a higher risk of nutrient deficiencies. This is especially true when vegan diets are not well planned. For vegans who want to stay healthy, consuming a nutrient-rich diet with whole and fortified foods is very important.

Here are 11 foods and food groups that should be part of a healthy vegan diet:

- *Legumes*— In an effort to exclude all forms of animal exploitation and cruelty, vegans avoid traditional sources of protein and iron such as meat, poultry, fish and eggs. Therefore, it's important to replace these animal products with protein- and iron-rich plant alternatives, such as legumes. Beans, lentils and peas are great options that contain 10–20 grams of protein per cooked cup. They're also excellent sources of fibre, slowly digested carbs, iron, folate, manganese, zinc, antioxidants and other health-promoting plant compounds. However, legumes also contain a good amount of anti-nutrients, which can reduce the absorption of minerals. For instance, iron absorption from plants is estimated to be 50% lower than that from animal sources. Similarly, vegetarian diets seem to reduce zinc absorption by about 35% compared to those containing meat. It's advantageous to sprout, ferment or cook legumes well because these processes can decrease the levels of antinutrients. To increase your absorption of iron and zinc from legumes, you may also want to avoid consuming them at the same time as calcium-rich foods. Calcium can hinder their absorption if you consume it at the same time. In contrast, eating legumes in combination with vitamin C-rich fruits and vegetables can further increase your absorption of iron.

Note: Beans, lentils and peas are nutrient-rich plant alternatives to animal-derived foods. Sprouting, fermenting and proper cooking can increase nutrient absorption.

- *Nuts, Nut Butters and Seeds*— Nuts, seeds and their by-products are a great addition to any vegan refrigerator or pantry. That's in part because a 1-oz (28-gram) serving of nuts or seeds contains 5–12 grams of protein. This makes them a good alternative to protein-rich animal products. In addition, nuts and seeds are great sources of iron, fibre, magnesium, zinc, selenium and vitamin E. They also contain a good amount of antioxidants and other beneficial plant compounds. Nuts and seeds are also extremely versatile. They can be consumed on their own, or worked into interesting recipes such as sauces, desserts and cheeses. Cashew cheese is one delicious option. Try to choose unblanched and unroasted varieties whenever possible, since nutrients can be lost during processing. Favour nut butters that are natural rather than heavily processed. These are usually devoid of the oil, sugar and salt often added to household brand varieties.

Note: Nuts, seeds and their butters are nutritious, versatile foods that are rich in protein and nutrients. Every vegan should consider adding them to their pantry.

- *Hemp, Flax and Chia Seeds*— These three seeds have special nutrient profiles that deserve to be highlighted separately from the previous category. For starters, all three contain larger amounts of protein than most other seeds. One ounce (28 grams) of hemp seeds contains 9 grams of complete, easily digestible protein — about 50% more protein than most other seeds. What's more, the omega-3 to omega-6 fatty acid ratio found in hemp seeds is considered optimal for human health. Research also shows that the fats found in hemp seeds may be very effective at diminishing symptoms of premenstrual syndrome (PMS) and menopause. It may also reduce inflammation and improve certain skin conditions. For their part, chia and flaxseeds are particularly high in alpha-linoleic acid (ALA), an essential omega-3 fatty acid your body can partly convert into eicosapentaenoic acid (EPA) and docosahexaenoic acid (DHA). EPA and DHA play important roles in the development and maintenance of the nervous system. These long-chain fatty acids also seem to play beneficial roles in pain, inflammation, depression and anxiety. Since EPA and DHA are primarily found in fish and seaweed, it might be challenging for vegans to consume enough through their diets. For this reason, it's important for vegans to eat enough ALA-rich foods, such as chia and flaxseeds. However, studies suggest that the body is only able to convert 0.5– 5% of ALA to EPA and DHA. This conversion may be increased somewhat in vegan. Regardless of this, both chia and flaxseeds are incredibly healthy for you. They also make great substitutes for eggs in baking, which is just one more reason to give them a try.

Note: The seeds of hemp, chia and flax are richer in protein and ALA than most other seeds. Flax and chia seeds are also great substitutes for eggs in recipes.

- *Tofu and Other Minimally Processed Meat Substitutes*— Tofu and tempeh are minimally processed meat substitutes made from soybeans. Both contain 16–19 grams of protein per 3.5-oz (100-gram) portion. They're also good sources of iron and calcium. Tofu, created from the pressing of soybean curds, is a popular replacement for meats. It can be sautéed, grilled or scrambled. It makes a nice alternative to eggs in recipes such as omelettes, frittatas and quiches. Tempeh is made from fermented soybeans. Its distinctive flavour makes it a popular replacement for fish, but tempeh can also be used in a variety of other dishes. The fermentation process helps reduce the amount of anti-nutrients that are naturally found in soybeans, which may increase the amount of nutrients the body can absorb from tempeh. The fermentation process of tempeh may produce small amounts of vitamin B12, a nutrient mainly found in animal foods that soybeans do not normally contain. However, it remains unclear whether the type of vitamin B12 found in tempeh is active in humans. The quantity of vitamin B12 in tempeh also remains low and can vary from one brand of tempeh to another. Therefore, vegans should not rely on tempeh as their source of vitamin B12. Seitan is another popular meat alternative. It provides about 25 grams of wheat protein per 3.5 oz. (100 grams). It is also a good source of selenium and contains small amounts of iron, calcium and phosphorus. However, individuals with celiac disease or gluten sensitivity should avoid seitan due to its high gluten content. More heavily processed mock meats, such as "vegan burgers" or "vegan chicken fillets," usually provide far fewer nutrients and can contain various additives. They should be eaten sparingly.

Note: Minimally processed meat alternatives including tofu, tempeh and seitan are versatile, nutrient-rich additions to a vegan diet. Try to limit your consumption of heavily processed vegan mock meats.

- *Calcium-Fortified Plant Milks and Yogurts—* Vegans tend to consume smaller amounts of calcium per day than vegetarians or meat eaters, which may negatively affect their bone health. This seems especially true if calcium intake falls below 525 mg per day. For this reason, vegans should attempt to make calcium-fortified plant milks and plant yogurts part

of their daily menu. Those looking to simultaneously increase their protein intake should opt for milks and yogurts made from soy or hemp. Coconut, almond, rice and oat milks are lower-protein alternatives. Calcium-fortified plant milks and yogurts are usually also fortified with vitamin D, a nutrient that plays an important role in the absorption of calcium. Some brands also add vitamin B12 to their products. Therefore, vegans looking to reach their daily intakes of calcium, vitamin D and vitamin B12 through foods alone should make sure to opt for fortified products. To keep added sugars to a minimum, make sure to choose unsweetened versions.

Note: Plant milks and yogurts fortified with calcium, vitamin D and vitamin B12 are good alternatives to products made from cows' milk.

- *Seaweed—* Seaweed is one of the rare plant foods to contain DHA, an essential fatty acid with many health benefits. Algae such as spirulina and chlorella are also good sources of complete protein. Two tablespoons (30 ml) of these provide about 8 grams of protein. In addition, seaweed contains magnesium, riboflavin, manganese, potassium, iodine and good amounts of antioxidants. The mineral iodine, in particular, plays crucial roles in your metabolism and in the function of your thyroid gland. The Reference Daily Intake (RDI) of iodine is 150 micrograms per day. Vegans can meet their requirements by consuming several servings of seaweed per week. That being said, some types of seaweed (such as kelp) are extremely high in iodine, so should not be eaten in large amounts. Other varieties, such as spirulina, contain very little iodine. Those who are having difficulty meeting their recommended daily intakes through seaweed alone should aim to consume half a teaspoon (2.5 ml) of iodized salt each day (31). Similar to tempeh, seaweed is often promoted as a great source of vitamin B12 for vegans. Although it does contain a form of vitamin B12, it is still not clear whether this form is active in humans. Until more is known, vegans who want to reach their daily recommended vitamin B12 intake should rely on fortified foods or use supplements.

Note: Seaweed is a protein-rich source of essential fatty acids. It is also rich in antioxidants and iodine, but should not be relied on as a source of vitamin B12.

- *Nutritional Yeast*— Nutritional yeast is made from a deactivated strain of Saccharomyces cerevisiae yeast. It can be found in the form of yellow powder or flakes in most supermarkets and health food stores. One ounce (28 grams) contains approximately 14 grams of protein and 7 grams of fibre. In addition, nutritional yeast is commonly fortified with zinc, magnesium, copper, manganese and B vitamins, including vitamin B12. Therefore, fortified nutritional yeast can be a practical way for vegans to reach their daily vitamin B12 recommendations. However, it's important to note that vitamin B12 is lightsensitive and may degrade if bought or stored in clear plastic bags. Non-fortified nutritional yeast should not be relied on as a source of vitamin B12.

Note: Fortified nutritional yeast is a protein-rich source of vitamin B12. However, nonfortified versions are not a reliable source of the vitamin.

- *Sprouted and Fermented Plant Foods*— Although rich in nutrients, most plant foods also contain varying amounts of anti-nutrients. These anti-nutrients can reduce your body's ability to absorb the minerals these foods contain. Sprouting and fermenting are simple and time-tested methods of reducing the amount of anti-nutrients found in various foods. These techniques increase the amount of beneficial nutrients absorbed from plant foods and can also boost their overall protein quality. Interestingly, sprouting may also slightly reduce the amount of gluten found in certain grains. Fermented plant foods are good sources of probiotic bacteria, which may help improve immune function and digestive health. They also contain vitamin K2, which may promote bone and dental health as well as help decrease the risk of heart disease and cancer. You can try sprouting or fermenting grains at home. Some can also be bought in stores, such as Ezekiel bread, tempeh, miso, natto, sauerkraut, pickles, kimchi and kombucha.

Note: Sprouting and fermenting foods helps enhance their nutritional value. Fermented foods also provide vegans with a source of probiotics and vitamin K2.

- *Whole Grains, Cereals and Pseudo cereals—* Whole grains, cereals and pseudo cereals are good sources of complex carbs, fibre, and iron, as well as B vitamins, magnesium, phosphorus, zinc and selenium. That said, some varieties are more nutritious than others, especially when it comes to protein. For instance, the ancient grains spelt and teff contain 10–11 grams of protein per cooked cup (237 ml). That's a lot compared to wheat and rice. The pseudo cereals amaranth and quinoa come in a close second with around 9 grams of protein per cooked cup (237 ml). They are also two of the rare sources of complete protein in this food group. Like many plant foods, whole grains and pseudo cereals contain varying levels of antinutrients, which can limit the absorption of beneficial nutrients. Sprouting is useful for reducing these antinutrients.

Note: Spelt, teff, amaranth and quinoa are flavourful, high-protein substitutes for betterknown grains such as wheat and rice. Sprouted varieties are best.

- *Choline-Rich Foods*— The nutrient choline is important for the health of your liver, brain and nervous system. Our bodies can produce it, but only in small amounts. That's why it's considered an essential nutrient that you must get from your diet. Choline can be found in small amounts in a wide variety of fruits, vegetables, nuts, legumes and grains. That said, the plant foods with the largest amounts include tofu, soymilk, cauliflower, broccoli and quinoa. Daily choline requirements increase during pregnancy. Endurance athletes, heavy drinkers and postmenopausal women may also be at increased risk of deficiency. Therefore, vegan individuals who fall into one of these categories should make a special effort to ensure they have sufficient choline-rich foods on their plates.

Note: Choline-rich plant foods such as soy, cauliflower, broccoli and quinoa are important for the proper functioning of your body.

- *Fruits and Vegetables*— Some vegans rely heavily on mock meats and vegan junk food to replace their favourite animal foods. However, these types of foods are often highly processed and unhealthy. Luckily, there are many ways to replace your favourite meals with vitamin- and mineral-rich fruits and vegetables instead. For instance, mashed banana is a great substitute for eggs in baking recipes. Banana ice cream is also a popular replacement for dairy-based ice cream. Simply blend a frozen banana until its smooth. Then you can add your preferred toppings. Eggplant and mushrooms, especially cremini or Portobello, are a great way to get a meaty texture in vegetable form. They're particularly easy to grill. Perhaps surprisingly, jackfruit is a great stand-in for meat in savoury dishes such as stirfries and barbecue sandwiches. Meanwhile, cauliflower is a versatile addition to many recipes, including pizza crust. Vegans should also aim to increase their intake of iron- and calcium-rich fruits and vegetables. This includes leafy greens such as bok choy, spinach, kale, watercress and mustard greens. Broccoli, turnip greens, artichokes and blackcurrants are also great options.

Note: Fruits and vegetables are very healthy and some of them can be used as alternatives for animal foods.

Helpful tip— Vegans avoid all foods of animal origin, including meat and foods containing animalderived ingredients. This can limit their intake of certain nutrients and increase their requirements for others. A well-planned plant-based diet that includes sufficient amounts of the foods discussed in this article will help vegans stay healthy and avoid nutrient deficiencies. Nevertheless, some vegans may find it difficult to eat these foods in sufficient quantities. In these cases, supplements are a good backup option to consider.

THRIVING ON THE VEGAN DIET.

Well-planned vegan diets contain all the nutrients we need to remain strong and healthy. When people go vegan, they often eat more fruit and vegetables, and enjoy meals higher in fibre and lower in saturated fat.

VEGAN LIFESTYLE GUIDE

The tips below will help you to get the most out of your vegan lifestyle:

- Make sure that your diet contains a variety of fruit and vegetables – eat a rainbow!

- Choose higher fibre starchy foods, such as oats, sweet potato, wholemeal bread, wholewheat pasta and brown rice

- Include good sources of protein in most meals, such as beans, lentils, chickpeas, tofu, soya alternatives to milk and yoghurt, or peanuts

- Eat nuts and seeds daily, especially those rich in omega-3 fat

- Eat calcium-rich foods daily, such as calcium-fortified products and calcium-set tofu

- Ensure that your diet contains a reliable source of vitamin B12 (either fortified foods or a supplement)

- Ensure that your diet contains a reliable source of iodine (arguably a supplement is the best option)

- Everyone in UK should consider a vitamin D supplement during autumn and winter, and year-round supplementation should be considered by people who do not regularly expose their skin to sunlight, and those with darker skin

- Use small amounts of spread and oil high in unsaturated fats, such as vegetable (rapeseed) and olive oils

- Season food with herbs and spices instead of salt

- Drink about six to eight glasses of fluid a day

- Consider a supplement containing long chain omega-3 fats from microalgae, particularly for infants and those who are pregnant or breastfeeding

- Check out our information about vitamins B12 and D, calcium, iron, zinc, selenium and omega-3 fats to make sure that you are getting enough

- Keep active

- Maintain a healthy weight, or lose some weight if it is above the healthy range.

30 DAY VEGAN MEAL PLAN.

Following a vegan diet is a healthy approach to eating when you fill your plate with a balance of vegetables, fruits, whole grains and legumes. These next-level vegan recipes are packed with wholesome ingredients and fantastic flavours that will leave you feeling nourished and satisfied. Even if you're not a full-time vegan, these recipes are a great way to start eating a more plantbased diet.

BEEFLESS VEGAN TACOS: Take taco night in a new direction with these healthy vegan tacos. We've swapped crumbled tofu for the ground beef, without sacrificing any of the savoury seasonings you expect in a taco. You can also use the filling in burritos, bowls, taco salads and to top nachos.

Ingredient: 1 (16 ounce) package extra-firm tofu, drained, crumbled and patted dry2 tablespoons reduced-sodium tamari or soy sauce1 teaspoon chili powder½ teaspoon garlic powder½ teaspoon onion powder1 tablespoon extra-virgin olive oil1 ripe avocado1 tablespoon vegan mayonnaise1 teaspoon lime juice Pinch of salt½ cup fresh salsa or Pico de gallo2 cups shredded iceberg lettuce8 corn or flour tortillas, warmed Pickled radishes for garnish.

Preparation: Combine tofu, tamari (or soy sauce), chili powder, garlic powder and onion powder in a medium bowl. Heat oil in a large non-stick skillet over medium-high heat. Add the tofu mixture and cook, stirring occasionally, until nicely browned, 8 to 10 minutes. Meanwhile, mash avocado, mayonnaise, lime juice and salt in a small bowl until smooth. Serve the taco "meat" with the avocado crema, salsa (or pico de gallo) and lettuce in tortillas. Serve topped with pickled radishes, if desired.

To make ahead: Prepare through Step 1 and refrigerate for up to 3 days.

Nutritional information: Serving size: 2 tacos

Per serving: 360 calories; 21 g fat(3 g sat); 8 g fiber; 33 g carbohydrates; 17 g protein; 64 mcg folate; 0 cholesterol; 4 g sugars; 0 g added sugars; 556 IU vitamin A; 8 mg vitamin C; 375 mg calcium; 4 mg iron; 610 mg sodium; 553 mg potassium

Nutrition Bonus: Calcium (38% daily value), Iron (22% dv)

Carbohydrate Servings: 2

Exchanges: 2½ fat, 1½ medium-fat protein, 1½ starch, 1 vegetable.

CITRUS LIME TOFU SALAD: This veggie-packed salad has plenty of protein and fibre, so you'll feel full and satisfied. Prep the ingredients ahead of time for an easy vegan lunch idea to pack for work.

Ingredient: 2 cups mixed greens1 cup roasted vegetables, chopped if desired (see associated recipes)1 cup roasted tofu (see associated recipes)1 tablespoon pumpkin seeds2 tablespoons Citrus-Lime Vinaigrette (see associated recipes).

Preparation: Arrange greens, veggies, tofu and pumpkin seeds in a 4-cup sealable container or bowl. Drizzle vinaigrette over the salad just before serving.

To make ahead: Refrigerate salad and dressing separately for up to 5 days.

Nutritional information: Serving size: 4 cups

Per serving: 390 calories; 27 g fat(5 g sat); 7 g fibre; 20 g carbohydrates; 25 g protein; 188 mcg folate; 0 cholesterol; 6 g sugars; 0 g added sugars; 10,634 IU vitamin A; 109 mg vitamin C; 302 mg calcium; 6 mg iron; 366 mg sodium; 843 mg potassium

Nutrition Bonus: Vitamin A (213% daily value), Vitamin C (182% dv), Folate (47% dv), Iron (33% dv), Calcium (30% dv).

Carbohydrate Servings: 1½

Exchanges: 2½ fat, 2 1/1 medium-fat protein, 1½ vegetable, ½ starch.

FALAFEL SALAD WITH LEMON-TAHINI DRESSING: Deep-fried falafel can be a total grease bomb. But these pan-seared falafel still get crispy in just a few tablespoons of oil with equally satisfying results. Be sure to use dried, instead of canned, chickpeas in this healthy recipe—canned chickpeas add too much moisture.

Ingredient: 1 cup dried chickpeas2 cups packed flat-leaf parsley, divided¼ cup chopped red onion plus ¼ cup thinly sliced, divided2 cloves garlic5 tablespoons extra-virgin olive oil, divided3 tablespoons lemon juice, divided1 tablespoon ground cumin1 teaspoon salt, divided5 tablespoons tahini5 tablespoons warm water6 cups sliced romaine lettuce2 cups sliced cucumbers and/or radishes1 pint grape tomatoes, quartered.

Preparation: Soak chickpeas in cold water for 12 to 24 hours. Drain the chickpeas and transfer to a food processor. Add 1 cup parsley, chopped onion, garlic, 1 tablespoon oil, 1 tablespoon lemon juice, cumin and ½ teaspoon salt; process until finely and evenly ground. Shape into 12 patties (1½ inches wide), using a generous 2 tablespoons each. Heat 2 tablespoons oil in a large nonstick skillet over medium-high heat. Reduce heat to medium. Cook the falafel until golden brown, 3 to 5 minutes. Turn, swirl in 1 tablespoon oil and cook until golden on the other side, 3 to 5 minutes more. Meanwhile, whisk tahini, water and the remaining 2 tablespoons lemon juice, 1 tablespoon oil and ½ teaspoon salt in a large bowl. Transfer ¼ cup to a small bowl. Add romaine and the remaining 1 cup parsley to the large bowl and toss to coat. Top with cucumbers and/or radishes, tomatoes, the sliced onion and the falafel. Drizzle with the reserved ¼ cup dressing.

Nutrition information

Serving size: 3 falafel & 2 cups salad

Per serving: 499 calories; 31 g fat(4 g sat); 13 g fibre; 45 g carbohydrates; 16 g protein; 358 mcg folate; 0 mg cholesterol; 10 g sugars; 0 g added sugars; 9,390 IU vitamin A; 63 mg vitamin C; 176 mg calcium; 7 mg iron; 626 mg sodium; 1,024 mg potassium

Nutrition Bonus: Vitamin A (188% daily value), Vitamin C (105% dv), Folate (90% dv), Iron (39% dv)

Carbohydrate Servings: 3

Exchanges: 2 starch, 1½ vegetable, 1 lean meat, 5½ fat.

CHINESE SWEET & SOUR TOFU STIR-FRY WITH SNOW PEAS

This healthy sweet and sour tofu stir-fry is easy to whip together on weeknights. Just be sure to plan ahead so that you can freeze the tofu in advance. It gives the tofu a meatier texture and helps it absorb the sauce.

Ingredient: 1 (14 ounce) package water-packed firm tofu⅔ cup pineapple juice½ cup ketchup1 tablespoon reduced-sodium soy sauce1 tablespoon cornstarch2 tablespoons vegetable oil1 tablespoon minced fresh ginger8 ounces snow peas (4¼ cups), trimmed2 tablespoons thinly sliced scallions.

Preparation: One to three days before cooking, drain and rinse tofu. Wrap in foil and freeze until solid, at least 3½ to 4 hours. One day before cooking, place the tofu in a bowl and transfer to the refrigerator to thaw overnight. Place the thawed tofu on a plate lined with a double layer of paper towels. Cover with another 2 paper towels, place a plate on top and set a weight, such as 2 cans of beans, on the plate. Let stand for 20 minutes. Combine pineapple juice, ketchup, and soy sauce in a small bowl; set aside. Cut the pressed tofu into 12 slices, a scant ½ inch thick. Lightly dust both sides with corn-starch. Heat a 12-inch stainless steel skillet (or 14-inch flat-bottomed carbonsteel wok; see Tip) over high heat until a drop of water vaporizes within 1 to 2 seconds of contact. Swirl in oil, reduce heat to medium, and add the tofu in an even layer. Cook until light golden on the bottom, about 1 minute. Turnover, sprinkle with ginger, and cook until the second side is light golden, 1 minute more. Remove from heat. Add snow peas and the reserved sauce. Cover and let stand until the sauce stops sputtering, about 30 seconds. Uncover, return the pan to medium heat, and stir-fry until the sauce is well distributed and the peas are tender-crisp, 1 to 2 minutes. Sprinkle with scallions.

Tip: Use a stainless-steel skillet for this recipe unless you have a well-seasoned carbon-steel wok. The acidity of the pineapple juice and ketchup will remove a new wok's patina; a well-seasoned wok's patina will return with more cooking.

Equipment: 12-inch stainless-steel skillet or well-seasoned 14-inch flat-bottomed carbon-steel wok.

Nutrition information

Serving size: 1 cup

Per serving: 225 calories; 11 g fat(2 g sat); 3 g fibre; 23 g carbohydrates; 11 g protein; 48 mcg folate; 0 mg cholesterol; 15 g sugars; 308 IU vitamin A; 33 mg vitamin C; 231 mg calcium; 3 mg iron; 504 mg sodium; 440 mg potassium

Nutrition Bonus: Vitamin C (55% daily value), Calcium (23% dv) Carbohydrate Servings: 1½.

VEGAN EGGPLANT PARMESAN: Classic eggplant Parm is filled with cheese, but this vegan eggplant Parmesan combines non-dairy mozzarella cheese with nutritional yeast for a dairy-free cheesy substitute that gives you the comfort food factor without animal products. For the breading, use egg replacer, which you can find in natural-foods stores and the special-diet section of large supermarkets.

Ingredient: Cooking spray3 tablespoons egg replacer⅔ cup water1 cup fine dry whole-wheat breadcrumbs1½ teaspoons dried basil, divided1½ teaspoons dried oregano, divided1 eggplant (about 1 pound), cut crosswise into 12 slices2 tablespoons extra-virgin olive oil1 28-ounce can nosalt-added crushed tomatoes1 teaspoon garlic powder¼ teaspoon salt¼ teaspoon ground pepper1 cup shredded vegan mozzarella cheese, divided3 teaspoons nutritional yeast, divided Chopped fresh basil for garnish.

Preparation: Place a large rimmed baking sheet in the oven. Preheat to 425°F. Spray an 8-inchsquare baking dish with cooking spray. Whisk egg replacer and water in a shallow dish. Combine breadcrumbs and ½ teaspoon each basil and oregano in another shallow bowl. Dip each eggplant slice in the liquid, then press in the breadcrumbs. Remove the heated baking sheet from the oven and add oil, tilting to coat. Arrange the prepared eggplant pieces on it (don't let the pieces touch). Generously coat the tops with cooking spray. Bake for 15 minutes. Flip the slices and continue baking until golden brown, about 15 minutes more. Meanwhile, combine tomatoes, garlic powder, salt, pepper and the remaining 1 teaspoon each basil and oregano. Spread 1 cup of the tomato sauce in the prepared baking dish. Arrange 6 eggplant slices on top (they may overlap). Spread 1 cup sauce over the eggplant. Sprinkle with ½ cup cheese and 1½ teaspoons nutritional yeast. Repeat with the remaining eggplant, sauce, cheese and nutritional yeast. Bake, uncovered, until the sauce is bubbling, 15 to 20 minutes. Garnish with fresh basil, if desired.

To make ahead: Prepare through Step 5 and refrigerate for up to 2 days before baking.

Nutrition information

Serving size: 1½ cups

Per serving: 407 calories; 20 g fat(8 g sat); 11 g fibre; 45 g carbohydrates; 9 g protein; 83 mcg folate; 0 cholesterol; 11 g sugars; 0 g added sugars; 1,664 IU vitamin A; 17 mg vitamin C; 68 mg calcium; 5 mg iron; 654 mg sodium; 927 mg potassium

Nutrition Bonus: Vitamin A (33% daily value), Iron (28% dv), Vitamin C (28% dv), Folate (21% dv)

Carbohydrate Servings: 3

Exchanges: 5 fat, 3½ vegetable, 1 starch.

EDAMAME & VEGGIE RICE BOWL: The

ingredients in this vegan grain bowl recipe can be prepped ahead for an easy lunch to pack for work. The tangy citrus dressing is a refreshing flavour with the sweet caramel of the roasted sheet-pan veggies.

Ingredient: ½ cup cooked brown rice (see associated recipes) 1 cup roasted vegetables (see associated recipes) ¼ cup edamame¼ avocado, diced2 tablespoons sliced scallions2 tablespoons chopped fresh cilantro2 tablespoons Citrus-Lime Vinaigrette (see associated recipes).

Preparation: Arrange rice, veggies, edamame and avocado in a 4-cup sealable container or bowl. Top with scallions and cilantro. Drizzle with vinaigrette just before serving. To make ahead: Refrigerate dressing and bowl separately for up to 5 days.

Nutrition information

Serving size: 2 cups

Per serving: 394 calories; 22 g fat(3 g sat); 9 g fibre; 44 g carbohydrates; 9 g protein; 202 mcg folate; 0 cholesterol; 6 g sugars; 0 g added sugars; 7,974 IU vitamin A; 101 mg vitamin C; 91 mg calcium; 2 mg iron; 240 mg sodium; 935 mg potassium

Nutrition Bonus: Vitamin C (168% daily value), Vitamin A (159% dv), Folate (50% dv)

Carbohydrate Servings: 3

Exchanges: 4 fat, 2 starch, 1 vegetable, ½ lean-protein.

VEGAN BLATS (BLTS WITH AVOCADO):

Roasted shiitake mushrooms doused in soy sauce with

a dash of smoked paprika become a natural, vegan alternative to bacon. Try them in this vegan version of a classic BLT with creamy avocado and eggless mayonnaise or on top of a salad as a substitute for bacon bits.

Ingredient: 1 tablespoon avocado oil2 tablespoons reduced-sodium tamari½ teaspoon smoked paprika8 ounces whole shiitake mushrooms, stems removed8 small slices whole-grain bread (or 4 large slices, halved)4 tablespoons vegan mayonnaise½ teaspoon finely grated or minced garlic1 avocado, halved and sliced8 thin slices tomato4 leaves romaine lettuce.

Preparation: Preheat oven to 375°F. Stir oil, tamari and paprika together in a medium bowl. Add shiitakes and stir until all the liquid is absorbed. Spread on a rimmed baking sheet and roast, turning once, until golden brown on both sides, about 30 minutes. Toast bread. Stir mayonnaise and garlic together in a small bowl. Spread 1 tablespoon of the mayonnaise mixture on each of 4 pieces of toast. Divide avocado, tomato, lettuce and the roasted shiitakes over the toasts. Top with the remaining toasts.

Nutrition information

Serving size: 1 sandwich

Per serving: 271 calories; 19 g fat(2 g sat); 6 g fibre; 21 g carbohydrates; 7 g protein; 109 mcg folate; 0 cholesterol; 4 g sugars; 2 g added sugars; 4,045 IU vitamin A; 8 mg vitamin C; 49 mg calcium; 2 mg iron; 541 mg sodium; 530 mg potassium

Nutrition Bonus: Vitamin A (81% daily value), Folate (27% dv)

Carbohydrate Servings: 1½

Exchanges: 3½ fat, 1½ vegetable, 1 starch.

VEGETARIAN LO MEIN WITH SHIITAKES, CARROTS & BEAN SPROUTS

VEGETARIAN LO MEIN WITH SHIITAKES, CARROTS & BEAN SPROUTS: A hit of Sriracha gives a sweet and spicy edge to this healthy vegetarian recipe. Traditional lo mein is made with fresh lo mein noodles, which can be found in Asian markets. You can also use fresh or dried linguine noodles—fresh linguine is in the refrigerated section of some grocery stores. This easy dinner comes together in just 30 minutes, so it's perfect for weeknights.

Ingredient: 8 ounces fresh lo mein noodles or fresh or dried linguine pasta2 teaspoons toasted sesame oil3 tablespoons reduced-sodium soy sauce2 teaspoons Sriracha2 tablespoons vegetable oil, divided2 tablespoons minced garlic1 large carrot, halved lengthwise and cut into ¼-inch-thick halfmoon slices (about 1 cup)4 ounces fresh shiitake mushrooms, stems removed, caps sliced ¼-inch thick1 cup thinly sliced celery2 cups bean sprouts3 tablespoons finely chopped fresh cilantro.

Preparation: Bring a large pot of water to a boil. Cook noodles according to package directions. Drain, rinse with cold water, and shake out excess water until the noodles are completely dry (pat noodles dry if needed). Transfer to a large bowl and toss with sesame oil; set aside. Combine soy sauce and Sriracha in a small bowl; set aside. Heat a 14-inch flat-bottomed carbon-steel wok (or 12-inch stainless-steel skillet) over high heat until a drop of water vaporizes within 1 to 2 seconds of contact. Swirl in 1 Tbsp. vegetable oil. Add garlic; stir-fry until just fragrant, about 10 seconds. Add carrot, mushrooms, and celery; stir-fry until the celery is bright green and the vegetables have absorbed all the oil, about 1 minute. Swirl in the remaining 1 Tbsp. vegetable oil. Add bean sprouts, the noodles, and the soy sauce mixture; stir-fry until the noodles are heated through and the vegetables are tender-crisp, 1 to 2 minutes. Add cilantro and toss to combine.

Equipment: 14-inch flat-bottomed carbon-steel wok or 12-inch stainless-steel skillet.

Nutrition information serving size: 1⅓ cups

Per serving: 319 calories; 12 g fat(1 g sat); 5 g fibre; 41 g carbohydrates; 10 g protein; 50 mcg folate; 27 mg cholesterol; 5 g sugars; 3,266 IU vitamin A; 10 mg vitamin C; 39 mg calcium; 2 mg iron; 553 mg sodium; 650 mg potassium Nutrition Bonus: Vitamin A (65% daily value) Carbohydrate Servings: 2½.

VEGAN KALE CAESAR SALAD WITH TOFU CROUTONS

: Swapping tofu for the bread in these meal-prep Caesar salad bowls bumps up the satiety factor with 18 grams of protein. These crispy tofu croutons originally appeared in Lauren Grant's recipe for Diabetic Living magazine (see Associated Recipes). Lacinato kale, also known as dinosaur kale or Tuscan kale, has flat, dark green-blue leaves—and its tenderness makes it perfect for eating raw, like in this salad.

Ingredient: Tofu Croutons1 (14 to 16 ounce) block extra-firm tofu, drained and cut into ¾-inch cubes¼ cup lemon juice¼ cup vegan Worcestershire sauce1 teaspoon garlic powder1 teaspoon onion powder3 teaspoons olive oil, dividedSalad8 cups chopped lacinato kale¼ cup nutritional yeast¼ cup toasted pumpkin seeds½ cup bottled vegan Caesar dressing1 avocado.

Preparation: To prepare tofu croutons: Arrange tofu on a baking sheet between layers of paper towels. Top with another pan, place a heavy can on top and let drain for 15 minutes. Whisk lemon juice, Worcestershire, garlic powder and onion powder in a large bowl. Add the tofu and toss to coat. Let stand for 15 minutes or refrigerate for up to 2 hours. Transfer the tofu to a plate, discarding liquid. Heat 1½ teaspoons oil in a large cast-iron skillet over medium heat until shimmering. Cook half the tofu until golden and crisp on all sides, 6 to 8 minutes; transfer to a paper-towel-lined plate to drain and cool. Repeat with the remaining oil and tofu. To prepare salad: Toss kale and nutritional yeast in a large bowl. Divide among 4 lidded single-serving containers. Top each with ½ cup of the croutons and 1 tablespoon pumpkin seeds. Divide dressing among 4 small lidded containers or jars. Seal the containers and refrigerate for up to 4 days. Toss each salad with the dressing and top with ¼ avocado (sliced) just before serving.

To make ahead: Refrigerate for up to 4 days.

Nutrition information

Serving size: 2¾ cups

Per serving: 400 calories; 28 g fat(4 g sat); 9 g fibre; 19 g carbohydrates; 20 g protein; 90 mcg folate; 6 mg cholesterol; 2 g sugars; 0 g added sugars; 3,340 IU vitamin A; 51 mg vitamin C; 137 mg calcium; 4 mg iron; 423 mg sodium; 670 mg potassium

Nutrition Bonus: Vitamin C (85% daily value), Vitamin A (67% dv), Folate (22% dv), Iron (22% dv)

Carbohydrate Servings: 1½

Exchanges: 5½ fat, 1½ medium-fat protein, 1 vegetable.

VEGAN CREAM OF MUSHROOM SOUP: This creamy vegan mushroom soup is thickened with walnuts, which give the soup a creamy texture—no cream required! Add sautéed mushrooms and walnuts on top for garnish and a little crunch, and a scattering of fresh chives for even more flavour.

INGREDIENT: Soup1 tablespoon extra-virgin olive oil, divided4 cups sliced shiitake mushroom caps4 cups sliced baby bella mushrooms1 cup diced onion or shallot½ cup diced celery3 cloves garlic, minced½ teaspoon dried thyme½ teaspoon salt½ cup dry sherry4 cups "no-chicken" broth or mushroom broth1 cup water1½ cups chopped walnuts2 teaspoons sherry vinegar½ teaspoon ground pepper Mushroom-Walnut Topping1 tablespoon extra-virgin olive oil1 cup coarsely chopped shiitake mushroom caps1 cup coarsely chopped baby Bella mushrooms½ cup chopped walnuts Pinch of salt2 tablespoons sliced fresh chives.

PREPARATION: To prepare soup: Heat 1 tablespoon oil in a large pot over medium-high heat. Add 4 cups shiitake mushrooms, 4 cups baby bella mushrooms, onion (or shallot), celery, garlic, thyme and ½ teaspoon salt and cook, stirring occasionally, until tender, 7 to 10 minutes. Add sherry; increase heat to high and simmer, stirring often, until the sherry has evaporated, 2 to 3 minutes. Add broth and bring to a simmer. Puree water and 1½ cups walnuts in a blender until completely smooth, about 1 minute. Pour into the soup; return to a simmer. Reduce heat to medium-low and cook, stirring often, until the vegetables are very soft, about 5 minutes longer. Meanwhile, prepare topping: Heat oil in a medium skillet over medium heat. Add mushrooms and cook, stirring often, until soft, about 2 minutes. Add walnuts and salt. Cook, stirring occasionally, until hot, about 1 minute more. Puree the soup with an immersion blender or in a regular blender (in batches, if necessary) until very smooth. (Use caution when blending hot liquids.) Stir in vinegar and pepper. Serve the soup topped with the mushroom-walnut mixture and chives.

To make ahead: Prepare through Step 4 and refrigerate for up to 2 days.

Nutrition information

Serving size: 2 cups

Per serving: 534 calories; 46 g fat(5 g sat); 7 g fibre; 23 g carbohydrates; 13 g protein; 98 mcg folate; 0 cholesterol; 7 g sugars; 0 g added sugars; 141 IU vitamin A; 6 mg vitamin C; 99 mg calcium; 3 mg iron; 410 mg sodium; 928 mg potassium

Nutrition Bonus: Folate (24% daily value)

Carbohydrate Servings: 1½

Exchanges: 10 fat, 3 vegetable.

WATERMELON RADISH & AVOCADO SUMMER ROLLS

: Consider the fillings in this vegan summer roll recipe as a starting point—papaya, snap peas and shrimp are all good alternatives. The first thing you layer on the rice paper will be what shows through on the finished roll, so vary what you start with for stunning, Instagram-worthy results.

Ingredient: Sauce¼ cup hoisin sauce¼ cup smooth natural peanut butter2 tablespoons water2 teaspoons reduced-sodium tamari2 teaspoons rice vinegar1 teaspoon chili-garlic sauce½ teaspoon toasted sesame oil Summer Rolls12 rice paper wrappers3 ounces thin rice noodles, prepared according to package directions2 Persian (mini) cucumbers, thinly sliced1 small watermelon radish, thinly sliced1 medium ripe mango, thinly sliced2 scallions, thinly sliced1½ cups fresh mint leaves1½ cups fresh basil leaves2 medium ripe avocados, halved and sliced into 12 pieces each4 large leaves butter lettuce, torn into 3 pieces each.

Preparation: To prepare sauce: Whisk hoisin, peanut butter, water, tamari, vinegar, chili-garlic sauce and oil in a small bowl. Set aside. To prepare rolls: Soak one wrapper at a time in a shallow dish of very hot water until softened, about 10 seconds. Lift out, let excess water drip off and lay the wrappers on a clean, dry cutting board. Layer 2 tablespoons rice noodles, a few slices each cucumber, radish and mango, 1 teaspoon scallions, 2 tablespoons each mint and basil, 2 avocado slices and 1 piece of lettuce on the bottom third of the wrapper. Fold the wrapper over the filling and roll into a tight cylinder, folding in the sides as you go. Repeat with the remaining wrappers and fillings. Serve with the sauce.

Nutrition information

Serving size: 1 roll and 1 tablespoon sauce

Per serving: 220 calories; 8 g fat(1 g sat); 5 g fiber; 32 g carbohydrates; 5 g protein; 65 mcg folate; 0 mg cholesterol; 7 g sugars; 0 g added sugars; 1,307 IU vitamin A; 18 mg vitamin C; 51 mg calcium; 2 mg iron; 181 mg sodium; 343 mg potassium

Nutrition Bonus: Vitamin C (30% daily value), Vitamin A (26% dv)

Carbohydrate Servings: 2

Exchanges: 1½ fat, 1½ starch, ½ fruit.

CREAMY VEGAN BUTTERNUT SQUASH CARBONARA:

Carbonara, traditionally bathed in eggs, gets a vegan makeover using roasted and pureed butternut squash instead to make it ultra-creamy. A topping of ground almonds, garlic and sage gives it texture and an herby, savoury flavour in place of the cheese and bacon.

Ingredient: 1 pound butternut squash, peeled, seeded and cut into 1-inch cubes (3 cups)1 medium onion, chopped4 garlic cloves, divided2 tablespoons tomato paste2 tablespoons extra-virgin olive oil, divided1 teaspoon salt, divided¼ teaspoon ground pepper1 pound whole-wheat spaghetti½ cup almonds, coarsely ground1 tablespoon chopped fresh sage1 cup "no-chicken" broth or vegetable broth, warmed3 tablespoons nutritional yeast.

Preparation: Preheat oven to 425°F. Bring a large pot of water to a boil for cooking spaghetti. Toss squash, onion, 2 garlic cloves, tomato paste, 1 tablespoon oil, ¼ teaspoon salt and pepper in a large bowl. Spread in an even layer on a large rimmed baking sheet and roast, stirring once halfway through, until the squash is tender, 25 to 30 minutes. Meanwhile, cook spaghetti according to package directions. Drain. Mince the remaining 2 cloves garlic. Heat the remaining 1 tablespoon oil in a small skillet over medium heat. Add almonds and the minced garlic. Cook, stirring frequently, until the almonds are toasted and fragrant, about 3 minutes. Add sage and ¼ teaspoon salt; cook, stirring, 1 minute more. Set aside. When the squash is tender, transfer the mixture to a blender. Add broth, nutritional yeast and the remaining ½ teaspoon salt. Puree until very smooth.

Return the spaghetti to the pot and toss with the squash sauce. Top each serving of pasta with a generous tablespoon of the almond mixture.

Nutrition information

Serving size: 1 cup

Per serving: 137 calories; 4 g fat(0 g sat); 2 g fibre; 21 g carbohydrates; 5 g protein; 72 mcg folate;

- cholesterol; 1 g sugars; 0 g added sugars; 2,164 IU vitamin A; 4 mg vitamin C; 25 mg calcium;

- mg iron; 156 mg sodium; 154 mg potassium

Nutrition Bonus: Vitamin A (43% daily value)

Carbohydrate Servings: 1½

Exchanges: 3½ starch, 1 fat, ½ vegetable.

RAINBOW VEGGIE SPRING ROLL BOWL:

With tons of colourful vegetables, sesame rice noodles and a healthy peanut sauce, this noodle bowl is a hit with adults and kids alike. Assemble the bowls before serving or let everyone make their own. Serve with Sriracha hot sauce, if desired.

Ingredient: Noodle Bowl4 ounces bean thread noodles (see Tip) or thin rice noodles1 tablespoon toasted (dark) sesame oil24 asparagus spears, trimmed2 cups shredded green or Napa cabbage2 tablespoons chopped fresh basil2 tablespoons chopped fresh mint2 teaspoons rice vinegar1 cup thinly sliced carrot1 cup thinly sliced beets1 cup thinly sliced red bell pepper1 cup thinly sliced yellow bell pepper Peanut Sauce½ cup smooth natural peanut butter¼ cup reduced-sodium tamari or soy sauce¼ cup water1 tablespoon rice vinegar1 tablespoon maple syrup1 teaspoon minced garlic¼ teaspoon crushed red pepper (optional).

Preparation: To prepare noodle bowl: Prepare noodles according to package directions. Rinse well with cold water. Toss with sesame oil. Bring 1 inch of water to a boil in a large pot. Place a medium bowl of ice water next to the stove. Cook asparagus in the boiling water for 30 seconds, then transfer to the ice water. Drain well, pat dry and cut into 2-inch pieces. Combine cabbage, basil, mint and rice vinegar in a medium bowl. Divide the noodles among 4 bowls. Top each bowl with ½ cup of the cabbage mixture, some asparagus, carrot, beet and red and yellow bell pepper. To prepare sauce: Whisk peanut butter, tamari (or soy sauce), water, rice vinegar, honey, garlic and crushed red pepper (if using) in a small bowl until smooth. Drizzle ¼ cup sauce over each bowl.

To make ahead: Refrigerate sauce for up to 2 days.

Tips: Bean Thread Noodles: Look for bean thread noodles, sometimes labelled vermicelli, mung bean or cellophane noodles, in the Asian section of large supermarkets or at an Asian market.

People with celiac disease or gluten-sensitivity should use soy sauces that are labelled "gluten-free," as soy sauce may contain wheat or other gluten-containing sweeteners and flavours.

Nutrition information.

Serving size: 1 cup noodles, 2 cups vegetables & ¼ cup peanut sauce each

Per serving: 434 calories; 20 g fat(3 g sat); 8 g fibre; 51 g carbohydrates; 12 g protein; 214 mcg folate; 0 cholesterol; 13 g sugars; 4 g added sugars; 7,005 IU vitamin A; 102 mg vitamin C; 68 mg calcium; 3 mg iron; 714 mg sodium; 626 mg potassium

Nutrition Bonus: Vitamin C (170% daily value), Vitamin A (140% dv), Folate (54% dv)

Carbohydrate Servings: 3½

Exchanges: 1½ starch, ½ other carbohydrate, 3 vegetables, 4 fat.

CURRIED SWEET POTATO & PEANUT SOUP

: In this flavourful soup recipe, sweet potatoes simmer in a quick coconut curry, resulting in a creamy, thick broth punctuated by notes of garlic and ginger. We love peanuts for their inexpensive price and versatile flavour. They're also a great source of protein—1 ounce has 7 grams.

Ingredient: 2 tablespoons canola oil1½ cups diced yellow onion1 tablespoon minced garlic1 tablespoon minced fresh ginger4 teaspoons red curry paste (see Tip)1 serrano chile, ribs and seeds removed, minced1 pound sweet potatoes, peeled and cubed (½-inch pieces)3 cups water1 cup "lite" coconut milk¾ cup unsalted dry-roasted peanuts1 (15 ounce) can white beans, rinsed¾ teaspoon salt¼ teaspoon ground pepper¼ cup chopped fresh cilantro2 tablespoons lime juice¼ cup unsalted roasted pumpkin seeds Lime wedges.

Preparation: Heat oil in a large pot over medium-high heat. Add onion and cook, stirring often, until softened and translucent, about 4 minutes. Stir in garlic, ginger, curry paste, and serrano; cook, stirring, for 1 minute. Stir in sweet potatoes and water; bring to a boil. Reduce heat to medium-low and simmer, partially covered, until the sweet potatoes are soft, 10 to 12 minutes. Transfer half of the soup to a blender, along with coconut milk and peanuts; puree. (Use caution when pureeing hot liquids.) Return to the pot with the remaining soup. Stir in beans, salt, and pepper; heat through. Remove from the heat. Stir in cilantro and lime juice. Serve with pumpkin seeds and lime wedges.

Tip: You can find red curry paste in the Asian section of many grocery stores, packaged in a small glass jar.

To make ahead: Refrigerate soup for up to 3 days. Reheat before serving.

Nutrition information

Serving size: 1 cup

Per serving: 345 calories; 19 g fat(4 g sat); 8 g fibre; 37 g carbohydrates; 13 g protein; 95 mcg folate; 0 mg cholesterol; 7 g sugars; 0 g added sugars; 10,785 IU vitamin A; 8 mg vitamin C; 88 mg calcium; 2 mg iron; 594 mg sodium; 699 mg potassium Nutrition Bonus: Vitamin A (216% daily value), Folate (24% dv) Carbohydrate Servings: 2½.

SUMMER VEGETABLE SESAME NOODLES:

Squash noodles elbow out some of the starchy ones to give this cool sesame noodle salad a veggie boost. This easy healthy recipe comes together in just 20 minutes, so it's great for weeknight dinners. Pack up any leftovers for lunch.

Ingredient: 1 medium yellow squash1 medium zucchini1 cup corn kernels, fresh or frozen8 ounces soba noodles¼ cup ponzu sauce (see Tip)2 tablespoons tahini2 tablespoons toasted sesame oil1 tablespoon rice vinegar¼ teaspoon salt1 pint cherry tomatoes, halved3 scallions, sliced2 teaspoons sesame seeds.

Preparation: Put a large saucepan of water on to boil. Spiralize squash and zucchini into mediumthick "noodles." (Alternatively, cut them lengthwise into long, thin strips with a vegetable peeler. Stop when you reach the seeds in the middle—seeds make the strips fall apart.) Place the vegetable noodles and corn in a large colander. Cook soba noodles in the boiling water according to package directions. Pour over the vegetables in the colander to drain. Meanwhile, combine ponzu, tahini, oil, vinegar and salt in a large bowl. Add the soba and vegetable noodles to the bowl along with tomatoes and scallions. Toss to combine. Serve topped with sesame seeds.

Tip: Ponzu, a Japanese soy sauce blend, gets complex flavour from tangy vinegar and citrus, plus some have added umami-packed fish flakes and seaweed. If you're vegan, look for a brand that skips the fish or make a substitute by combining 2 Tbsp. each soy sauce and lemon juice with a splash of rice vinegar. Equipment: Spiralizer.

Nutrition information

Serving size: 2 cups

Per serving: 387 calories; 13 g fat(2 g sat); 6 g fibre; 61 g carbohydrates; 15 g protein; 76 mcg folate; 0 mg cholesterol; 6 g sugars; 0 g added sugars; 947 IU vitamin A; 27 mg vitamin C; 61 mg calcium; 2 mg iron; 629 mg sodium; 621 mg potassium

Nutrition Bonus: Vitamin C (45% daily value)

Carbohydrate Servings: 4

Exchanges: 3½ starch, 2 fat, 1 vegetable.

MUSHROOM-QUINOA VEGGIE BURGERS WITH SPECIAL SAUCE

MUSHROOM-QUINOA VEGGIE BURGERS WITH SPECIAL SAUCE: These hearty mushroom, black bean and quinoa veggie burgers are a healthy and satisfying homemade alternative to store-bought veggie burgers. And they take just 25 minutes of active time to prep, so while they're special enough for entertaining, they're quick enough for weeknight dinners.

Ingredient: 1 large Portobello mushroom, gills removed, roughly chopped1 cup no-salt-added canned black beans, rinsed2 tablespoons unsalted creamy almond butter3 tablespoons canola mayonnaise, divided1 teaspoon ground pepper¾ teaspoon smoked paprika¾ teaspoon garlic powder, divided½ teaspoon salt½ cup cooked quinoa¼ cup old-fashioned rolled oats1 tablespoon ketchup1 teaspoon Dijon mustard1 tablespoon extra-virgin olive oil4 whole-wheat hamburger buns, toasted2 leaves green-leaf lettuce, halved4 slices tomato4 thin slices red onion.

Preparation: Place mushroom, black beans, almond butter, 1 tablespoon mayonnaise, pepper, paprika, ½ teaspoon garlic powder and salt in a food processor. Pulse, stopping once or twice to scrape down the sides, until a coarse mixture forms that holds together when pressed. Transfer to a bowl and add quinoa and oats; stir well to combine. Refrigerate for 1 hour. Meanwhile, whisk ketchup, mustard and the remaining 2 tablespoons mayonnaise and ¼ teaspoon garlic powder in a small bowl until smooth. Shape the mushroom mixture into 4 patties. Heat oil in a large grill pan or non-stick skillet over medium-high heat. Add the patties and cook until golden and beginning to crisp, 4 to 5 minutes. Carefully flip and cook until golden brown, 2 to 4 minutes more. Serve the burgers on buns with the special sauce, lettuce, tomato and onion.

To make ahead: The burger patties and special sauce can be made in advance. Prepare through Step 3; cover and refrigerate separately for up to 24 hours.

Nutrition information

Serving size: 1 burger

Per serving: 394 calories; 20 g fat(2 g sat); 9 g fibre; 46 g carbohydrates; 12 g protein; 51 mcg folate; 4 mg cholesterol; 7 g sugars; 0 g added sugars; 974 IU vitamin A; 4 mg vitamin C; 122 mg calcium; 3 mg iron; 659 mg sodium; 561 mg potassium

Carbohydrate Servings: 3

Exchanges: 3 fat, 2½ starch, ½ lean protein, ½ vegetable.

VEGAN WHITE BEAN CHILI: Fresh Anaheim (or poblano) chiles add mild heat to this classic white bean chili and contribute lots of smoky flavor. Quinoa adds body to the chili, while diced zucchini provides pretty flecks of green and increases the veggie content.

Ingredient: ¼ cup avocado oil or canola oil2 cups chopped seeded Anaheim or poblano chiles (about 3)1 large onion, chopped4 cloves garlic, minced½ cup quinoa, rinsed4 teaspoons dried oregano4 teaspoons ground cumin1 teaspoon salt½ teaspoon ground coriander½ teaspoon ground pepper4 cups low-sodium vegetable broth2 (15 ounce) cans no-salt-added white beans, rinsed1 large zucchini, diced (about 3 cups) ¼ cup chopped fresh cilantro2 tablespoons lime juice, plus wedges for serving.

Preparation: Heat oil in a large pot over medium heat. Add chiles, onion and garlic. Cook, stirring, until the vegetables are softened, 5 to 7 minutes. Add quinoa, oregano, cumin, salt, coriander and pepper; cook, stirring, until aromatic, about 1 minute. Stir in broth and beans. Bring to a boil. Reduce heat to a simmer. Partially cover and cook, stirring occasionally, for 20 minutes. Add zucchini; cover and continue cooking until the zucchini is soft and the chili has thickened, 10 to 15 minutes more. Stir in cilantro and lime juice. Serve with lime wedges, if desired. To make ahead: Refrigerate chili for up to 4 days. Reheat before serving.

Nutrition information

Serving size: 1⅓ cups

Per serving: 283 calories; 12 g fat(1 g sat); 8 g fibre; 37 g carbohydrates; 10 g protein; 78 mcg folate; 0 cholesterol; 7 g sugars; 0 g added sugars; 757 IU vitamin A; 135 mg vitamin C; 96 mg calcium; 4 mg iron; 529 mg sodium; 671 mg potassium

Nutrition Bonus: Vitamin C (225% daily value), Iron (22% dv), Folate (20% dv)

Carbohydrate Servings: 2½

Exchanges: 2 fat, 2 vegetable, 1½ starch, ½ lean protein.

ROASTED BUTTERNUT SQUASH & PEAR QUINOA SALAD

ROASTED BUTTERNUT SQUASH & PEAR QUINOA SALAD: This roasted vegetable and fruit salad gets infused with flavour from quinoa that's cooked with fresh ginger, garlic and a hit of turmeric. Serve it alongside a roast chicken, then mix the leftovers together for lunch. Your future self will thank you.

Ingredient: 3 cups diced peeled butternut squash (½-inch pieces)5 tablespoons extra-virgin olive oil, divided½ teaspoon salt, divided½ teaspoon ground pepper, divided¼ teaspoon crushed red pepper1 firm ripe pear, sliced into 8 wedges2 teaspoons finely chopped fresh ginger1 clove garlic, finely chopped⅛ teaspoon ground turmeric½ cup quinoa1 cup no-chicken or vegetable broth1 scallion, sliced3 tablespoons pear vinegar or cider vinegar2 teaspoons minced red onion1 teaspoon Dijon mustard1 teaspoon chopped fresh rosemary Minced fresh red chili to taste2 cups baby arugula.

Preparation: Preheat oven to 400°F. Toss squash in a large bowl with 1 tablespoon oil, ¼ teaspoon each salt and pepper and crushed red pepper. Spread on a large rimmed baking sheet. Roast for 15 minutes. Stir the squash, add pear and roast until browned and tender, about 15 minutes more. Meanwhile, heat 1 tablespoon oil in a large saucepan over medium heat and add ginger, garlic and turmeric; cook until sizzling, about 1 minute. Add quinoa and cook, stirring, for 30 seconds. Add broth and bring to a boil over high heat. Reduce heat to a simmer, cover and cook until the broth is absorbed, about 15 minutes. Remove from heat and let stand, covered, for 5 minutes. Stir in scallion and the remaining ¼ teaspoon each salt and pepper and let cool. Whisk vinegar, onion, mustard, rosemary and chile in a large bowl. Slowly whisk in the remaining 3 tablespoons oil. Stir half the dressing into the quinoa. Add the pears and squash to the bowl with the remaining dressing; gently stir to coat. Let stand, stirring occasionally, for 15 minutes or refrigerate separately for up to 1 day. Fold arugula into the squash and pears and serve over the quinoa. To make ahead: Prepare through Step 4 and refrigerate for up to 1 day.

Nutrition information Serving size: 1 cup

Per serving: 210 calories; 13 g fat(2 g sat); 4 g fiber; 22 g carbohydrates; 3 g protein; 42 mcg folate; 0 mg cholesterol; 5 g sugars; 0 g added sugars; 7,051 IU vitamin A; 15 mg vitamin C; 64 mg calcium; 1 mg iron; 309 mg sodium; 313 mg potassium

Nutrition Bonus: Vitamin A (141% daily value), Vitamin C (25% dv)

Carbohydrate Servings: 1½

Exchanges: 2½ fat, 1 starch, ½ fruit.

DAN DAN NOODLES WITH SPINACH & WALNUTS

In this riff on Asian dan dan noodles, spinach and red bell peppers are tossed with a sesame-chile-soy sauce and topped with walnuts. If you want to bump up the protein, add tofu, seitan or even chopped egg.

Ingredient: 1½ cups low-sodium vegetable broth4 scallions, chopped, divided1 tablespoon chopped fresh ginger1 teaspoon toasted sesame oil¼ teaspoon ground pepper10 ounces baby spinach (about 12 cups) 12 ounces Chinese flat noodles (see Tips) or linguine¼ cup Chinese sesame paste (see Tips) or tahini3 tablespoons reduced-sodium soy sauce1 tablespoon hot chile oil¼ teaspoon sugar1 medium red bell pepper, diced1 cup toasted chopped walnuts3 tablespoons toasted sesame seeds.

Preparation: Combine broth, 1 scallion, ginger, sesame oil and pepper in a medium saucepan. Bring just to a boil over high heat. Stir and set aside for 20 minutes. Meanwhile, bring a large pot of water to a boil. Cook spinach for 1 minute. Transfer with a slotted spoon to a colander (leave the water in the pot) and drain, pressing on the spinach to remove excess water. Add noodles to the boiling water and cook according to package directions. Drain and rinse well. Chop the spinach. Gently combine the noodles and spinach in a large shallow serving bowl, separating the spinach so it doesn't clump together. Place the saucepan of broth over medium heat. Add sesame paste (or tahini), soy sauce, chile oil and sugar; whisk until thoroughly combined. Bring to a low boil and remove from heat. Pour the sauce over the noodles. Top with bell pepper, walnuts, sesame seeds and the remaining 3 scallions. Toss together at the table before serving.

Any type of flat wheat noodle can be used for this recipe; for the most authentic taste and texture, seek out a Chinese brand of noodles from an Asian market or a supermarket with a large selection of ingredients used in Chinese cooking.

Look for Chinese sesame paste—similar to tahini with a more prominent roasted-sesame flavour— in Asian markets.

Nutrition information

Serving size: 1⅓ cups

Per serving: 488 calories; 25 g fat(3 g sat); 7 g fibre; 54 g carbohydrates; 16 g protein; 305 mcg folate; 0 mg cholesterol; 3 g sugars; 0 g added sugars; 5,163 IU vitamin A; 41 mg vitamin C; 149 mg calcium; 5 mg iron; 347 mg sodium; 567 mg potassium

Nutrition Bonus: Vitamin A (103% daily value), Folate (76% dv), Vitamin C (68% dv), Iron (28% dv)

Carbohydrate Servings: 3½

Exchanges: 3 starch, ½ vegetable, 4½ fat.

THAI TOFU & VEGETABLE CURRY WITH ZUCCHINI NOODLES

THAI TOFU & VEGETABLE CURRY WITH ZUCCHINI NOODLES: For this quick Thai curry recipe, we've combined tofu and plenty of veggies with a flavourful sauce made with red curry paste, lime juice and coconut milk. Serve the curry over lightly warmed zucchini noodles to get even more veggies in your weeknight dinner. Bonus: Everything is cooked in one skillet, so there's only one pan to wash after dinner.

Ingredient: 2 tablespoons toasted sesame oil1 (14 ounce) package extra-firm tofu, cut into ½-inch pieces1 (14 ounce) can coconut milk2 tablespoons red curry paste1 tablespoon lime juice2 medium cloves garlic, grated½ teaspoon salt1 tablespoon avocado oil1 (8 ounce) package sliced mushrooms1 bunch scallions, cut into 1-inch pieces6 cups chopped kale2 (10 ounce) packages zucchini noodles.

Preparation: Heat sesame oil in a large non-stick skillet over medium-high heat. Pat tofu dry and add to pan. Cook in a single layer, without stirring, until the pieces turn golden, about 4 minutes. Gently stir and continue cooking, stirring occasionally, until golden all over, 4 minutes more. Transfer to a plate. Meanwhile, whisk coconut milk, curry paste, lime juice, garlic and salt in a small bowl. Add avocado oil, mushrooms and scallions to the pan. Cook, stirring, until the mushrooms have released their liquid and started to brown, about 5 minutes. Add kale, the sauce mixture and the tofu and cook, stirring, until the kale is wilted, the sauce has thickened and the tofu is heated through, about 2 minutes. Transfer to a bowl. Add zucchini noodles to the pan and cook, stirring, until heated through, about 1 minute. Serve the curry over the noodles.

Nutrition information

Serving size: 1 cup noodles & 1 cup sauce each

Per serving: 428 calories; 37 g fat(21 g sat); 5 g fibre; 17 g carbohydrates; 16 g protein; 125 mcg folate; 0 cholesterol; 7 g sugars; 0 g added sugars; 2,907 IU vitamin A; 62 mg vitamin C; 297 mg calcium; 6 mg iron; 518 mg sodium; 1,106 mg potassium

Nutrition Bonus: Vitamin C (103% daily value), Vitamin A (58% dv), Iron (33% dv), Folate (31% dv), Calcium (30% dv)

Carbohydrate Servings: 1

Exchanges: 5½ fat, 2 vegetable, 1½ medium-fat protein.

USE-ALL-THE-BROCCOLI STIR-FRY:

Spiralized broccoli stems transform into tender noodles in this lo mein-inspired vegetarian recipe. Serve on top of brown rice or buckwheat soba noodles.

Ingredient: 2½ pounds large broccoli heads with stems at least 1 inch thick (4-5 heads)1 medium red onion½ cup water, divided2 tablespoons Shaoxing rice wine or dry sherry2 tablespoons reducedsodium tamari1 tablespoon chile-garlic sauce4 teaspoons toasted sesame oil, divided2 teaspoons cornstarch1 teaspoon light brown sugar2 tablespoons peanut oil, divided⅛ teaspoon salt2 small red chiles, sliced (seeded if desired)1 tablespoon minced fresh ginger2 tablespoons chopped roasted unsalted peanuts.

Preparation: Remove florets from broccoli stems. Cut the florets into 1-inch pieces and set aside. Trim the stem ends. Using a vegetable spiralizer with the thin-noodle blade, spiralize as much of each stem as possible. Chop any remaining stem into ½-inch pieces. Switch to the thick-noodle blade and spiralize onion. Whisk ¼ cup water, rice wine (or sherry), tamari, chili-garlic sauce, 2 teaspoons sesame oil, corn-starch and brown sugar in a small bowl. Set by the stove. Heat 1 tablespoon peanut oil in a large flat-bottom carbon-steel wok over medium-high heat. Add the broccoli noodles, stem pieces and onion; cook, stirring, until tender, about 5 minutes. Transfer the mixture to a large bowl and toss with the remaining 2 teaspoons sesame oil and salt. Add the remaining 1 tablespoon peanut oil, chilies and ginger to the pan. Cook, stirring constantly, for 15 seconds. Add the reserved florets and cook, stirring, until starting to brown, about 1 minute. Add the remaining ¼ cup water, cover and cook until the florets are tender, about 3 minutes more.

Uncover and add the reserved sauce. Cook, stirring, until the sauce is thick, about 1 minute. Arrange the noodle mixture on a platter with the florets on top. Serve sprinkled with peanuts. Equipment: Spiralizer.

Nutrition information

Serving size: about 2 cups

Per serving: 252 calories; 14 g fat(2 g sat); 9 g fibre; 24 g carbohydrates; 11 g protein; 215 mcg folate; 0 mg cholesterol; 9 g sugars; 2 g added sugars; 5,109 IU vitamin A; 299 mg vitamin C; 150 mg calcium; 3 mg iron; 590 mg sodium; 1,066 mg potassium

Nutrition Bonus: Vitamin C (498% daily value), Vitamin A (102% dv), Folate (54% dv) Carbohydrate Servings: 1½.

ROASTED ROOT VEGGIES & GREENS OVER SPICED LENTILS

: This earthy bowl of lentils bursting with Middle Eastern flavours is topped with leftover roasted root veggies from a large batch for an easy weeknight dinner. Keep it vegan or add a drizzle of plain yogurt for extra richness.

Ingredient: Lentils1½ cups water½ cup black beluga lentils or French green lentils (see Tip)1 teaspoon garlic powder½ teaspoon ground coriander½ teaspoon ground cumin¼ teaspoon ground allspice¼ teaspoon kosher salt2 tablespoons lemon juice1 teaspoon extra-virgin olive oilVegetables1 tablespoon extra-virgin olive oil1 clove garlic, smashed1½ cups roasted root vegetables (see associated recipes)2 cups chopped kale or beet greens1 teaspoon ground coriander⅛ teaspoon ground pepper Pinch of kosher salt2 tablespoons tahini or low-fat plain yogurt Fresh parsley for garnish.

Preparation: To prepare lentils: Combine water, lentils, garlic powder, ½ teaspoon coriander, cumin, allspice, ¼ teaspoon salt and sumac (if using) in a medium pot. Bring to a boil. Reduce heat to maintain a simmer, cover and cook until tender, 25 to 30 minutes. Uncover and continue simmering until the liquid reduces slightly, about 5 minutes more. Drain. Stir in lemon juice and 1 teaspoon oil. Meanwhile, to prepare vegetables: Heat oil in a large skillet over medium heat. Add garlic and cook until fragrant, 1 to 2 minutes. Add roasted root vegetables and cook, stirring often, until heated through, 2 to 4 minutes. Stir in kale (or beet greens) and cook until just wilted, 2 to 3 minutes. Stir in coriander, pepper and salt. Serve the vegetables over the lentils, topped with tahini (or yogurt). Garnish with parsley, if desired.

Tip: We like black beluga lentils or French green lentils instead of brown when we want lentils that hold their shape (instead of breaking down) when cooked. Look for them in natural-foods stores and some supermarkets.

Nutrition information

Serving size: Generous 1 cup vegetables & ⅔ cup lentils

Per serving: 453 calories; 22 g fat(3 g sat); 14 g fibre; 50 g carbohydrates; 18 g protein; 81 mcg folate; 0 cholesterol; 5 g sugars; 0 g added sugars; 5,939 IU vitamin A; 35 mg vitamin C; 114 mg calcium; 5 mg iron; 346 mg sodium; 465 mg potassium

Nutrition Bonus: Vitamin A (119% daily value), Vitamin C (58% dv), Iron (28% dv), Folate (20% dv)

Carbohydrate Servings: 3½

Exchanges: 4 fat, 2½ starch, 2 lean protein, 1 vegetable.

HOMEMADE KIMCHI: If you are looking to start fermenting your own vegetables, kimchi is a great place to start. It is easy to make, and fermentation takes just a few days. Once you have kimchi on hand, use this healthy Asian condiment to liven up brown rice, soups, stir-fries, grilled cheese sandwiches, tacos—and the list goes on!

Ingredient: 2 pounds napa cabbage, cored and cut into 1-inch pieces¼ cup kosher salt8 ounces daikon radish, cut into matchstick strips (2 cups)4 scallions, trimmed and cut into 1-inch pieces24 tablespoons Korean-style red pepper flakes (gochugaru)2 tablespoons fish sauce¾ ounce fresh ginger, cut into matchstick strips (¼ cup)2 cloves garlic, quartered1 teaspoon sugar.

Preparation: Combine cabbage and salt in a large bowl. Add enough water to cover the cabbage. Keep the cabbage submerged with a plate or a sealable bag filled with water. Cover the bowl and let stand at room temperature overnight or up to 24 hours. Drain the cabbage, saving the brine. Rinse and squeeze the cabbage dry. Return to the bowl and add daikon and scallions. Place red pepper flakes, fish sauce, ginger, garlic and sugar in a mini food processor. Process until almost smooth. Transfer to the large bowl with the cabbage. Using a disposable food-safe glove, massage the vegetables and the red pepper mixture together until well coated. Pack into a 2-quart glass jar. Add enough of the reserved brine to just cover the vegetables. Screw on the lid. Place the jar on a rimmed baking sheet and let stand in a cool place. Make sure that the vegetables are always covered with brine. Taste after 3 to 5 days. The kimchi is ready when it tastes good to you. Reseal the jar and store in the refrigerator.

To make ahead: Refrigerate the finished kimchi for up to 3 weeks

Nutrition information.

Serving size: ¼ cup

Per serving: 9 calories; 0 g fat(0 g sat); 1 g fiber; 2 g carbohydrates; 1 g protein; 19 mcg folate; 0 cholesterol; 0 g sugars; 0 g added sugars; 428 IU vitamin A; 7 mg vitamin C; 14 mg calcium; 0 mg iron; 104 mg sodium; 97 mg potassium Carbohydrate Servings: 0 Exchanges: Free food.

VEGAN CAULIFLOWER FRIED RICE:
Substituting riced cauliflower for rice trims calories and carbs in this veggie-packed dish. Use the vibrant flavors of traditional fried rice—ginger, scallions and tamari—to create a low-carb fried rice version of the classic take-out meal.

Ingredient: 3 tablespoons peanut oil, divided3 scallions, sliced1 tablespoon grated fresh ginger1 tablespoon minced garlic½ cup diced red bell pepper1 cup trimmed and halved snow peas1 cup shredded carrots1 cup frozen shelled edamame, thawed4 cups riced cauliflower (see Tips)⅓ cup unsalted roasted cashews3 tablespoons reduced-sodium tamari or soy sauce (see Tips)1 teaspoon toasted sesame oil.

Preparation: Heat 1 tablespoon peanut oil in a large wok or skillet over high heat. Add scallions, ginger and garlic; cook, stirring, until scallions have softened, 30 to 40 seconds. Add bell pepper, snow peas, carrots and edamame; cook, stirring, until just tender, 2 to 4 minutes. Transfer everything to a plate. Add the remaining 2 tablespoons peanut oil to the pan. Add cauliflower and stir until mostly softened, about 2 minutes. Return the cooked vegetables to the pan, along with cashews, tamari (or soy sauce) and sesame oil. Stir until well combined.

Tips: You can find riced cauliflower in the produce aisle or your supermarket, or you can prepare it yourself. Place cauliflower florets in a food processor and pulse until it breaks down into ricesize pieces.

People with celiac disease or gluten sensitivity should use soy sauces that are labelled "gluten-free," as soy sauce may contain wheat or other gluten-containing ingredients.

Nutrition information

Serving size: scant 1½ cups

Per serving: 287 calories; 19 g fat(3 g sat); 6 g fibre; 18 g carbohydrates; 10 g protein; 157 mcg folate; 0 cholesterol; 6 g sugars; 0 g added sugars; 5,426 IU vitamin A; 80 mg vitamin C; 77 mg calcium; 3 mg iron; 451 mg sodium; 449 mg potassium

Nutrition Bonus: Vitamin C (133% daily value), Vitamin A (109% dv), Folate (39% dv)

Carbohydrate Servings: 1

Exchanges: 3½ fat, 2 vegetable, ½ lean protein, ½ starch.

FALAFEL: Tuck these tasty chickpea patties into whole-wheat pitas and top with tahini sauce (see associated recipe, below). Be sure to soak the chickpeas overnight for the creamiest mixture. The quick-soak method won't work for these pan-fried falafel patties.

Ingredient: 1 cup dried chickpeas, soaked overnight½ cup packed flat-leaf parsley¼ cup chopped onion2 medium cloves garlic4 tablespoons extra-virgin olive oil, divided1 tablespoon lemon juice1 tablespoon ground cumin½ teaspoon salt¼ teaspoon baking soda1-3 tablespoons water, if needed.

Preparation: Drain chickpeas and transfer to a food processor. Add parsley, onion, garlic, 1 tablespoon oil, lemon juice, cumin, salt and baking soda; process, adding water as needed, until finely ground and the mixture just holds together. Using about 3 tablespoons per patty, shape into twelve 1½-inch patties. Heat 2 tablespoons oil in a large non-stick skillet over medium-high heat. Reduce heat to medium. Add the patties and cook until golden brown on the bottom, 3 to 5 minutes. Turn, swirl in the remaining 1 tablespoon oil and cook until golden, 2 to 4 minutes more.

Nutrition information

Serving size: 3 patties

Per serving: 331 calories; 17 g fat(2 g sat); 7 g fibre; 34 g carbohydrates; 11 g protein; 293 mcg folate; 0 cholesterol; 6 g sugars; 0 g added sugars; 673 IU vitamin A; 15 mg vitamin C; 57 mg calcium; 3 mg iron; 389 mg sodium; 425 mg potassium Nutrition Bonus: Folate (73% daily value), Vitamin C (25% dv)

Carbohydrate Servings: 2½

Exchanges: 2½ fat, 2 starch, 1½ lean protein, ½ vegetable.

VEGAN BUTTERNUT SQUASH SOUP

VEGAN BUTTERNUT SQUASH SOUP: Thai spices and creamy coconut milk distinguish this version from traditional butternut squash soup. Curry paste is a convenient way to add complex flavour, but if you want to make sure this soup is vegan or if you are allergic to shellfish, check the ingredient list carefully— some brands contain shellfish.

Ingredient: 2 tablespoons avocado oil1 cup chopped onion1 tablespoon minced garlic1 tablespoon minced ginger2 tablespoons Thai curry paste4 cups low-sodium vegetable broth1 small butternut squash (about 2 pounds), peeled and cubed (about 5 cups)½ teaspoon salt1 (14 ounce) can coconut milk1 tablespoon lime juice, plus lime wedges for serving Chopped fresh cilantro for garnish.

Preparation: Heat oil in a large saucepan over medium heat. Add onion, garlic and ginger; cook, stirring, until starting to soften, about 3 minutes. Add curry paste and cook for another minute. Add broth, squash and salt; bring to a boil. Reduce heat to maintain a simmer and cook, stirring occasionally, until the squash is tender, 20 to 25 minutes. Stir in coconut milk and lime juice and cook until heated through, 1 to 2 minutes more. Remove from heat. Puree the soup in the pot using an immersion blender or in batches in a blender. (Use caution when blending hot liquids.) Serve garnished with cilantro and a squeeze of lime, if desired.

To make ahead: Refrigerate soup for up to 4 days. Reheat before serving.

Nutrition information

Serving size: 1 cup

Per serving: 183 calories; 14 g fat(10 g sat); 3 g fibre; 13 g carbohydrates; 2 g protein; 25 mcg folate; 0 cholesterol; 4 g sugars; 0 g added sugars; 8,298 IU vitamin A; 14 mg vitamin C; 54 mg calcium; 2 mg iron; 313 mg sodium; 355 mg potassium

Nutrition Bonus: Vitamin A (166% daily value), Vitamin C (23% dv)

Carbohydrate Servings: 1

Exchanges: 3 fat, ½ starch, ½ vegetable.

VEGAN PESTO SPAGHETTI SQUASH WITH MUSHROOMS & SUN-DRIED TOMATOES:

Low-carb spaghetti squash stands in for wheat noodles in this updated twist on a classic pesto pasta dish. Cashews lend richness to the pesto, while nutritional yeast, mushrooms and sun-dried tomatoes contribute satisfying umami to this vegan dinner recipe.

Ingredient: 1 2½- to 3-pound spaghetti squash, halved lengthwise and seeded4 tablespoons extravirgin olive oil, divided8 ounces cremini mushrooms, sliced½ cup julienned sun-dried tomatoes½ teaspoon salt, divided1 cup packed fresh basil leaves2 cloves garlic, coarsely chopped⅓ cup unsalted raw cashews3 tablespoons lemon juice2 teaspoons nutritional yeast½ teaspoon ground pepper.

Preparation: Place squash halves, cut-side down, in a microwave-safe dish; add 2 tablespoons water. Microwave, uncovered, on High until tender, 10 to 14 minutes. (Alternatively, place squash halves, cut-side down, on a rimmed baking sheet. Bake in a 400°F oven until tender, 40 to 50 minutes. You can also cook the squash in a pressure cooker/multicooker. Meanwhile, heat 1 tablespoon oil in a large skillet over medium heat. Add mushrooms, tomatoes and ¼ teaspoon salt; cook, stirring, until the mushrooms are soft and starting to brown, 5 to 6 minutes. Remove from heat. Combine basil, the remaining 3 tablespoons oil, garlic, cashews, lemon juice, nutritional yeast, the remaining ¼ teaspoon salt and pepper in a food processor. Process until mostly smooth. Use a fork to scrape the squash flesh from the shells into a colander. Press lightly on the flesh to remove some of the liquid. Divide the squash among 4 plates. Top each serving with mushroom mixture and then a dollop of basil pesto.

Nutrition information Serving size: 1 cup

Per serving: 310 calories; 22 g fat(3 g sat); 5 g fibre; 27 g carbohydrates; 7 g protein; 74 mcg folate; 0 cholesterol; 8 g sugars; 0 g added sugars; 1,003 IU vitamin A; 29 mg vitamin C; 96 mg calcium;

3 mg iron; 377 mg sodium; 895 mg potassium

Nutrition Bonus: Vitamin C (48% daily value), Vitamin A (20% dv)

Carbohydrate Servings: 2

Exchanges: 4½ vegetable, 4 fat.

QUINOA AVOCADO SALAD: Protein-packed quinoa pairs with creamy avocado in this refreshing grain salad. It's the perfect make-ahead side dish to bring on a picnic or take to a potluck. Or pack it for lunch or enjoy it as a light dinner.

Ingredient: 3 tablespoons lime juice2 tablespoons avocado oil¾ teaspoon garlic powder½ teaspoon salt¼ teaspoon ground pepper3 cups cooked quinoa, cooled2 medium avocados, chopped1 cup grape tomatoes, halved1 cup diced cucumber½ cup chopped fresh cilantro1 scallion, sliced.

Preparation: Whisk lime juice, oil, garlic powder, salt and pepper in a medium bowl. Add quinoa, avocados, tomatoes, cucumber, cilantro and scallion; stir gently until combined.

To make ahead: Refrigerate for up to 4 hours.

Nutrition information

Serving size: 1½ cups

Per serving: 414 calories; 25 g fat(3 g sat); 12 g fibre; 44 g carbohydrates; 9 g protein; 156 mcg folate; 0 cholesterol; 4 g sugars; 0 g added sugars; 722 IU vitamin A; 22 mg vitamin C; 58 mg calcium; 3 mg iron; 313 mg sodium; 968 mg potassium

Nutrition Bonus: Folate (39% daily value), Vitamin C (37% dv)

Carbohydrate Servings: 3

Exchanges: 5 fat, 2 starch, 1 vegetable.

FRENCH RATATOUILLE: Ratatouille, a classic French dish with tomatoes, eggplant, zucchini, bell pepper and onion, is frequently cooked low and slow until it turns silky and luscious. We kept the classic flavour but gave it a makeover by thinly slicing the vegetables and layering them in a cast-iron pan. We brighten up the flavour at the end with a splash of red-wine vinegar.

Ingredient: 4 tablespoons extra-virgin olive oil, divided1 small onion, thinly sliced1 red bell pepper, thinly sliced½ teaspoon salt, divided1 large eggplant (about 1 pound), thinly sliced2 small zucchini and/or summer squash (about 12 ounces), thinly sliced3 medium tomatoes, thinly sliced¼ teaspoon ground pepper1 tablespoon red-wine vinegar1 tablespoon chopped fresh marjoram.

Preparation: Preheat oven to 425°F. Heat 1 tablespoon oil in a large cast-iron skillet over medium heat. Add onion, bell pepper and ¼ teaspoon salt. Cook, stirring frequently, until the pepper is soft and the onion is beginning to brown, about 10 minutes. Remove the pan from the heat. Carefully layer eggplant, zucchini (and/or summer squash) and tomatoes in an alternating shingle pattern over the pepper and onion. (They will overlap quite a bit.) If you have extra vegetable slices, save them for another use. Drizzle with 2 tablespoons oil and sprinkle with pepper and the remaining ¼ teaspoon salt. Place the pan in the oven and bake until the vegetables are tender, about 1 hour. Drizzle vinegar and the remaining 1 tablespoon oil over the top and sprinkle with marjoram. Let cool for about 5 minutes before serving. Leftovers can be refrigerated for up to 4 days.

Nutrition information.

Serving size: 1 cup

Per serving: 200 calories; 15 g fat(2 g sat); 6 g fibre; 16 g carbohydrates; 3 g protein; 71 mcg folate;

• cholesterol; 9 g sugars; 0 g added sugars; 1,881 IU vitamin A; 65 mg vitamin C; 45 mg calcium;

• mg iron; 305 mg sodium; 731 mg potassium

Nutrition Bonus: Vitamin C (108% daily value), Vitamin A (38% dv)

Carbohydrate Servings: 1

Exchanges: 3 fat, 3 vegetable.

SAUCE AND CONDIMENT RECIPE.

There's just something about a saucy, juicy, savoury meal, especially when you know where all the ingredients in the sauce come from. When cooks boast about their secret ingredients, those unexpected flavours are often part of the sauce. The ingredients in these vegan sauces aren't secret, though, just a great way to change up your day to day flavours, or reinvent leftovers. What we love about sauce is how easy they make sticking to the whole foods we promised ourselves we'd eat. Of course, the dishes under the sauce are worth a try, too.

HOMEMADE SPICY RED WINE TOMATO SAUCE

: If you eat plant-based, you probably are used to marinara, because unlike most sauces, it's usually meat and dairy free. This sauce is no prosaic marinara, however. With an array of zesty spices, a bit of a burn, and red wine in the mix, this tomato sauce will rescue any pasta dish.

Ingredient: 1 can (28oz) puree of whole peeled tomatoes (I used no salt added) OR 1 lb 12oz- 2 lb whole plum tomatoes, juice of 1/2 lemon glug or two of red wine (around 1/4 cup) (I used no sulfites added Tree-Hugger Wine) 2-3 tsp. palm sugar (any mild-tasting sweetener should do)

4-5 cloves garlic Italian spices (basil, oregano, rosemary, sage, thyme, marjoram)* ground black pepper red pepper flakes (optional for spicy, spiciness yum).

Preparation: For fresh tomatoes, you're going to want to Blanche them. This removes the skin easily and makes for a smoother sauce texture. Real easy though, fill a large pot with enough water to cover tomatoes, boil water, drop tomatoes in for a minute or two (when skin starts to separate), then transfer to another pot filled with ice water. Then peel tomatoes! I would recommend keeping the seeds unless they really bother you. You can either squeeze or cut them out. Set stove to simmer (or lowest setting). Add blanched tomatoes (smooch them) or canned tomatoes to a large sauce pan. Add rest of ingredients to pan, to taste

Let simmer for as long as you like (I've seen even an hour or two), or simply until heated and pleases your palate. Take note: the longer you simmer, the more time the flavours will have to meld and sauce will thicken a bit.

Serve over your favourite pasta (gluten-free brown rice pasta recommended :)), veggies, or any dish!

VEGAN 'FISH' SAUCE: A staple in Thai and Vietnamese cooking, 'fish' sauce will also come in handy for giving other dishes more flavour, with mushroom soy sauce, garlic and peppercorns.

Ingredient: 1/2 cups shredded wakame (see notes), 2 cups filtered water, 2 large garlic cloves, crushed, 1 teaspoon whole peppercorns, 1/3 cup mushroom-flavoured dark soy sauce, regular soy sauce, or gluten-free tamari, 1 teaspoon of genmai miso (it's already pretty salty so this is optional).

Preparation: Combine wakame, garlic, peppercorns, and water in a large sauce pan and bring to a boil. Lower heat and simmer about 20 minutes. Strain and return the liquid back to the pot. Add soy sauce, bring back to a boil, and cook until mixture is reduced and almost unbearable salty. Remove from heat and stir in miso.

Decant into a bottle and keep in the refrigerator. Use one-for-one to replace fish sauce in vegan recipes.

DELICIOUS VEGAN VODKA CREAM SAUCE:

This lush-ious sauce is heavy on the cashews and marinara, making a creamy yet familiar sauce for pasta, whole grains or baked veggies.

Ingredient: 1/4 cup raw cashews, 1/4 cup water, 1 24-ounce jar fat-free marinara or pasta sauce, 2 tablespoons vodka.

Preparation: In a blender or food processor, purée cashews and water until smooth.

Stir cashew cream into pasta sauce in pot over medium heat.

Add vodka and simmer for 2-3 minutes, stirring constantly.

Serve over whole-grain or gluten-free pasta, spaghetti squash, rice, polenta, steamed spinach, or whatever you like.

SPAGHETTI SQUASH WITH ALFREDO SAUCE

SAUCE: Cashews form the base of this creamy Alfredo sauce, while kelp and nutmeg refresh the usual spice blend of garlic and basil.

Ingredient: 1 medium to large spaghetti squash, 2 cups cherry tomatoes, 15 shiitake or cremini mushrooms, 2 Tbsp. olive oil, ¼ tsp. sea salt + sprinkle, Black pepper, Raw Alfredo Sauce:, ½ cup cashew nuts, soaked for 2 hours, ½ cup filtered water, ½ lemon, juiced + ½ tsp. zest, 1 garlic clove, 1.5 Tbsp. nutritional yeast, 5 fresh basil leaves, ¼ tsp. dried basil, ¼ tsp. sea salt, ¼ tsp. kelp powder, Pinch nutmeg, Pinch cayenne pepper.

Preparation: Preheat oven to 400F. Cut squash in half and remove seeds with a soup spoon. Place squash cut side down in the baking with and add about 2 centimetres of water. Place in the oven for 40 minutes. Clean and trim mushrooms, then chop roughly. On a baking sheet mix cherry tomatoes and mushrooms with olive oil, sea salt and pepper. Place in the oven for 30 minutes. Take tomatoes, mushrooms and squash out of the oven. Turn squash cut side up, sprinkle with a dash of sea salt and olive oil and put back in the oven for 5 minutes.

When squash is ready, use a fork to scrape out squash into a serving dish. To make alfredo sauce, drain and rinse nuts in the sieve. Add all ingredients into a blender and buzz until smooth. Mix all ingredients and serve!

TEMPEH 'FISH' N' CHIPS WITH TARTAR SAUCE

SAUCE: Sour and creamy, tartar sauce is a familiar comfort food to some and exotic to others. Either way, with only four ingredients this tartar sauce is quick and easy, but no less satisfying.

Ingredient: For the Tempeh "Fish"—2 packages of tempeh, 2 cups chickpea flour, 1 Tbs. baking powder, 1 Tbs. garlic powder, 1 Tbs. chili powder, 2 tsp. Old Bay seasoning, ¼ cup cider vinegar, 12 oz. seltzer, 1 cup corn starch, 1 Tbs. kelp flakes, Safflower oil for frying

For the Chips—4 large russet potatoes cut into wedges, Cooking oil spray, Salt and pepper to taste, ½ tsp. garlic powder, ½ tsp. paprika

For the Tartar Sauce—1 cup Vegan mayonnaise, 2 Tbs. unsweetened pickle relish, 1 tsp. lemon zest, Juice of half a lemon.

Preparation: Split the tempeh in half so that you have two thin rectangles. The way I do this is to lay the tempeh on a cutting board, hold the top steady with the palm of your hand and with a knife, and slice through it like you are splitting open a bagel. If you like your tempeh less chewy, steam it for a few minutes to soften it. Cut each piece of tempeh into 4 pieces so you will have 16 pieces in total. In a bowl, add the flour, baking powder, garlic powder, chili powder, and Old Bay seasoning. Mix well. Add in the vinegar and slowly mix in the seltzer until the batter is the desired consistency (like pancake batter). In another bowl, mix the corn starch and the kelp flakes. Heat 2 inches of oil in a large skillet. Dredge the tempeh pieces into the corn starch-kelp mixture, shake off the excess, and then coat with the batter. If you want an extra crunchy, thicker battered covering, re-dredge the tempeh a second time. Fry the tempeh in the skillet in batches, turning once, until golden brown. Place the pieces on paper towels to drain and sprinkle with salt. Serve while hot with chips and tartar sauce on the side. Add lemon wedges for garnish, if desired.

For the Chips— preheat oven to 425ºF with a baking sheet in the oven. Pull the hot sheet pan out of the oven and put potato wedges on it in a single layer. Spray with cooking spray, sprinkle the spices onto the potatoes and put them back into the oven. Bake the potatoes, turning occasionally, until golden brown and tender, about 40 minutes.

For the Tartar Sauce— in a bowl, mix the Vegan mayonnaise with the unsweetened pickle relish. Add some lemon zest and the juice of half a lemon. Mix well. Refrigerate until ready to serve.

GREATEST HOMEMADE HOT SAUCE: This hot sauce claims to be the greatest. If you find that hard to believe, you'll have to challenge the sauce for its trophy. Your other option is to eat all of it, and worry about whether or not it was the greatest later. Either way, it is definitely hot!

Ingredient: 6 cloves garlic, unpeeled, 1 cup apple cider vinegar, 1 cup water, 1 carrot, chopped, 1/2 onion, chopped, 10 habanero chilies, stems removed, 4 Serrano peppers, stems removed, 2 teaspoons sea salt, 1/2 teaspoon brown rice syrup.

Preparation: In a skillet over medium heat add unpeeled garlic. Roast the garlic for 10 to 15 minutes, turning every few minutes to roast evenly on all sides. When the garlic becomes softer and blacked in spots it is done. Set aside to cool. Meanwhile, to a saucepan add apple cider vinegar, water, chopped carrot, and onion, along with the habanero chilies and Serrano peppers.

Cover saucepan half way with a lid, and simmer over medium-low heat for 12 minutes, until the carrots are nice and tender. Carefully pour into a blender. *For me, it's easiest to scoop the solids into the blender, and then pour the liquid in. Peel the cooled garlic and add to the blender.

Lastly, add the sea salt and brown rice syrup to the blender. Blend until the hot sauce is smooth.*

Note -With hot liquids use caution and keep one corner of the lid up to prevent the vacuum effect that creates heat explosions. Place a towel over the top of the machine, pulse a few times then process on high speed until smooth. Also note – The fumes from blending the peppers are powerful so don't put your face over it.

Allow to cool. Pour hot sauce into jars or bottles and store in the refrigerator.

RAW HOT SAUCE: For the raw foodies, and anyone who wants to give raw food a fair shake in their diet, hot sauce is just as easy and delicious raw, not to mention just as spicy.

Ingredient: 10 – 15 Hot peppers of choice – de-stemmed (The number of peppers will vary due to the variety you choose, their size, and desired consistency. For bigger peppers, fewer; smaller peppers, more.) 1 cup taw apple cider vinegar, 4 garlic cloves, 1/2 tsp. sea salt, 1/2 tsp. chili powder, 1/2 tsp. coriander, 1/4 tsp. cumin, juice of 1/2 lime, zest of 1/2 lime, chia seed gel (optional) for thicker sauce.

Preparation: Chop peppers into chunk sized pieces.

If you want a hotter sauce, leave those seeds in. For a milder sauce, remove seeds and white skin membrane (they pack the HEAT!) This is a HOT sauce, so let's make it CALIENTE! Since jalapenos aren't super-hot and Scott likes the heat, we added a couple of habanero peppers to the mix to spice it up! Measure out all the other ingredients. Toss all ingredients into a high-powered blender and blend till you reach desired consistency. Taste and adjust seasonings to liking or add chia gel to thicken. If it's too thin, add more peppers or chia gel to thicken and give it a few buzzes. If it's too thick, add some more vinegar.

HOMEMADE HEALTHY BARBECUE SAUCE:

The store bought barbecue sauce might sometimes be cruelty free, but the ingredient list isn't exactly inspiring. This healthy barbecue sauce, on the other hand, will taste amazing without the gross additives.

Ingredient: 1 (8 ounce) can tomato sauce, 2 Tablespoons dijon mustard, 2 Tablespoons low sodium tamari (You can use regular soy sauce if you want, or coconut aminos for a soy and grain free option.), 1 teaspoon molasses, 1 Tablespoon apple cider vinegar, 1 teaspoon garlic powder, 3 packets stevia (You can use more or less, depending on how sweet you want your sauce.), 1 teaspoon liquid aminos, salt and pepper, to taste.

Preparation: In a medium-large bowl, whisk all ingredients together until thoroughly combined. Add salt and pepper to taste.

LEMON-CANNELINI SAUCE: A cannelini bean-based sauce comes to life with garlic and nutritional yeast.

Ingredient: For the vegetables—1 sweet yellow onion, diced, 2 cups peeled and diced butternut or other winter squash, 2 cups Brussels sprouts, halved lengthwise, 2 carrots, cut diagonally into 1/2-inch slices, 1 large Yukon gold potato, cut into 1-inch chunks, 1 tablespoon olive oil, Salt and freshly ground black pepper.

For the sauce—2 cups cooked or canned cannelini beans, 2 tablespoons nutritional yeast, 1/2 teaspoon garlic powder, 1/2 cup vegetable broth, 1/2 teaspoon salt, 1/8 teaspoon cayenne pepper, 2 tablespoons fresh lemon juice, 1 tablespoon fresh minced basil, parsley, tarragon, cilantro, chives, or sage (optional).

Preparation: Preheat the oven to 425 degrees F. Line a rimmed baking sheet with parchment paper or spray it with cooking spray. Combine the vegetables with the oil and salt and pepper to taste, tossing to coat. Arrange the vegetables in a single layer on the prepared baking sheet. Roast the vegetables until tender and slightly caramelized, about 45 minutes, turning once about halfway through.

For the sauce— while the vegetables are roasting, combine all the sauce ingredients (except for the optional herbs) in a food processor or blender and process until smooth. The amount of salt needed will depend on the saltiness of your broth. Transfer the sauce to a small saucepan and heat until hot, stirring so it doesn't stick. Keep warm. To serve, transfer the vegetables to a large serving bowl and drizzle with the sauce. Sprinkle with herb of choice, if using. Serve hot.

VEGAN BOLOGNESE SAUCE: While normally meat-heavy, one clever vegan has found a way to make the legendary Bolognese sauce transcend into the realm of meat-free sauces just in time to take over your taste buds and your dinner table. Tempeh, mushrooms and lentils give this sauce an excellent texture.

Ingredient: 3 tablespoons extra virgin olive oil, 3 large cloves garlic, minced, 1 medium yellow onion, finely chopped, 1/2 small green bell pepper, finely chopped, 1 small carrot, finely chopped, 1 stalk celery, finely chopped, 1 8-ounce package tempeh, crumbled, 8 ounces cremini or white mushrooms, chopped, 1/2 teaspoon crushed red pepper flakes, 1 6-ounce can tomato paste, 1 bay leaf, 1 teaspoon dried oregano, 1 teaspoon dried basil, 1/2 cup dried red lentils, 1 28-ounce can crushed tomatoes, 1 28-ounce can whole tomatoes, undrained, chopped, 1 cup dry red wine, 1/4 cup chopped flat-leaf parsley, 1/2 teaspoon freshly ground black pepper, 1/2 teaspoon fennel seed, 1/2 teaspoon salt, or up to 1 teaspoon, to taste.

Preparation: Heat the oil over medium heat in a large Dutch oven. Add the garlic, onion, bell pepper, carrot, celery and crushed red pepper, and sauté for 5 minutes, stirring occasionally. Turn the heat up a bit, add the mushrooms and tempeh and cook for 3 minutes, stirring constantly. Lower the heat back to medium, stir in the tomato paste and cook for 2 minutes more. Add the herbs, tomatoes, parsley and wine, and bring to a boil. Reduce heat and simmer, partially covered, for 10 minutes. Add the lentils and cook until they just tender. This usually takes 20 minutes, but I've had some lentils take a lot longer. So keep tasting it along the way to determine when it's done. If the sauce gets too dry, add a bit of water. Add salt at the end of the cooking time. Serve on whole wheat spaghetti or use in lasagna.

BREAKFAST RECIPES.

Just because you're vegan doesn't mean breakfast is limited to smoothies, oatmeal, or energy bars. You're not limited to chia pudding, granola, or peanut butter toast either. Let's look at some great breakfast ideas.

CHIVE WAFFLES WITH MAPLE & SOY MUSHROOMS: These delicious vegan pancakes can be sweet or savoury and are super adaptable to every taste. A great low-calorie breakfast or brunch option.

Ingredient: 1 tsp. cider vinegar or lemon juice, 2 tbsp. rapeseed oil, 100g cooked, mashed sweet potato, 150g polenta, 130g plain flour, 1 tbsp. baking powder, small bunch chives, snipped, 1 tbsp. maple syrup, 2 tsp. light soy sauce, 6 large mushrooms, thickly sliced, olive oil for frying soya yogurt, to serve (optional).

Preparation: Heat the waffle iron. Mix the soya or rice milk with the vinegar and rapeseed oil (don't worry if it starts to split), then whisk in the sweet potato mash. Tip the polenta, flour and baking powder into a bowl, mix and make a well in the centre. Add a large pinch of salt, then slowly pour in the milk mixture and whisk to make a batter. Stir in half the chives. Pour enough batter into the waffle iron to fill and cook for 4-5 mins. Lift out the waffle, keep it warm and repeat with the remaining mixture until you have six waffles.

Meanwhile, mix the maple syrup with the soy sauce. Brush it over the mushrooms and season with pepper. Heat a little oil in a frying pan and fry the mushrooms on both sides until they are browned and cooked through – make sure they don't burn at the edges. Serve the waffles topped with mushrooms, add a spoonful of soya yogurt, if you like, and scatter over the remaining chives.

TOFU BREKKIE PANCAKES: Silken tofu is the secret to making a stack of fluffy, thick, American-style vegan pancakes without gluten, eggs or dairy.

Ingredient: 50g Brazil nuts, 3 sliced bananas, 240g raspberries maple syrup or honey, to serve.

For the batter—349g pack firm silken tofu, 2 tsp. vanilla extract, 2 tsp. lemon juice

400ml unsweetened almond milk, 1 tbsp. vegetable oil, plus 1-2 tbsp. extra for frying, 250g buckwheat flour, 4 tbsp. light muscovado sugar, 1½ tsp. ground mixed spice, 1 tbsp. gluten-free baking powder.

Preparation: Heat oven to 180C/160C fan/gas 4. Scatter the nuts over a baking tray and cook for 5 mins until toasty and golden. Leave to cool, then chop. Turn the oven down low if you want to keep the whole batch of pancakes warm, although I think they are best enjoyed straight from the pan. Put the tofu, vanilla, lemon juice and 200ml of the milk into a deep jug or bowl. Using a stick blender, blend together until liquid, and then keep going until it turns thick and smooth, like yogurt. Stir in the oil and the rest of the milk to loosen the mixture. Put the dry ingredients and 1 tsp. salt in a large bowl and whisk to combine and aerate. If there are any lumps in the sugar, squish them with your fingers. Make a well in the centre, pour in the tofu mix and bring together to make a thick batter.

Heat a large (ideally non-stick) frying pan and swirl around 1 tsp. oil. For golden pancakes that don't stick, the pan and oil should be hot enough to get an enthusiastic sizzle on contact with the batter, but not so hot that it scorches it. Test a drop. Using a ladle or large serving spoon, drop in 3 spoonful's of batter, easing it out gently in the pan to make pancakes that are about 12cm across. Cook for 2 mins on the first side or until bubbles pop over most of the surface. Loosen with a palette knife, then flip over the pancakes and cook for 1 min more or until puffed up and firm. Transfer to the oven to keep warm, if you need to, but don't stack the pancakes too closely. Cook the rest of the batter, using a little more oil each time. Serve warm with sliced banana, berries, toasted nuts and a good drizzle of maple syrup or honey.

CARDAMOM & PEACH QUINOA PORRIDGE:
A healthy breakfast of oats and quinoa with fresh ripe peach. Almond milk makes its suitable for dairy-free and vegan diets.

Ingredient: 75g quinoa, 25g porridge oats, 4 cardamom pods, 250ml unsweetened almond milk, 2 ripe peaches, cut into slices, 1 tsp. maple syrup.

Preparation: Put the quinoa, oats and cardamom pods in a small saucepan with 250ml water and 100ml of the almond milk. Bring to the boil, then simmer gently for 15 mins, stirring occasionally. Pour in the remaining almond milk and cook for 5 mins more until creamy. Remove the cardamom pods, spoon into bowls or jars, and top with the peaches and maple syrup.

PROTEIN PANCAKES: With 29g of protein in each serving, this delicious breakfast stack is the perfect fuel after exercise. Complete with layers of yogurt, seeds and blueberry chia jam.

Ingredient: For the batter, 2 tbsp. ground flaxseeds, 20g ground almonds, 300ml soya milk

200g quinoa flour, 1 medium banana, mashed, 2 tbsp. maple syrup, coconut oil, for frying.

For the blueberry chia jam (makes 200ml), 200g blueberries, mashed. 2 tbsp. chia seeds

1-2 tbsp. maple syrup, to taste. 2 tsp. lemon juice. For the stack—100g coconut yogurt or Greek yogurt, 1 tbsp. pistachio nuts or pumpkin seeds, chopped, toasted if you like, 2 tsp. hulled hemp seeds, mixed berries.

Preparation: In a small bowl stir the flaxseeds with 6 tbsp water and set aside to soak while you make the jam. Mash the blueberries with a fork in a pan then set over a low-medium heat until syrupy and bubbling. Remove from the heat and stir in the chia seeds, maple syrup and lemon juice. Leave to cool slightly then transfer to a small serving jar. Put the ground almonds, milk, flour, banana, maple syrup and a pinch of salt in a blender. Stir the flax to make sure it has become thick and gloopy, like an egg, then tip into the mix and blitz until smooth and thick.

Heat 1 tsp. of coconut oil in a large frying pan over a medium heat and add tablespoon dollops of batter into the pan. Cook for a couple of mins on one side until the edges are browning, and bubbles have formed on top. Once the pale, white batter has turned a sandy colour, flip over with a spatula and cook for another few mins till dark golden brown. Set aside and keep warm while you repeat the process with the remaining batter, adding another tsp of coconut oil with each batch. You should make about 16 pancakes. Pile the pancakes high between two plates, alternating the layers with spoonful of jam and yogurt. Dollop any remaining yogurt and another spoonful of jam on top then scatter over the nuts, seeds and berries to serve. Leftover jam will keep in the fridge for up to 1 week.

BLACKCURRANT COMPOTE: A simple fruity compote to dollop onto your breakfast bowl, taking it from bland to berry beautiful.

Ingredient: juice ½ lemon, 500g blackcurrants, and 100g golden caster sugar.

Preparation: Put 2 tbsp. water and the lemon juice in a large saucepan, bring to the boil, then add the blackcurrants and simmer until broken down. Tip in the golden caster sugar and bring to 105C on a temperature probe. Pour into sterilised jars and leave to cool. Will keep in the fridge for up to 3 weeks.

"SHAMROCK" VEGAN BREAKFAST SANDWICH

: This vegan breakfast sandwich is a gorgeously green spin on your usual morning meal. This "Shamrock" Breakfast Sandwich is loaded with kale, pepitas and a flavourful veggie sausage patty.

Ingredient: Skillet Ingredients: 1 vegan sausage patty, 1 cup kale, 2 tsp. extra virgin olive oil, 1 Tbsp. pepitas, salt and pepper, to taste

Special Sauce: 1 tbsp. vegan mayo, 1/8 tsp. chipotle powder, or sub with smoky paprika, 1 tsp. jalapeno, chopped – optional

Other Items: 1 English muffin, toasted, 1/4 avocado, sliced – use more if desired.

Preparation: Toast English muffin. Set aside when done. Add a drizzle of oil to a sauté pan. Turn heat to high. Add the patty. Cook 1-2 minutes, flip. Add the kale and pepitas to the pan to toast the pepitas and wilt the kale. Add salt and pepper to the kale to taste. When the patty is browned and the kale soft, turn off heat. Mix together the special spicy sauce.

Assemble! Spread the vegan jalapeno sauce/mayo on the inside of each toasted English muffin. Add sliced avocado, patty, then top with kale and pepitas. Serve warm.

RASPBERRY RIPPLE CHIA PUDDING: Fancy raspberry ripple for breakfast? Well now you can with our vegan chia pudding bowl.

Ingredient: 50g white chia seeds, 200ml coconut drinking milk, 1 nectarine, or peach, cut into slices, 2 tbsp. goji berries, For the raspberry purée, 100g raspberries, 1 tsp. lemon juice, 2 tsp. maple syrup.

Preparation: Divide the chia seeds and coconut milk between two serving bowls and stir well. Leave to soak for 5 mins, stirring occasionally, until the seeds swell and thicken when stirred. Meanwhile, combine the purée ingredients in a small food processor, or blitz with a hand blender. Swirl a spoonful into each bowl, then arrange the nectarine or peach slices on top and scatter with the goji berries. Will keep in the fridge for 1 day. Add the toppings just before serving.

SUMMER PORRIDGE: A healthy, summery vegan porridge with jumbo oats and bright pink pomegranate seeds.

Ingredient: 300ml almond milk, 200g blueberries, ½ tbsp. maple syrup, 2 tbsp. chia seeds, 100g jumbo oats, 1 kiwi fruit, cut into slices. 50g pomegranate seeds, 2 tsp. mixed seeds.

Preparation: In a blender, blitz the milk, blueberries and maple syrup until the milk turns purple. Put the chia and oats in a mixing bowl, pour in the blueberry milk and stir very well. Leave to soak for 5 mins, stirring occasionally, until the liquid has absorbed, and the oats and chia thicken and swell. Stir again, then divide between two bowls. Arrange the fruit on top, then sprinkle over the mixed seeds. Will keep in the fridge for 1 day. Add the toppings just before serving.

VEGAN GRANOLA: Create your own crunchy toasted granola with a hint of spice and a touch of sweetness from maple syrup.

Ingredient: 400g jumbo oats, 2 tsp. cinnamon, 150g dried apple, roughly chopped

150g coconut oil, melted, 250g pack mixed nuts, roughly chopped, 100ml maple syrup.

Preparation: Heat oven to 180C/160C fan/gas 4. Line two large baking trays with baking parchment. Mix all the ingredients together except the maple syrup. Spread the granola out on the trays and drizzle over the maple syrup. Bake in the oven for 20 mins, stirring the granola well halfway through so that it cooks evenly. Leave to cool before storing in a Kilner jar or airtight container.

VEGAN FRY-UP: Try this vegan take on the classic English breakfast that boasts vegan sausages with hash browns, mushrooms, tomatoes, scrambled tofu and baked beans.

Ingredient: For the hash browns—1 large potato, unpeeled. 1 ½ tbsp. peanut butter

For the tomatoes and mushrooms— 14 cherry tomatoes, sunflower oil, 2 tsp. maple syrup, 1 tsp. soy sauce, ¼ tsp. smoked paprika, 1 large Portobello mushroom, sliced.

For the scrambled tofu—349g pack silken tofu, 2 tbsp. nutritional yeast, ½ tsp. turmeric, 1 clove garlic, crushed. To serve— 4 vegan sausages (we used Dee's leek & onion), 1 x 200g can baked beans.

Preparation: Cook the potato whole in a large pan of water, boil for 10 mins then drain and allow to cool. Peel the skin away then coarsely grate. Mix with the peanut butter and season well. Set aside in the fridge until needed. Heat oven to 200C/180C fan/gas 6. Put the cherry tomatoes onto a baking tray, drizzle with 2 tsp. sunflower oil, season and bake for 30 mins or until the skins have blistered and start to char. Cook the beans and sausages following the instructions on the pack so they're ready to serve at the same time as the scrambled tofu. Meanwhile, mix the maple syrup, soy sauce and ¼ tsp. smoked paprika together in a large bowl, add the sliced mushroom and toss to coat in the mixture. Leave to stand while you pour 2 tsp. sunflower oil into a non-stick frying pan and bring it up to a medium high heat. Fry the mushroom until just starting to turn golden but not charred. Scoop onto a plate and keep warm until serving.

Put 1 tbsp. oil into the frying pan and add spoonful of the potato mixture – you should get about

4. Fry for 3-4 mins each side then drain onto kitchen paper. Crumble the tofu into your frying pan and sprinkle over the remaining ingredients and a good pinch of salt and pepper. If the pan looks a little dry add a splash more oil. Fry for 3-4 mins or until the tofu is broken into pieces, well coated in the seasoning and hot through. Divide everything between 2 plates and serve with a hot mug of tea made using soy milk.

VEGAN LUNCH RECIPES.

Lunch time could be anytime and you need to refuel your body. Whether you need to take something for just the moment or for the kids at school, or even a proper lunch date, these ideas are great for you. Packed with large nutritional content— you can make any of these lunch ideas and have a swell time. Veganism provides treats as well!

VEGAN BANH MI: Make this decadent vegan sandwich using veggies and hummus with an Asian dressing and hot sauce all stuffed inside a baguette. Great for a filling lunch.

Ingredient: 150g leftover raw veggies, (such as red cabbage and carrots), shredded, 3 tbsp goodquality vegan white wine vinegar, 1 tsp golden caster sugar, 1 long French baguette, 100g hummus, 175g cooked tempeh, very finely sliced. ½ small pack coriander, leaves picked, to serve, ½ small pack mint, leaves picked, to serve hot sauce, to serve (we used sriracha).

Preparation: Put the shredded veg in a bowl and add the vinegar, sugar and 1 tsp salt. Toss everything together, then set aside to pickle quickly while you prepare the rest of the sandwich. Heat oven to 180C/160C fan/gas 4. Cut the baguette into four, then slice each piece horizontally in half. Put the baguette pieces in the oven for 5 mins until lightly toasted and warm. Spread each piece with a layer of hummus, then top four pieces with the tempeh slices and pile the pickled veg on top. To serve, sprinkle over the herbs and squeeze over some hot sauce, then top with the other baguette pieces to make sandwiches.

CHEESY' VEGAN SCONES: Try these dairy-free vegan scones that use nutritional yeast for a cheesy flavour, pepped up by mustard and smoked paprika. Serve with vegan onion chutney.

Ingredient: 3 tbsp. olive oil, plus extra for the tray, 1 tsp. white wine vinegar, 250ml almond milk, 1 cauliflower stalk (around 100g), 300g self-rising flour, plus extra for dusting, ½ tsp. baking powder. 3 tbsp. nutritional yeast, ¼ tsp. mustard powder, ¼ tsp. smoked paprika, 3 thyme sprigs, leaves picked, vegan onion chutney, to serve.

Preparation: Heat oven to 220C/200C fan/gas 7 and lightly oil a baking tray. Mix the vinegar with the almond milk and set aside. Bring a saucepan of water to the boil, add the cauliflower stalk and cook for 5 mins until almost tender. Drain well, leave to cool, then finely chop. Mix the flour, baking powder, nutritional yeast, spices, thyme leaves and 1 tsp. salt in a large bowl. Add the cauliflower, then add the oil and pour in 230ml of the soured almond milk. Working quickly, bring the mixture together with a wooden spoon; if there is any dry mixture in the bowl, add more almond milk to make a soft but not sticky dough. Tip the dough onto a floured work surface and pat to a thickness of about 2.5cm. Cut out rounds with a 6cm fluted cutter and transfer to the baking tray. Gather together any offcuts and cut out more rounds. Bake on the top shelf of the oven for 10-12 mins until golden. Serve warm with onion chutney.

Bean, tomato & watercress salad: Try this gluten-free, vegan salad with filling beans and fresh watercress for a quick, light meal. It has just four ingredients and three of your five-a-day.

Ingredient: 2 x 400g can cannellini beans, 100g watercress, 1 lemon, zested and juiced. 250g pack sundried tomatoes and olives.

Preparation: Drain and rinse the beans, then combine in a bowl with the watercress, zest and juice of the lemon, tomatoes and olives, including the oil from the pack. Toss well and season to taste.

BEETROOT & LENTIL TABBOULEH: Serve this tasty beetroot, chickpea and lentil tabbouleh as a side dish or vegan main. It's healthy, gluten-free, low-calorie and three of your five-a-day.

Ingredient: 1 small pack flat-leaf parsley, plus extra leaves to serve (optional), 1 small pack mint, 1 small pack chives, 200g radishes, 2 beetroot, peeled and quartered. 1 red apple, cored, quartered and sliced, 1 tsp. ground cumin, 4 tbsp. olive oil, 250g pack cooked quinoa, 400g can chickpeas, drained and rinsed, 400g can green lentils, drained, 2 lemons, juiced.

Preparation: Put the herbs, radishes and beetroot in a food processor and blitz until chopped into small pieces. Stir in the rest of the ingredients, adding the lemon juice a bit at a time to taste – you may not need all of it. Season, then place on a large platter topped with a few parsley leaves, if you like, and serve straight away.

VEGAN CHICKPEA CURRY JACKET POTATOES

: Get some protein into a vegan diet with this tasty chickpea curry jacket. It's an easy midweek meal, or filling lunch that packs a lot of flavour.

Ingredient: 4 sweet potatoes, 1 tbsp. coconut oil, 1 ½ tsp. cumin seeds, 1 large onion, diced. 2 garlic cloves, crushed, thumb-sized piece ginger, finely grated. 1 green chilli, finely chopped, 1 tsp garam masala, 1 tsp. ground coriander, ½ tsp. turmeric, 2 tbsp. tikka masala paste, 2 x 400g can chopped tomatoes, 2 x 400g can chickpeas, drained, lemon, wedges and coriander leaves, to serve.

Preparation: Heat oven to 200C/180C fan/gas 6. Prick the sweet potatoes all over with a fork, then put on a baking tray and roast in the oven for 45 mins or until tender when pierced with a knife. Meanwhile, melt the coconut oil in a large saucepan over medium heat. Add the cumin seeds and fry for 1 min until fragrant, then add the onion and fry for 7-10 mins until softened. Put the garlic, ginger and green chilli into the pan, and cook for 2-3 mins. Add the spices and tikka masala paste and cook for a further 2 mins until fragrant, then tip in the tomatoes. Bring to a simmer, then tip in the chickpeas and cook for a further 20 mins until thickened. Season. Put the roasted sweet potatoes on four plates and cut open lengthways. Spoon over the chickpea curry and squeeze over the lemon wedges. Season, then scatter with coriander before serving.

MEZE BENTO: Be the envy of your work colleagues with this tasty lunchbox meze featuring hummus, pitta, stuffed vine leaves, tabbouleh, chopped carrot and olives.

Ingredient: 2 tbsp. hummus, handful of olives, 1 sliced wholemeal pitta, 1 chopped carrot, 1 chopped baby fennel bulb, 2-3 ready-made stuffed vine leaves, 4 tbsp. tabbouleh.

Preparation: Put 2 tbsp. hummus in a compartment in a bento box. Fill the other sections with other meze ingredients – we used a handful of olives, 1 sliced wholemeal pitta, 1 chopped carrot, 1 chopped baby fennel bulb, 2-3 ready-made stuffed vine leaves and 4 tbsp. tabbouleh.

VEGGIE OLIVE WRAPS WITH MUSTARD VINAIGRETTE

VEGGIE OLIVE WRAPS WITH MUSTARD VINAIGRETTE: Eat the rainbow with our simple, healthy, veggie wrap. This olive and veg sandwich makes an easy vegan, low-calorie lunch option to eat al-desko.

Ingredient: 1 carrot, shredded or coarsely grated. 80g wedge red cabbage, finely shredded, 2 spring onions, thinly sliced, 1 courgette, shredded or coarsely grated, handful basil leaves, 5 green olives, pitted and halved, ½ tsp. English mustard powder, 2 tsp. extra virgin rapeseed oil, 1 tbsp., cider vinegar, 1 large seeded tortilla.

Preparation: Mix all the ingredients except for the tortilla and toss well. Put the tortilla on a sheet of foil and pile the filling along one side of the wrap – it will almost look like too much mixture, but once you start to roll it firmly it will compact. Roll the tortilla from the filling side, folding in the sides as you go. Fold the foil in at the ends to keep stuff inside the wrap. Cut in half and eat straight away. If taking to work, leave whole and wrap up like a cracker in baking parchment.

GUACAMOLE & MANGO SALAD WITH BLACK BEANS

BLACK BEANS: Get four of your five-a-day with this healthy salad of mango, avocado and beans. It's a nutritional powerhouse that's also vegan and gluten free.

Ingredient: 1 lime, zested and juiced. 1 small mango, stoned, peeled and chopped, 1 small avocado, stoned, peeled and chopped. 100g cherry tomatoes, halved, 1 red chilli, deseeded and chopped, 1 red onion, chopped, ½ small pack coriander, chopped, 400g can black beans, drained and rinsed.

Preparation: Put the lime zest and juice, mango, avocado, tomatoes, chilli and onion in a bowl, stir through the coriander and beans.

ROASTED BEETS, PLUM & PECAN SALAD:

The earthiness of beetroot complements the sweet yet tart plums and toasted pecans in this side salad. Pair with lamb for an autumnal feast.

Ingredient: 4 large beetroot (about 500g), peeled, ends trimmed and spiralized into thick noodles, 1 tbsp. olive oil, 4 ripe plums, (about 200g), cut into wedges, 60g pecans, toasted and roughly chopped, 1 small pack mint, leaves picked, some reserved for garnish.

For the dressing— 1 ½ tbsp. extra virgin olive oil, ½ tbsp. red wine vinegar, ½ tbsp. pomegranate molasses.

Preparation: Heat oven to 200C/180C fan/gas 6.Toss the spiralized beetroot in the olive oil and some seasoning in a roasting tin then spread out into an even layer. Roast for 15 mins until tender. While the beetroot is roasting, combine the dressing ingredients together in a jug with a little seasoning. To assemble the salad, toss the rest of the ingredients in the roasting tin with the cooked beetroot and dressing. Serve on a sharing platter, garnished with a few reserved mint leaves.

EASY FALAFELS: Pair John Torode's easy falafels with soft flatbreads, well-spiced humous and crunchy pickles for a magnificent meze of a lunch, or a shareable starter.

Ingredient: 250g dried chickpeas or dried split broad beans, ½ tsp. bicarbonate of soda, 3 garlic cloves, 1 onion, roughly chopped. 1 leek, roughly chopped, 1 celery stick, roughly chopped, 1 small chilli, roughly chopped (deseeded if you don't like it too hot). 1 tsp. ground cumin, 1 tsp. cayenne pepper, 1 tsp. sumac, good handful chopped coriander, and good handful chopped parsley, 80g gram flour, 100ml vegetable oil.

Preparation: Soak the chickpeas in cold water for 8 hrs. Or overnight. Drain the chickpeas and pulse with the bicarb in a food processor until roughly chopped. Remove 3/4 of the mixture and set aside. Add the garlic, vegetables, spices and herbs to the remaining mixture in the processor and purée to a paste. Stir the paste into the rough purée of chickpeas, add the gram flour, season and mix well. Heat oven to 110C/90C fan/gas 1/4. Heat a large, non-stick frying pan over a medium heat and add some of the oil. Use your hands to form the mixture into patties (there should be enough to make about 16). Fry for 2 mins each side until crisp. Keep in a warm oven while you fry the remainder of the mixture, continuing to add a little oil to the pan with each batch. Serve wrapped in flatbreads, if you like, alongside the houmous, tabbouleh and pickled red onion & radish.

VEGAN DINNER RECIPES.

Dinners are naturally light foods with a good amount of nourishment to replenish the body and help it recover; the vegan diet also provides awesome meals you can go for that wouldn't even be that time consuming or make you break the bank. Check out these ones_

VEGAN PIE: Make this fantastic beetroot, sweet potato, chard and celeriac rainbow-layered pie as a stunning centrepiece for a vegan Christmas or dinner party.

Ingredient: 80ml olive oil, plus extra for brushing. 2 tsp. ground cumin, ½ tsp. ground cinnamon, 1 tbsp. vegan red wine vinegar (we used Aspall), 3 beetroots (about 400g), peeled and sliced into rounds about ½ cm thick, 1 small celeriac (about 750g), peeled, cut into quarters and then sliced into triangles about 1 cm thick, 4 thyme sprigs, leaves picked, 4 fat unpeeled garlic cloves, 3 large sweet potatoes (about 600g), peeled and sliced into rounds about ½ cm thick, 2 tsp. smoked paprika, 1 tbsp. semolina, 250g Swiss chard, leaves only (save the stalks to add to soups, stews and risottos).

For the pastry— 150g coconut oil, plus extra for the tin, 500g spelt flour, almond milk, for brushing.

Preparation: First, make the filling. Heat oven to 220C/200C fan/gas 7. Mix together 1½ tbsp. oil with the cumin, cinnamon and vinegar, and rub the mixture all over the beetroot. Put the beetroot into a small roasting tin, season well, then cover with foil and roast for 20 mins. Meanwhile, toss the celeriac with 2½ tbsp. oil, the thyme, garlic and some seasoning in a second roasting tin. Separate out the slices so they cook evenly, then cover the tin in foil. In a third roasting tin, mix the sweet potato with the remaining oil, the smoked paprika and some seasoning, and cover with foil. Once the beets have cooked for 20 mins, add the celeriac and sweet potato to the oven alongside them, and roast all the veg for 40 mins further or until tender. Remove the thyme sprigs, squeeze the garlic cloves out of their skins and mash them in with the celeriac, then leave all the veg to cool. All the veg can be cooked the day before and kept in the fridge.

For the pastry, boil the kettle and use some coconut oil to grease a deep 20cm springform cake tin. Pour the flour into a bowl and add 1 tsp. salt. Mix the coconut oil with 200ml boiling water, stir until melted (put it in the microwave if need be), then pour into the flour and mix with a wooden spoon to form a dough. Working as quickly as you can (it's best to roll the pastry when it's warm), cut off a ¼ of the dough and set aside under a tea towel. Roll out the rest to 0.5cm thick, then use it to line the cake tin, pressing the dough into the corners and leaving any excess pastry overhanging the sides. Don't worry if the pastry breaks – it's very forgiving, so you can patch it up as you go. Heat oven to 200C/180C fan/gas 6.

Now build the pie. Cover the base with chard leaves, then scatter over the semolina (which will absorb the beet juices), press in the beetroot, and season. Add another layer of chard, followed by the sweet potato, and season. Add a final layer of chard leaves, then top with the celeriac and season again. Roll out the pastry you set aside to a thickness of 0.5cm to use as the lid. Put the lid on top of the pie and, using a fork, press together the overhanging pastry to create a crimped edge. Make a steam hole, then brush the top with a little almond milk mixed with a spoonful of oil (this will help to colour the pastry). Bake in the centre of the oven for 45 mins until the pastry is a deep golden brown. Leave to cool for 15 mins, then remove from the tin and serve in the middle of the table. Will keep for up to three days in the fridge (the pie is also delicious cold).

BRUSSELS SPROUTS PAD THAI: Vegans will love this pad Thai that you can make on Boxing Day to use up leftover Brussels sprouts. You could also cook the dish using fresh sprouts.

Ingredient: 250g flat rice noodles (check the packet to make sure they're vegan), 1 tbsp. soy sauce or tamari. 1 tbsp. tamarind paste (or 2 limes, juiced), 2 tsp. palm sugar (or soft brown sugar), 2 tbsp. vegetable oil, 1 garlic clove, thinly sliced, 2 spring onions, thinly sliced on a diagonal, 1 red chilli, sliced, 200g charred Brussels sprouts, left over from Christmas Day, or cook from raw, 100g beansprouts, 30g salted peanuts (or any other nuts you might have), roughly chopped, to serve, lime, wedges, to serve.

Preparation: First, put the noodles in a large heatproof bowl, cover in boiling water and leave for 10 mins. Drain and rinse with cold water, then set aside. In a bowl, mix the soy sauce or tamari, tamarind or lime juice and sugar. Heat the oil in a large frying pan or wok. Fry the garlic, spring onions, chilli and the cooked or leftover sprouts for around 2 mins (to cook the sprouts from raw, boil for 8-10 mins until tender). Then, add the noodles and beansprouts and fry for 1 min more. Pour over the sauce and toss well, working quickly to coat all the vegetables and noodles. Once everything is heated through, season and divide between four bowls. Scatter with the nuts and serve with lime wedges to squeeze over.

Beetroot & red onion tarte tatin: Bake my vegan tart for a showstopper at a dinner party. The bold red of beetroot against the green salad also makes it ideal for a meat-free Christmas Day.

Ingredient: 400g beetroot, cut into wedges. 1 red onion, cut into wedges, 3 tbsp. olive oil, 2 tbsp. rice wine vinegar, 2 tbsp. soft brown sugar, 2 star anise, flour, for rolling. 500g block puff pastry (we used vegan Jus-Rol), 1 orange, zested. Peppery green salad, to serve.

Preparation: Heat oven to 200C/180C fan/gas 6. In a bowl, toss the beetroot and onion in 2 tbsp. of the oil, the vinegar and sugar. Add the star anise and season well. Heat the rest of the oil in a large, ovenproof non-stick frying pan, then nestle in the veg so that they cover the surface of the pan. Cover with foil and cook in the oven for 45 mins. On a well-floured surface, roll the pastry to a thickness of 0.5cm and cut out a circle the same size as your frying pan. Carefully take the pan out of the oven, remove the foil and wiggle the beets and onion around in the pan to make a compact layer. Put the pastry on top, tucking it in all around the edges, then return the pan to the oven and bake for 35 mins or until the pastry has puffed up and is a deep golden brown.

Slide a palate knife around the edge of the tart, then put a plate on top of the pastry, serving side down. Flip the pan over to turn the tart out onto the plate – be careful not to burn yourself with the handle. Top with the orange zest and a sprinkle of sea salt, then serve with a peppery salad on the side.

STUFFED PUMPKIN: Throwing a vegan dinner party in the autumn or winter months? Bake a pumpkin with a gorgeous stuffing of rice, fennel, apple, pomegranate seeds and pecans.

Ingredient: 1 medium-sized pumpkin, or round squash (about 1kg), 4 tbsp. olive oil, 100g wild rice, 1 large fennel bulb, 1 Bramley apple, 1 lemon, zested and juiced. 1 tbsp. fennel seeds, ½ tsp. chilli flakes, 2 garlic cloves, crushed, 30g pecans, toasted and roughly chopped. 1 large pack parsley, roughly chopped. 3 tbsp. tahini, pomegranate seeds, to serve.

Preparation: Heat oven to 200C/180C fan/gas 6. Cut the top off the pumpkin or squash and use a metal spoon to scoop out the seeds. Get rid of any pithy bits but keep the seeds for another time (see our pumpkin seed recipe ideas). Put the pumpkin on a baking tray, rub with 2 tbsp. of the oil inside and out, and season well. Roast in the centre of the oven for 45 mins or until tender, with the 'lid' on the side. Meanwhile, rinse the wild rice well and cook following pack instructions, then spread out on a baking tray to cool. Thinly slice the fennel bulb and apple, then squeeze over ½ the lemon juice to stop them discolouring. Heat the remaining 2 tbsp oil in a frying pan. Fry the fennel seeds and chilli flakes, then, once the seeds begin to pop, stir in ½ the garlic and the fennel. Cook for 5 mins until softened, then mix through the apple, pecans and lemon zest. Remove from the heat. Add the mixture to the cooked rice, then stir in the chopped parsley and taste for seasoning.

Pack the mixture into the cooked pumpkin and return to the oven for 10-15 mins until everything is piping hot. Meanwhile, whisk the remaining lemon juice with the tahini, the rest of the garlic and enough water to make a dressing. Serve the pumpkin in the middle of the table, topped with pomegranate seeds and the dressing.

BUTTERNUT, CHESTNUT & LENTIL CAKE:

This stunning cake is a modern take on the classic nut roast, and the ideal vegan centrepiece, accompanied by all the usual trimmings.

Ingredient: 1 large butternut squash, 3 tbsp. sunflower oil, plus extra for greasing. 3 onions, chopped. 15g pack of sage, 12 leaves reserved, rest finely chopped, 2 sprigs rosemary, leaves stripped and chopped, plus a few springs to serve, 3 garlic cloves, crushed, 1 tsp. ground mace, 2 tbsp. ground chia seeds or linseeds (flaxseeds), 2 x 200g packs cooked chestnuts, 2 x 400g cans brown lentils, rinsed and drained, 200g wholemeal vegan breadcrumbs, 3 tbsp. rapeseed oil.

Preparation: First, use a veg peeler to peel the butternut squash and heat oven to 200C/180C fan/gas 6. Then using, a large, sharp knife cut a few 1cm thick ring-slices from the bulbous end, and a few small solid slices from the top end. Set aside the slices, and dice the rest into 1-2cm chunks. Toss the chunks with 1 tbsp. of the sunflower oil on a baking parchment-lined tray and roast for 20-30 mins until tender and golden. Meanwhile prepare the tin. It's worth taking some time to do this, as it'll be the top of your cake in the end – and the bit you want to look impressive! Line the base of a deep, round, 25cm tin with a sheet of baking parchment. Brush the new base and sides with some oil, then start to arrange the rings in the base. You want to get in as many as you can, overlapping a bit like the Olympic rings. Snuggle in as many flat as you can, then sit your overlapping ones on top, cutting out bits of the squash, so they'll also sit flat too. Any leftover trimmings, put in a microwave-proof bowl with a splash of water, cover with cling film and microwave on High at 2 min intervals until tender – around 5-6 minutes.

In a separate pan, soften the onion in the last 2 tbsp. of sunflower oil, over a very low heat so it doesn't brown. Stir in the chopped sage, half the rosemary, and the garlic and mace, and cook for another few mins until fragrant. Mix the ground chia seeds or linseeds with 4 tbsp. of water, and set aside with the cooling onions, until gluey. Meanwhile, roughly chop half the chestnuts but keep them chunky. Put the other half in a food processor with half the lentils, the microwaved squash and one-third of the roasted squash. Pulse to a mashed mixture. Tip this into a large mixing bowl with the softened onions, breadcrumbs, ground seed mixture and 1 tsp salt. Mash everything together really well to thoroughly mix, then more gently stir in the chopped chestnuts, followed by the whole lentils, and finally the remaining roasted squash chunks. Carefully press this mixture around and over the squash rings in the prepared tin. Level off the top, making sure it is tightly packed, then cover with foil. The cake can now be chilled for up to 24 hours before continuing.

To bake, heat the oven to 180C/160C fan/gas 4. Put the cake (still foil covered), into the oven on a middle shelf and bake for 1 hr. To serve, heat the rapeseed oil in a small frying pan and sizzle the reserved sage leaves with the remaining rosemary sprigs for a minute. Loosen around the sides of the cake with a round-bladed knife, then sit a serving plate inverted on top, and carefully flip the plate to turn out the cake. Spoon over the sizzled sage and rosemary leaves and herby oil, and serve at the table – for cutting into wedges in front of everyone.

CURRIED TOFU WRAPS: This spicy vegan supper is big on taste. It's simple to make and packed with chunky tandoori-spiced tofu on a cool mint, yogurt and red cabbage relish.

Ingredient: ½ red cabbage, (about 500g), shredded, 4 heaped tbsp. dairy-free yogurt (we used Alpro Plain with Coconut), 3 tbsp. mint sauce, 3 x 200g packs tofu, each cut into 15 cubes, 2 tbsp. tandoori curry paste, 2 tbsp. oil, 2 onions, sliced. 2 large garlic cloves, sliced, 8 chapatis, 2 limes, cut into quarters.

Preparation: Mix the cabbage, yogurt and mint sauce, season and set aside. Toss the tofu with the tandoori paste and 1 tbsp. of the oil. Heat a frying pan and cook the tofu, in batches, for a few mins each side until golden. Remove from the pan with a slotted spoon and set aside. Add the remaining oil to the pan, stir in the onions and garlic, and cook for 8-10 mins until softened. Return the tofu to the pan and season well. Warm the chapatis following pack instructions, then top each one with some cabbage, followed by the curried tofu and a good squeeze of lime.

CHILLI & AVOCADO SALSA SWEET POTATOES

: A fresh, summery vegan recipe that won't break the bank. Get 5 of your 5 a day the easy way.

Ingredient: 2 large sweet potatoes, 1 tbsp. vegetable oil, 1 onion, finely chopped, 2 garlic cloves, crushed. 1 tsp. paprika, 400g can chopped tomatoes, 1 small avocado, chopped. 1 red chilli, finely chopped. ½ small pack coriander, chopped, 400g can mixed beans, drained, ½ x 460g jar roasted red peppers, sliced, 1 tbsp. coconut yogurt, to serve (optional).

Preparation: Heat oven to 200C/180C fan/gas 6. Prick the sweet potatoes with a fork and bake for 40-45 mins, or until tender and cooked. Meanwhile, heat the oil in a deep frying pan and cook the onion for about 10 mins until softening. Add the garlic and paprika, and stir for 1 min. Tip in the tomatoes, then bring to a gentle simmer, season well and leave to bubble away for 10-15 mins. To make the salsa, combine the avocado, chilli and coriander in a small bowl. Pour the mixed beans into the pan with the red peppers. Warm through for 5 mins and taste. Halve each baked potato, ladle over the chilli and spoon on the salsa. Add a dollop of coconut yogurt to each half before serving, if you like.

SWEET POTATO & COCONUT CURRY: Prep your veggies and let the slow cooker do the work with our filling sweet potato curry.

Ingredient: 4 tbsp. olive oil, 2 large onions, halved and sliced. 3 garlic cloves, crushed

Thumb-sized piece root ginger, peeled. 1 tsp. paprika, ½ tsp. cayenne, 2 red chillies, deseeded and sliced, 2 red peppers, deseeded and sliced, 250g red cabbage, shredded. 1kg sweet potatoes, peeled and chopped into chunks. 300g passata, 400ml coconut milk, 2 tbsp. peanut butter

To serve— small bunch fresh coriander, chopped, cooked couscous (or gluten-free alternative).

Preparation: Heat 1 tbsp. olive oil in a large non-stick frying pan and add the onion. Fry gently for 10 mins until soft then add the garlic and grate the ginger straight into the pan. Stir in the paprika and the cayenne and cook for another minute then tip into the slow cooker. Return the pan to the heat and add another 1 tbsp. oil along with the chilli, red pepper and shredded cabbage.

Cook for 4-5 mins then tip into the slow cooker. Use the remaining oil to fry the sweet potatoes, you may have to do this in 2 or 3 batches depending on the size of your pan. Cook the sweet potatoes for around 5 mins or just until they start to pick up some colour at the edges then put them in the slow cooker too. Pour the passata and the coconut milk over the sweet potatoes, stir to mix everything together and cover the slow cooker with a lid and cook for 6-8hrs or until the sweet potatoes are tender. Stir the peanut butter through the curry, season well with salt and pepper and serve with couscous and chopped coriander scattered over the top.

LENTIL RAGU WITH COURGETTE: A healthy tomato 'pasta' dish that makes full use of your spiralizer. This vegan-friendly supper is five of your five-a-day and will fill you to the brim.

Ingredient: 2 tbsp. rapeseed oil, plus 1 tsp. 3 celery sticks, chopped, 2 carrots, chopped. 4 garlic cloves, chopped, 2 onions, finely chopped, 140g button mushrooms from a 280g pack, quartered, 500g pack dried red lentils, 500g pack passata, 1l reduced-salt vegetable bouillon (we used Marigold), 1 tsp. dried oregano, 2 tbsp. balsamic vinegar, 1-2 large courgettes, cut into noodles with a spiraliser, julienne peeler or knife.

Preparation: Heat the 2 tbsp. oil in a large sauté pan. Add the celery, carrots, garlic and onions, and fry for 4-5 mins over a high heat to soften and start to colour. Add the mushrooms and fry for 2 mins more. Stir in the lentils, passata, bouillon, oregano and balsamic vinegar. Cover the pan and leave to simmer for 30 mins until the lentils are tender and pulpy. Check occasionally and stir to make sure the mixture isn't sticking to the bottom of the pan; if it does, add a drop of water. To serve, heat the remaining oil in a separate frying pan, add the courgette and stir-fry briefly to soften and warm through. Serve half the ragu with the courgetti and chill the rest to eat on another day. Can be frozen for up to 3 months.

VEGGIE TAHINI LENTILS: Quick, easy and packed with healthy veg, this is a great midweek meal for vegans and veggies.

Ingredient: 50g tahini, zest and juice 1 lemon, 2 tbsp. olive oil, 1 red onion, thinly sliced, 1 garlic clove, crushed, 1 yellow pepper, thinly sliced, 200g green beans, trimmed and halved, 1 courgette, sliced into half-moons, 100g shredded kale, 250g pack pre-cooked puy lentils.

Preparation: In a jug, mix the tahini with the zest and juice of the lemon and 50ml of cold water to make a runny dressing. Season to taste, then set aside. Heat the oil in a wok or large frying pan over a medium-high heat. Add the red onion, along with a pinch of salt, and fry for 2 mins until starting to soften and colour. Add the garlic, pepper, green beans and courgette and fry for 5 min, stirring frequently. Tip in the kale, lentils and the tahini dressing. Keep the pan on the heat for a couple of mins, stirring everything together until the kale is wilted and it's all coated in the creamy dressing.

VEGAN DESSERT AND SNACK RECIPES.

No matter how much more popular veganism is becoming these days, some people can't shake the perception that all egg- and dairy-free desserts must taste like flavourless slabs of sandpaper. Clearly, these people have never tried any of these 100 percent vegan recipes. The cookies in this roundup don't contain butter, the pies have no eggs, and you won't find cream cheese frosting anywhere near the cupcakes, but thanks to a few simple yet clever swaps, they're all delicious examples of how a purely plant-based diet can translate to some pretty mind-blowing sweet treats. So don't let the vegan label throw you off

VEGAN TIFFIN: Make our vegan tiffin squares as a festive treat, packed with Christmas ingredients like ginger nuts, dried cranberries and pistachios. They're great for a party.

Ingredient: 75g coconut oil, plus extra for the tin, 200g vegan dark chocolate (at least 70%), roughly chopped, 2 tbsp. golden syrup, 200g vegan ginger nuts, 100g dried cranberries, 50g pistachios, toasted and chopped.

Preparation: Lightly oil a 20cm square brownie tin with coconut oil and line the base with baking parchment. Melt the chocolate with the coconut oil and golden syrup in the microwave in 30second bursts until smooth and glossy. Break the ginger nuts into small pieces in a bowl, then add the dried cranberries and pistachios. Scrape in the chocolate mixture and give everything a good mix to combine, then spoon the tiffin into the tin. Use the back of the spoon to smooth out the top and press it down, then chill in the fridge for 2 hrs or until set hard. Once set, cut into 25 mini squares. Will keep for a week in the fridge.

VEGAN VANILLA ICE CREAM: Indulge in our dairy-free and egg-free vanilla ice cream, the perfect dessert for summer as part of a vegan menu. Serve on its own or try with fresh berries.

Ingredient: 2 x 400g cans coconut milk (not light), 175g caster sugar, 1 tsp. sea salt flakes, 1 vanilla pod or 1 tbsp. vanilla bean paste, 2 tbsp. corn flour, a pinch turmeric.

Preparation: Pour most of the coconut milk into a saucepan, reserving a splash in a small bowl for later. Add the sugar, salt and turmeric (for colour) to the pan. Cut the vanilla pod in half lengthways (if using) and scrape the seeds out of both sides with the side of the knife. Put the seeds and the pod, or vanilla paste, into the pan. Warm on a low heat for 10 mins until the sugar has melted and the mixture starts to steam.

Mix the corn flour with the reserved coconut milk in a small bowl until smooth. Pour into the hot milk, and continually whisking, heat for another 5-10 mins until the mixture thickens to a pourable custard consistency. Strain into a bowl, and cover. Leave to cool, then chill for at least 2 hrs. Pour the chilled mix into an ice cream maker, and churn for 20-30 mins until you get a soft scoop ice cream. Transfer to a sealable container and freeze for up to 3 months until ready to serve. If you don't have an ice cream maker, pour the chilled mix into a wide-based plastic tub or dish. Freeze for 2-3 hrs. Stirring the mix every 20 mins with a fork, to break up any large ice crystals, until soft ice cream. Transfer to a smaller tub and freeze until ready to serve. You should be able to scoop the ice cream easily from the freezer, or leave for a few mins at room temperature to soften, if you need to.

VEGAN ETON MESS: Nothing says summer like a sweet, berry-filled Eton mess and this vegan version swaps the egg whites in the meringues for an ingenious alternative.

Ingredient: Drained liquid from a 400g can chickpeas (aquafaba), 100g golden caster sugar, 500g

mixed berries, 2 tbsp. icing sugar, ½ tbsp. rose water, 400ml vegan coconut yogurt (we used COYO, vanilla flavoured) rose petals, to serve.

Preparation: Heat oven to 110C/90C fan/gas 1 and line a baking tray with parchment. Whisk the drained chickpea liquid with an electric whisk until white, fluffy and just holding its shape – be persistent, this will take longer than you imagine. Gradually whisk in the caster sugar until your chickpea meringue reaches stiff peaks. Spoon the vegan meringue onto the baking parchment and bake for 1hr 30 mins, or until they come off the paper easily. Leave to cool. Meanwhile, mix the berries with the icing sugar and rose water. Set aside for 30 mins so the flavours infuse and the berries release some of their juices. Put the yogurt into a large bowl, crush in the meringues then stir through 1/3 of the fruit, rippling it through the yogurt. Spoon into 4 serving dishes then top with the remaining fruit and the rose petals.

STICKY TOFFEE PEAR PUDDING: A lighter version of sticky toffee pudding, rich with dates and spices, and the juicy texture of poached pears, this vegan dessert is sure to please a crowd.

Ingredient: 8 small firm pears (we used Conference), 200g golden caster sugar, 2 cinnamon sticks, 1 star anise, 6 cloves, 1 lemon, zest pared. 1 orange, zest pared, vegan ice cream, to serve (optional)

For the sponge— 250g pitted dates, 2 tbsp. linseeds, 300ml unsweetened almond milk 200ml vegetable oil, plus extra for greasing, 175g dark muscovado sugar, 200g self-rising flour

1 tsp. bicarbonate of soda, 1 tsp. ground mixed spice.

Preparation: Peel the pears and cut the bottom off each to give a flat base – cut them to a height that will fit snugly in your tin. Use a melon baller or small knife to cut out the pips from the base. Roughly chop the pear scraps, discarding the pips, and set aside. Tip the sugar, cinnamon, star anise, cloves, zests and 600ml water into a saucepan large enough to fit all the pears. Bring to the boil, then simmer until the sugar has dissolved. Add the pears, cover with a lid or a piece of baking parchment, and poach gently for 15 mins until a knife easily slides into a pear. Leave to cool in the liquid. Now make the sponge. Put the dates and linseeds in a saucepan and add the almond milk. Bring to a gentle simmer, then cook for 2-3 mins until the dates are soft. Pour into a food processor and blitz until smooth. Add the oil and blend again, then scrape into a bowl and set aside to cool a little. Heat oven to 180C/160C fan/gas 4. Grease and line a 20 x 30cm baking tin (a loose -bottomed one if possible) with a strip of baking parchment.

419

Put the dry ingredients in a large mixing bowl with 1/ 2 tsp. salt. Mix well, breaking up any lumps of sugar with your fingers, and shaking the bowl a few times to encourage any remaining lumps to come to the surface. Add the date and oil mixture, and stir well. Fold in the chopped pear scraps. Scrape the cake mixture into the tin, then nestle in the pears, standing straight up, so that the bottom halves are covered. Bake for 35-40 mins until the cake is cooked through. Insert a skewer to the centre to check – it should come out clean. If there is any wet cake mixture on the skewer, return the cake to the oven and bake for 10 mins more, and then check again. Meanwhile, bring the pear poaching liquid back to the boil and simmer until reduced to a glossy syrup. When the pudding is cooked, cool for 5-10 mins, then brush all over with the syrup, saving a little extra to serve alongside, with vegan ice cream, if you like.

VEGAN LEMON CHEESECAKE: An easy no-cook cheesecake that's dairy-free and gluten-free with just a little agave syrup to sweeten. A lusciously lemony vegan dessert the family will love.

Ingredient: 30g coconut oil, plus extra for greasing, 100g blanched almonds, 100g soft pitted date

For the topping— 300g cashew nuts, 2 ½ tbsp. agave syrup, 50g coconut oil, 150ml almond milk, 2 lemons, zested and juiced.

Preparation: Put the cashews in a large bowl, pour over boiling water and leave to soak for 1 hr.

Meanwhile, blitz the ingredients for the base with a pinch of salt in a food processor. Grease a

23cm tart tin with coconut oil, then press the mix into the base and pop in the fridge to set (about 30 mins). Drain the cashews and tip into the cleaned out food processor. Add all the remaining topping ingredients, reserving a quarter of the lemon zest in damp kitchen paper to serve, then blitz until smooth. Spoon onto the base and put in the fridge to set completely (about 2 hrs). Just before serving, scatter over the reserved lemon zest.

AVOCADO & STRAWBERRY ICES: Replace dairy with creamy avocado, full of healthy fat, in these delicious ices and bring out the flavour of strawberries with balsamic vinegar.

Ingredient: 200g ripe strawberries, hulled and chopped, 1 avocado, stoned, peeled and roughly chopped. 2 tsp. balsamic vinegar, ½ tsp. vanilla extract, 1-2 tsp. maple syrup (optional).

Preparation: Put the strawberries (save four pieces for the top), avocado, vinegar and vanilla in a bowl and blitz using a hand blender (or in a food processor) until as smooth as you can get it. Have a taste and only add the maple syrup if the strawberries are not sweet enough.

Pour into containers, add a strawberry to each, cover with cling film and freeze. Allow the pots to soften for 5-10 mins before eating.

VEGAN CUPCAKES: Make vegan cupcakes with buttercream topping using dairy-free and egg-free ingredients. They make the perfect treat for afternoon tea or a mid-morning snack.

Ingredient: 150ml non-dairy milk, (such as almond or soy), ½ tsp. cider vinegar, 110g vegan butter or sunflower spread, 110g caster sugar, 1 tsp. vanilla extract, 110g self-rising flour, ½ tsp. baking powder.

For the buttercream— 125g vegan butter, 250g icing sugar, 1¼ tsp. vanilla extract, a few drops of vegan food colourings (check the label).

Preparation: Heat the oven to 180C/160C fan/gas 4. Line the holes of a 12-hole cupcake tin with paper cases. Stir the milk and vinegar in a jug and leave to thicken slightly for a few mins. Beat the butter and sugar with an electric whisk until well combined. Whisk in the vanilla, then add the milk a splash at a time, alternating with spoonful of the flour. Fold in any remaining flour, the baking powder and a pinch of salt until you get a creamy batter. Don't worry if it looks a little curdled at this stage. Divide between the cupcake cases, filling those, two-thirds full, and bake for 20 mins until golden and risen. Leave to cool on a wire rack.

To make the buttercream, beat the butter, icing sugar and vanilla with an electric whisk until pale and creamy. Divide between bowls and colour with different food colourings until you get desired strength. Spoon or pipe onto the cooled cupcakes.

VEGAN SHORTBREAD: Make our vegan shortbread with olive oil for a buttery flavour and corn flour to get the crumbliness of traditional versions. They taste great with nut butter.

Ingredient: 250g plain flour, plus extra for dusting, 75g caster sugar, plus 1 tbsp., ½ tbsp. corn flour, 1 tsp. vanilla extract, 125ml light olive oil.

Preparation: Whizz the flour, sugar and corn flour in a food processor to sieve and mix briefly, then add the vanilla and drizzle in the olive oil, pulsing the food processor blades until you get a soft, golden dough. Wrap and chill for 30 mins to rest. Heat the oven to 180C/160C fan/gas 4, and line a baking sheet with parchment or a baking mat. Roll the dough out on a lightly floured work surface to a 5mm thickness and use a round or fluted cutter, about 6cm diameter, to cut out shortbread rounds. Use a small palette knife to transfer to the baking sheet. Can be frozen on the baking tray, then transferred to a box when solid. Will keep for up to three months. Sprinkle the 1 tbsp. sugar over the biscuits and bake for 15-20 mins until golden brown. Leave to cool for a few mins to firm up on the tray, then transfer to a cooling rack to cool completely. Add 2-4 mins to the cooking time if baking from frozen.

CHEAT'S PINEAPPLE, THAI BASIL & GINGER SORBET: An easy blended sorbet with vibrant Thai basil and spicy ginger. Try serving with a drizzle of vodka or white rum.

Ingredient: 1 large pineapple, peeled, cored and cut into chunks. Juice and zest 1 lime, 1 small piece of ginger, sliced. Handful Thai basil leaves, plus a few extra little ones to serve, 75g white caster sugar, vodka or white rum (optional).

Preparation: A couple of days before eating, tip everything into a blender or smoothie maker with 200ml water and blitz until very smooth. Pour into a freezable container and freeze overnight until solid. A few hours before serving, remove from the freezer and allow to defrost slightly so it slides out of the container in a block. Chop the block into ice cube-sized chunks and blitz in the blender or smoothie maker again until you have a thick, slushy purée. Tip back into the container and refreeze for 1 hr. or until it can be scooped out.

To serve, scoop the sorbet into chilled bowls or glasses and top with extra basil. If you want you can drizzle with something a little more potent, such as vodka or white rum.

VEGAN CHOCOLATE BANANA ICE CREAM: A low-fat chocolate ice cream? It really does exist! Our blitzed banana creation is gluten and dairy-free and ready in minutes.

Ingredient: 1 frozen banana, 1 tsp. cocoa powder.

Preparation: In a blender, blitz the frozen banana with the cocoa powder until smooth. Eat straight away.

CONCLUSION

Becoming a vegan isn't as tough as people think, and it certainly doesn't make you sick or weak.

It's simply a decision you make to improve your health and protect animals from needless slaughter. Many people go about the wrong believe and get scared off— no, as you must have discovered here, there's no need to.

All that's needed is the right understanding of veganism, the types, what it entails and benefits; the you go about how to become one, the right way off course.

We hope that this guide gives you everything or almost, to satisfactorily get you on the go with being a vegan. While it may be weird to some people, you could actually be having the best meals of your life while maintaining awesome health and achieve your body goals.

Vegan Instant Pot Cookbook

101 Easy And Healthy Vegan Instant Pot Recipes for Your Pressure Cooker

INTRODUCTION:

One unexpected benefit of exploring a plant-based diet is that it can inspire you to discover the joy of cooking. Most hobbies cost money, but learning how to cook will save you piles of cash. Doing your own cooking is much cheaper than eating at restaurants or buying frozen foods, plus you'll be eating fresher, tastier meals made with higher-quality ingredients.

This edition of our cookbook actually covers a lot and we've included newly discovered recipes that would serve you a kind of savoury that you've never had; both new and long existing vegans. You really don't have to miss anything because you're vegan, in fact, you are advantaged because these meals gives you the best nutritional benefits and keeps you much healthier.

Vegan made easy.

Whatever brought you as far as getting this cookbook, you've already taken the all-important first step on your vegan journey. There's an absolute, fantastic journey for you ahead as you journey to becoming a vegan. It's actually very easy, easier for some though, like every other transitional step in life, it takes a little bit of time, patience and the right guidance.

A vegan lifestyle is compatible with the highest levels of health and fitness, protects huge numbers of animals, and is a potent way to combat climate change. Plus, the food is insanely delicious and it becomes more widely available every year.

Keep your end goal in mind, but go at your own pace. Some people manage to go vegan overnight and if that's the right approach for you, fantastic. But don't be concerned if you feel you need more time. Like any other lifestyle change, going vegan not only takes getting used to, but it takes time to determine what will work best for you. It's not a one size fits all experience and there are numerous approaches you can take.

Making small changes to your everyday meals is one of the easiest ways to increase the amount of plant-based foods in your diet. You could start by removing meat or dairy one day a week and go from there. Or you could try changing one meal at a time, having vegan breakfasts during your first week, adding a vegan lunch during week two and so on. You could even try changing one product at a time by swapping cow's milk for almond or soya milk or butter for coconut oil or margarine. There's a plant-based alternative for almost every type of food you can think of, so you don't have to miss out on any of your favourite foods.

Make sure you don't miss out on essential nutrients. Just because you're vegan that doesn't mean you're 100% healthy, as there are vegan versions of almost every type of junk food you can think of. As long as you eat a wide variety of tasty plant foods, planning a healthy diet that incorporates all the vitamins and nutrients you need will be a breeze.

People commonly assume that going vegan requires enormous discipline and dedication. Luckily, nothing could be further from the truth. Switching to a vegan diet is surprisingly easy—and just a little reading puts you halfway there. Most new vegans end up being shocked by how little effort the transition takes.

Let's start by looking at how to construct a smart overall approach. The most obvious way to become vegan is to focus on eliminating animal products from your diet. Surprisingly, however, this method of transitioning is needlessly difficult. The truth is that gritting your teeth and exerting willpower makes the task of becoming vegan needlessly difficult. So let's look at a better way

Go Vegan by Crowding, Not Cutting— Instead of trying to cut animal products out of your diet, crowd them out. Constantly seek out new vegan foods. Every time you discover one you adore, it'll push the animal-based foods in your life further to the fringes. The more vegan foods you sample, the easier it becomes to eat vegan most of the time.

So cultivate the habit of trying new foods at every opportunity. The payoff is huge, and the commitment required is tiny. Just make a point of sampling at least five new vegan foods each week, and you'll discover a steady stream of foods you love. Week by week, these items will begin crowding out the animal products that are currently in your diet. Before long, anytime you get hungry the first food that comes to mind will be vegan.

You'll Find a Vast Assortment of Delicious Vegan Foods— Does going vegan mean you'll need to spend loads of time in the kitchen? Absolutely not. You'll be amazed by how many instant and near-instant options exist. THIS COOKBOOK is a large step in the right direction to soothing that.

How Fast Should You Go?— Since a key part of learning how to go vegan involves discovering new foods, you're always in control of how fast or slow you go. You certainly don't need to go vegan all at once. Some people do it overnight, while others ease into it over months or even years. How fast you go is not nearly as important as whether the approach you take feels easy and comfortable. Use whatever stepping-stones work for you. The goal, after all, is not just to go vegan but to stay vegan long-term. You want fill your diet with delicious vegan foods that you're delighted to eat every day.

Dipping in Your Toe— some people get intimidated by the thought of becoming absolutely, positively vegan—with no room for slips or exceptions. If making a 100 percent commitment sounds too much for you right now, no problem. There are always smaller steps that still accomplish a great deal of good.

One of America's most influential food writers, Mark Bittman, has long followed what he calls a "Vegan before 6:00," approach. That is, he follows a totally vegan diet from morning through afternoon, and then eats whatever he likes for dinner and the rest of the evening. Bittman's approach can easily get you past the halfway point towards becoming vegan. Simply by following Vegan before 6:00, you'll doubtless eat far fewer animal products than most people. If this approach sounds appealing, you can get hold of Bittman's book on the topic.

Buying Vegan Foods Online— If you live in a community that lacks a good natural foods store, don't despair. Amazon.com can pick up the slack. They carry all sorts of essential vegan items, from energy bars to hot cereals to cookies to nutritional yeast. You can find every imaginable vegan food product on Amazon.com. The trouble is that many items listed by third parties sell for exorbitant prices. But Amazon itself fulfils dozens of great vegan foods, at prices that are remarkably competitive.

We maintain a grocery page listing Amazon's best vegan food deals. It's worth checking out even if you have a good natural foods store nearby, since you will certainly find items unavailable locally. Amazon won't carry every vegan grocery item you need, but you can save a lot of time and money by ordering some of your groceries through them.

INSTANT POT BASICS.

The Instant Pot isn't nearly as simple or "instant" as you might think it is. In fact, they are pretty complicated and many folks never use half of the functions available.

What is the Instant Pot?

It is one appliance that has many functions: electric pressure cooker, rice cooker, steamer, yogurt maker, sauté pan, slow cooker and warmer. The function that most people praise the Instant Pot for is the electric pressure cooker feature, but I personally LOVE its slow cooker feature.

Are electric pressure cookers safe?

Yes and no. They still have a danger factor, but knowing how to use yours will prevent injury. The Instant Pot has a safety feature of locking until the pressure is released an safe to open so there is no guessing. However, the "quick release" function, also known as "venting" or QR, releases some pretty hot steam that could easily cause harm or injury. Your Instant Pot is locked when the little metal piece right next to the valve is UP.

Do I need to use liquid?

Yes, by definition, pressure cookers need some amount of liquid to build pressure. You need at least 1/2 cup to 1 cup of liquid for your Instant Pot to work. For dry foods, more is needed, but if you are using water containing foods, like vegetables, less is needed.

What can I make in the Instant Pot?

Most people think of fried chicken when they think of electric pressure cookers, but you can make so many things. Chuck roasts will be fork tender, chicken will shred in just 10 minutes and seafood will be done in 4 minutes. You can also make desserts, such as cakes and puddings, cheese, yogurt, broths, stocks and stubborn grains like quinoa, sorghum and steel cut oats in just minutes.

Why isn't the timer starting right away on my Instant Pot?

I think one of the things that frustrates me the most about recipe writers for the Instant Pot, they never include the amount of time it takes for the pot to build pressure or heat. If you are starting with cold or frozen foods, it will take longer to come to pressure (see what this means below), whereas hot or previously simmered/sautéed foods won't take as long. Plan for anywhere between 10-15 minutes additional time for the Instant Pot to come to pressure.

What is NPR or natural pressure release?

Natural pressure release is sometimes abbreviated to NP or NPR. It basically means you are going to gradually (and naturally) allow the pressure to release.

This process takes about 15-20 minutes. Food will continue to cook while on natural pressure release.

What is QR or quick pressure release?

It is the opposite of NPR. Instead of allowing the pressure to gradually release, you vent it out super-fast. Be careful though, this steam is HOT and can cause injury. Also, don't do it under your cabinets or around anything that has a painted finish- it will literally peel the paint. Release pressure in an open space on the counter.

What is venting and sealing?

The knob on the Instant Pot has two settings: venting and sealing. Venting means that you are not building up pressure at all, instead the pressure and steam is releasing during the cooking process. This is used for steaming. Sealing means that you are pressure cooking and all of that good stuff is staying inside the Instant Pot.

What is PIP?

PIP stands for "pot in pot" cooking. Basically, another pot that goes into the inner pot. You need this for casseroles, cakes and if you want to cook multiple things at once. The Instant makes some fabulous cheesecakes! These are the ones I use the most:

- 1 quart casserole dish
- 7 inch spring form pan
- Steamer basket.

Do I still need a slow cooker if I have an Instant Pot?

Technically, no, the Instant Pot is also a slow cooker. One of the things I love about the Instant Pot as a slow cooker is that I can use the Sauté function either before slow cooking to brown the meat or at the very end to reduce or thicken sauces, eliminating the need to use even more dishes.

How do I use the trivet?

The trivet can be used in multiple ways. Put the "legs" down and you can cook two things at once- meat on the and set the steam basket on top or vice versa or... put the "legs" up and now you can use them as handles to pull out things like the spring form pan.

Why does my Instant Pot smell?

It is most likely due to the silicone sealing ring. This ring holds in smells like no other. You can buy extras and use one for savoury dishes and another for sweet meals. I have one I use just for curry. Also, make sure to rinse the lid of the Instant Pot to get out smells. Many folks wash the inner pot, but not the lid! The rings are cheap.

What is the difference between low and high pressure?

The quick and dirty answer is that high pressure is better for cooking heartier items, like meats, chicken and pasta, while low pressure is better suited for delicate items like eggs, fish and some desserts. Why? First understand PSI, pounds per square inch. The PSI determines just how hot the cooker is going to get beyond the regular 212 Fahrenheit temperature, the boiling point of water at sea level.

A high pressure could get up to 10 or 12 PSI and as hot as 239 to 245 Fahrenheit, while a low pressure setting is between 5.5 to 7 PSI, with a temperature range from 229 to 233 Fahrenheit. Low pressure items might need to cook longer, but will benefit in the texture from lower pressure.

How do I use the Instant Pot at high altitude?

Some say that a pressure cooker defies nature and that altitude doesn't matter, but anyone who lives in a high altitude area (3,000 feet above sea level) will tell you that isn't true. According to the New High Altitude Cookbook, cooking time under pressure should be increased by 5% for every 1,000 feet after 2,000 feet above sea level.

Is it necessary to do the Water Test?

Yes! To make sure your Instant Pot is safe and comes to correct temperatures for cooking, do the water test. It really doesn't take long.

Pantry basics, sauces and dips.

Spaghetti Sauce: This rich and tasty homemade spaghetti sauce is made with fresh tomatoes! Just what you need for any pasta dish, and so quick and easy to make in the Instant Pot.

Ingredient: 2 tablespoons olive oil, 2 yellow onions, chopped, 2 cloves garlic, minced. 1 carrot, chopped. 1 celery stalk, chopped. 3 pounds plum tomatoes, 1 teaspoon dried oregano, 1 teaspoon Italian seasoning, 1 teaspoon sea salt, 1 teaspoon dried basil, 1/2 teaspoon ground black pepper.

Preparation: Turn on a multi-functional pressure cooker (such as Instant Pot(R)) and select Sauté function. Heat olive oil and stir in onions and garlic; cook until soft and translucent, about 5 minutes. Add carrot, celery, and tomatoes; cook until tender, about 4 minutes. Season with oregano, Italian seasoning, salt, basil, and pepper. Close and lock the lid. Select high pressure according to manufacturer's instructions; set timer for 25 minutes. Allow 10 to 15 minutes for pressure to build.

Release pressure using the natural-release method according to manufacturer's instructions, 10 to 40 minutes. Unlock and remove the lid. Blend with an immersion blender to desired consistency.

Instant Pot Vegan Cheese Sauce: This vegan cheese sauce recipe is so simple to make in the Instant Pot. You just need to dump everything together, cook it on high pressure and then puree it in a blender to a smooth sauce. So easy and tasty!

Ingredient: 1 large russet potato, 320 grams, cubed, 1 large sweet potato, 300 grams, cubed 2 large carrots, 170 grams, cut into rounds, 1/4 cup cashews, raw, 35 grams, 1 cup water, 8 oz., 1/2 cup nutritional yeast, 3/4 teaspoon smoked paprika, 1 teaspoon garlic powder. 1.25 teaspoon salt, or to taste, 1/4 teaspoon turmeric powder, 1 tablespoon white vinegar, 1.5 tablespoons lemon juice, 1/4 cup water or almond milk, 2 oz.

Preparation: To your instant pot add cubed potatoes, sweet potatoes, carrots, cashews and 1 cup water. Close the pot with its lid. Press the manual/pressure cook button and cook on high pressure for 5 minutes. The pressure valve should be in the sealing position. Let the pressure release naturally for 5 minutes and then do a quick pressure release by manually moving the valve from sealing to venting position. Let the veggies cool down a bit and then transfer them to a high speed blender. Add nutritional yeast, smoked paprika, garlic powder, salt, turmeric, white vinegar, lemon juice and 1/4 cup of either water or almond milk.

Pulse for 30 seconds or until the sauce is super creamy and smooth. Transfer vegan cheese sauce to serving bowl. Enjoy with chips or veggies!

Vegan Cheese Sauce: what truly makes this THE BEST Vegan Cheese Sauce Ever, is how quick and simple it is to make! Just throw all the ingredients into the INSTANT POT and in about 20 minutes you'll have a hot, delicious plant-based CHEESE SAUCE! Now how easy is that!

Ingredient: 2 cups water, 1/2 yellow or white onion, peeled and quartered, 2 cloves garlic, peeled, 1 cup carrots, peeled and sliced, 1 & 1/2 cups peeled and chopped Yukon Gold potatoes, 1/2 cup raw cashews (optional, but recommended for maximum creaminess.), 1/2 cup nutritional yeast (Different from baking yeast), 2 Tablespoons mellow white miso, 1 teaspoon smoked or sweet paprika, 1 1/2 Tablespoons lemon juice, 1 1/2 Tablespoons apple cider vinegar, 2 teaspoons sea salt (optional, but recommended to achieve a true cheese-like taste.)

Preparation: Place all ingredients in the Instant Pot in the order listed. (No need to soak the cashews- the Instant Pot will soften them.) Put the lid on the Instant Pot and twist it to the lock position. Select MANUAL with HIGH pressure, then set the cook time to 5 MINUTES. While the cheese sauce is coming up to pressure and cooking in the Instant Pot, prepare the food you would like to serve with it, such as elbow macaroni, broccoli, baked potatoes, tortilla chips, etc. When the Instant Pot has finished cooking, manually release the pressure and open the lid.

Using hot pads and avoiding the steam, lift the stainless steel pot out of the cooker. Carefully pour the entire contents of the pot into a high speed blender. Puree using the whole juice setting, or use the highest speed setting for about 2 minutes, until sauce is super smooth, thick and creamy. (If sauce is too thick, add 1/4 to 1/2 cup plant milk and blend again to thin. Sauce will continue to thicken as it cools, so you may want to make it a little thinner to start.) Alternately, you can use a hand-held immersion blender directly in the Instant Pot to blend all ingredients together for 2-3 minutes, or until cheese sauce is super smooth, thinning with a little additional plant milk as needed. Serve hot cheese sauce immediately by pouring over cooked macaroni, steamed broccoli, baked potatoes, or stir in spices and serve over baked corn tortilla chips as nachos.

If not serving right away, allow cheese sauce to cool completely and then store covered in the refrigerator for up to one week, or in the freezer for up to three months. (Sauce will thicken when chilled, so you may need to thin it down again before serving, by adding a bit of plant milk or water while re-heating) When ready to serve the previously refrigerated or frozen sauce, heat in the microwave till super-hot, stirring every 2-3 minutes.

Continue heating and stirring until all the cold clumps have melted, and the sauce once again has a super smooth consistency.) Alternately, you can heat the thawed sauce in a saucepan on the stovetop, stirring constantly, until very hot and no lumps remain, and thinning with a bit of plant milk as needed (The heating process will thicken the sauce, so you may need to add even more plant milk to thin it out again before serving.)

Penne in Cajun Mustard Cream Sauce: Make this Instant Pot Penne in Cajun Mustard Cream Sauce for a quick and easy weeknight meal. With options to prepare it with Andouille sausage or meatless you can make everyone happy.

Ingredient: 12 ounces penne rigate pasta, uncooked, 2 1/2 cups chicken broth (for more flavour) or water, 2–3 tsp. Cajun seasoning, 1 tsp. garlic powder, 1 Tbsp. butter, 1 (14.5 oz.) can petite diced tomatoes, 1 (13 oz.) package Cajun-style Andouille smoked sausage (optional), 4 oz. cream cheese, 1 Tbsp. lemon juice, 1 1/2 tsp. Dijon mustard.

Preparation: Add pasta to the Instant Pot. Pour broth/water over the top, try to cover pasta as much as possible. Sprinkle in 2 tsp. of the Cajun seasoning and add in the garlic powder. Add in the butter and petite diced tomatoes. If using sausage, slice it into 1/2 inch pieces and add it into the pot. Cover the pot and secure the lid. Make sure valve is set to sealing. Set the manual/pressure cook button to 5 minutes. When time is up move valve to venting for a quick release (you can also use a natural pressure release).

Turn the pot to the sauté setting and stir in the cream cheese, until it is melted. Turn off the sauté setting. Stir in the lemon juice and Dijon mustard. Taste and if needed add in another teaspoon of Cajun seasoning. Salt and pepper to taste as needed.

Serve and enjoy. Store leftovers in an airtight container in the refrigerator for up to 3 days.

Easy Instant Pot Spaghetti Sauce: Easy Instant Pot Spaghetti Sauce–this spaghetti sauce is so delicious you'll be licking your plate. The funny part is that it only takes a handful of easy ingredients and a few minutes in your pressure cooker. Bonus–if you want to cook a spaghetti squash at the same time as the sauce you can!

Ingredient: 1 (28 oz.) can crushed tomatoes, 4 Tbsp. butter, 1 tsp. onion powder, 1 tsp. garlic powder, 1/2 tsp. kosher salt, Optional: 1 small spaghetti squash.

Preparation: Add tomatoes, butter, onion powder, garlic powder and salt to Instant Pot.

Optional: If making a spaghetti squash, use a paring knife to cut your spaghetti squash in half crosswise (not lengthwise). Use a spoon to scoop out all the seeds and gunk. Place a trivet inside the pot and then arrange the 2 squash halves to fit in the pot. Cover the pot and secure the lid. Make sure valve is set to sealing. Set the manual/pressure cook button to 7 minutes. Once the time has counted down and the pot beeps you can perform a quick release by moving the valve to venting. Remove the lid. Use tongs to remove the squash to a cutting board. Once it has cooled, use a fork to shred the flesh of the squash into long spaghetti-like strands. Use an immersion blender to blend the sauce to desired consistency. Salt and pepper the sauce to taste.

Serve the sauce over spaghetti or spaghetti squash and top with generous amounts of parmesan cheese.

Instant-Pot Vegan Cauliflower Queso:
Cauliflower is a magical vegetable. It's tasty on its own, but it can transform into oil-free creamy sauces and even replace meat. In this recipe, it's the base for my favourite creamy, cheesy queso sauce. This is great on chips but even better on top of burritos and enchiladas. Best of all, you can get the pickiest of eaters to eat their veggies this way.

Ingredient: 2 cups (214 g) cauliflower florets (about 1/2 head small cauliflower), 1 cup (237 ml) water, 3/4 cup (96 g) thick-cut carrot coins, 1/4 cup (34 g) raw cashews, 1/4 cup (24 g) nutritional yeast, Liquid drained from 1 (10-oz [283-g]) can diced tomatoes with green chillies (I like Rotel), 1/2 tsp. smoked paprika, 1/2 tsp. salt (or to taste), 1/4 tsp. chili powder, 1/4 tsp. jalapeño powder, optional, 1/8 tsp. mustard powder.

Preparation: For the Instant Pot, add the cauliflower, water, carrots and cashews to your Instant Pot and cook on high pressure for 5 minutes, then carefully do a quick pressure release by moving the valve to release the pressure. Pour the cooked mixture into a strainer over the sink and drain the extra water. For the blender, put the drained mixture along with the nutritional yeast, liquid drained from the canned tomatoes, smoked paprika, salt, chili powder, jalapeño powder (if using) and mustard powder into your blender. Blend until smooth.

For the mix-ins, scrape out the blender contents into a mixing bowl and stir in the tomatoes and green chillies, bell pepper (if using), minced onion (if using) and cilantro.

You can serve this at room temperature or keep it warm on the lowest slow cooker setting.

INSTANT POT BLACK BEAN DIP: Instant Pot Black Bean Dip is a total breeze to throw together! No cans needed! Simply grab a bag of dried beans and get ready for a party-perfect vegetarian dip that's easy, make-ahead, and SO delicious!

Ingredient: 1.5 cups dried black beans, 1 medium onion, diced, 4 cloves garlic, peeled + minced, 2 medium jalapeños (approx. 1/3 cup chopped), 14.5 oz. can diced or crushed tomatoes, 1 + 3/4 cup vegetable broth, 1.5 TBSP avocado oil, juice of 1 lime, 2 tsp. ground cumin, 1 tsp. smoked paprika, 3/4 tsp. sea salt, 1/2 tsp. chili powder, 1/2 tsp. ground coriander, 4 ounces softened cream cheese, 1 cup freshly grated pepper jack and/or cheddar cheese, chopped tomatoes, sliced jalapeños, diced bell pepper, chopped red onion, cilantro, sour cream, Greek yogurt, salsa, Pico de Gallo, guacamole.

Preparation: Rinse your black beans and toss them in your Instant Pot. Dice and chop your veggies and mince your garlic. Add veggies, garlic, tomatoes, broth, oil, lime juice, and spices to the pot and mix. Press the bean button and cook for 30 minutes high pressure. Allow a natural release (NR) for 10 minutes then quick release (QR) remaining pressure. Use an immersion blender (or a blender or food processor) to blend the tip into creamy deliciousness and once cooled slightly, give it a taste. You can adjust the spiciness by adding anything from hot sauce, spicy salsa, red pepper flakes, or cayenne to the mix and add any extra spices/salt to suit your tastes. As written, it's on the mild side. Serve piled high with all your favourite toppings and dig in!

Vegetarian Dinners You Can Make in an Instant Pot.

The Instant Pot is awesome at cooking some of our favourite vegetarian staples, from perfectly cooked dried beans to tender, well-seasoned spaghetti squash. But it can just as easily deliver complete weeknight dinners. Here are 10 vegetarian dinner recipes using both the pressure cooker and slow cooker functions of your Instant Pot, proving it isn't just for basics.

Instant Pot sweet potatoes: If you've never made an Instant Pot sweet potato, are you in for a treat! Thanks to the Instant Pot, you won't have to wait over an hour for sweet potatoes to bake in the oven.

Ingredients: 1 cup water, 4 sweet potatoes (should be between 3-4 inches in diameter)

Topping ideas: Black beans, Corn, Pico de Gallo, Cilantro, Jalapeno peppers, Green onions, Red onion, Sautéed bell peppers, Sour cream, Shredded cheese.

Preparation: Add 1 cup of water to Instant Pot. Add trivet, then add sweet potatoes. Place lid on Instant Pot and make sure valve is set to seal. Press the pressure cook button and set to high, then cook for 15 minutes. Instant Pot will take about 10 minutes to come to pressure then pressure cook the 15 minutes.

Allow the pressure to release naturally (about 10-15 minutes), then open the lid when pressure gauge has dropped and the lid opens easily. Let cool about 5-10 minutes, then remove sweet potatoes and slice in half. Load with toppings of choice, adding the cheese first if using to ensure it melts. Serve and enjoy! Sweet potato leftovers can be refrigerated up to 5 days.

To freeze sweet potatoes: wrap in foil once cooled for 30-40 min and freeze up to 3 months. Reheat in the microwave for 7-8 minutes to defrost and serve.

PORTOBELLO POT ROAST: This hearty pot roast has all the savoury flavours of a beefy dish, but without the beef. Using the Instant Pot's slow-cook function gives the flavours plenty of time to meld.

Ingredient: 1.25 pounds Yukon gold potatoes, cut into bite-sized pieces, 1 pound baby belle mushrooms (if they are large, cut them in half), 2 large carrots, peeled and cut into bite-sized pieces, 2 cups frozen pearl onions, 4 cloves garlic, peeled and minced, 3 sprigs fresh thyme, 3, cups vegetable stock, divided, 1/2 cup dry red or white wine, 3 tablespoons tomato paste, 2 tablespoons vegetarian Worcestershire sauce, 2 tablespoons corn-starch, Kosher salt and freshly-cracked black pepper, Optional garnish: finely-chopped fresh parsley.

Preparation: Add potatoes, mushrooms, carrots, onions, garlic, thyme, 2.5 cups vegetable stock, wine and Worcestershire together in the bowl of a pressure cooker, and gently toss to combine. Close lid securely and set vent to "Sealing". Press "Manual", then press "Pressure" until the light on "High Pressure" lights up, then adjust the up/down arrows until time reads 20 minutes. Cook. Then let the pressure release naturally, about 15 minutes. Carefully turn the vent to "Venting", just to release any extra pressure that might still be in there. Remove the lid.

In a separate bowl, whisk together the remaining 1/2 cup vegetable stock and corn-starch until combined. Add to the roast mixture, and gently toss to combine. Continue to cook for 1-3 minutes, until the sauce thickens up a bit.

Serve immediately, garnished with fresh parsley if desired

Note: be sure to use vegan Worcestershire sauce.

Instant Pot Minestrone: Here, Instant Pot basics like beans and broth come together to make a wondrous version of the soup we all know and love: minestrone!

Ingredient: 2 tablespoons olive oil, 3 cloves garlic, minced, 1 onion, diced, 2 carrots, peeled and diced, 2 stalks celery, diced, 1 1/2 teaspoons dried basil, 1 teaspoon dried oregano, 1/2 teaspoon fennel seed, 6 cups low sodium chicken broth, 1 (28-ounce) can diced tomatoes, 1 (16-ounce) can kidney beans, drained and rinsed, 1 zucchini, chopped, 1 (3-inch) Parmesan rind, 1 bay leaf, 1 bunch kale, stems removed and leaves chopped, 2 teaspoons red wine vinegar, Kosher salt and freshly ground black pepper, to taste, 1/3 cup freshly grated Parmesan, 2 tablespoons chopped fresh parsley leaves.

Preparation: Set a 6-qt Instant Pot to the high sauté setting. Add olive oil, garlic, onion, carrots and celery. Cook, stirring occasionally, until tender, about 2-3 minutes. Stir in basil, oregano and fennel seed until fragrant, about 1 minute. Stir in chicken stock, diced tomatoes, kidney beans, zucchini, Parmesan rind and bay leaf. Select manual setting; adjust pressure to high, and set time for 5 minutes. When finished cooking, quick-release pressure according to manufacturer's directions. Stir in kale until wilted, about 2 minutes. Stir in red wine vinegar; season with salt and pepper, to taste.

Serve immediately, garnished with Parmesan and parsley, if desired.

Ethiopian-Style Spinach & Lentil Soup: This simple-looking lentil soup comes together quickly and is packed with warm spices and bright, lemony flavour.

Ingredient: 2 tablespoons unsalted butter, 1 tablespoon olive oil, 1 medium red onion, finely chopped, 1 teaspoon garlic powder, 2 teaspoons ground coriander, 1/2 teaspoon cinnamon powder, 1/2 teaspoon turmeric powder, 1/4 teaspoon clove powder, 1/4 teaspoon cayenne pepper, 1/4 teaspoon cardamom powder, 1/4 teaspoon fresh grated nutmeg, 2 cups brown lentils, 8 cups water, 2 teaspoons salt, 1/4 teaspoon pepper, 6 ounces fresh spinach or baby spinach (about 4 packed cups), 4 tablespoons lemon juice.

Preparation: Preheat the pressure cooker (by pressing brown/sauté mode). Add the butter, oil, onion, garlic, coriander, cinnamon, turmeric, clove, cayenne, cardamom, and nutmeg. Sauté three minutes. Add the lentils and water. Close the lid and pressure-cook for 10 minutes at high pressure. When time is up, open the pressure cooker with natural release: Turn off the pressure cooker and wait for pressure to come down naturally, about 15 to 20 minutes. Remove the lid, tilting it away from you. Add the salt and pepper, and mix in the spinach leaves to wilt them into the soup.

Stir in the fresh lemon juice and serve.

Chana Masala: Chana masala — dried chickpeas slow-cooked with tomatoes and spices — is one of those dinners that an Instant Pot or other slow cooker excels at. Assemble it in the morning and come home to a comforting dinner that will have everyone asking for seconds.

Ingredient: 2 cups dried chickpeas, 5 to 6 1/2 cups hot water, depending on desired consistency, 2 black cardamom pods, 2 (1-inch) pieces cassia, 4 to 6 cloves, 2 bay leaves, 1/4 teaspoon turmeric, 1/4 teaspoon ground Indian red chili, 1 1/2 to 2 teaspoon salt

For the masala: 3 tablespoons canola oil, 1 large yellow onion, diced small, 6 cloves garlic, coarsely chopped, 1 (2-inch) piece fresh ginger, peeled and coarsely chopped, about 1 tablespoon, 3 whole peeled tomatoes (canned or fresh) or 8 ounces diced canned tomatoes, 1 1/2 tablespoons ground coriander, 2 teaspoons ground cumin, 1/4 teaspoon turmeric, 1/4 teaspoon ground Indian red chili, 3/4 teaspoon green mango powder, 1/2 teaspoon black salt, 1/2 teaspoon ground black pepper, 2 Serrano chillies, halved lengthwise, 1/4 cup water, Chopped cilantro, for garnish.

Instant Pot Potato and Corn Chowder: Potato and corn chowder is a family favourite. Just make sure to use veggie stock instead of chicken, and of course skip the bacon. And since the Instant Pot does all the work here, don't skimp on the toppings.

Ingredient: 2 slices thick cut bacon chopped, 1/2 medium onion finely chopped, 1 rib celery finely chopped, 1 teaspoon minced garlic, 1 teaspoon salt, 1/4 teaspoon dried thyme, 1/8 teaspoon black pepper, 2 1/2 cups low sodium chicken broth, 3/4 pound Little potatoes any varietal (about 15 potatoes), 4 ears corn, 1/2 cup half and half cream, 1 tablespoon corn starch, shredded cheese or green onions for garnish.

Preparation: Turn the Instant Pot (mine is a 6 quart) to sauté. Add the bacon and onions and cook for 3-4 minutes until browned. Add the celery, garlic, salt, thyme and pepper and cook and stir 1 minute. Add the broth and scrape any browned bits off of the bottom (this helps to prevent a burn message and adds lots of flavour). Turn off the Instant Pot. Roughly chop the little potatoes. Use a knife to remove the corn kernels from the ears. Add potatoes and corn to the Instant Pot. Put the lid on, turn the valve to sealing, and select Manual or Pressure Cook for 2 minutes. It will take about 10-15 minutes to come to pressure and begin counting down. When the cook time is over, let the pressure release naturally for a few minutes, and then open the valve to release remaining pressure. Turn the Instant Pot to sauté, whisk together cream and corn starch and stir into soup to thicken slightly.

Serve with shredded cheese and green onions as desired.

Chickpea Tomato Soup: This Chickpea Tomato Soup is an easy, hearty soup, loaded with chickpeas and vegetables in every bite.

Ingredient: 1 tsp. olive oil, 1/2 cup chopped onion, 1/2 cup diced carrots, 1/2 cup diced celery, 2 garlic cloves, minced, 2 15 oz. cans chickpeas, rinsed and drained, 1 28 oz. can crushed tomatoes, 3 cups reduced sodium chicken broth, or vegetable broth for vegetarians, 1 fresh rosemary sprig, 2 bay leaves, 2 tbsp. chopped fresh basil, fresh black pepper, to taste, 2 cups fresh baby spinach, 1/4 cup shredded parmesan cheese, plus extra optional for garnish.

Preparation: Heat oil in a large non-stick skillet over medium heat. Add the carrots, celery, onion, garlic and sauté until tender and fragrant, about 6 to 8 minutes. Transfer to the instant pot along with the broth, tomatoes, chickpeas, parmesan cheese, and pepper. Add the rosemary, bay leaves and basil, cover and cook on low for 6 hours. When done add the spinach. Remove bay leaves, rosemary sprig and season to taste with salt and black pepper. Ladle soup into bowls and top with extra parmesan cheese if desired.

Slow Cooker Baked Ziti: If you haven't already discovered the pleasure of slow-cooking baked pasta, let me introduce you via the Instant Pot. This cheesy baked ziti is a hit with the whole family.

Ingredient: Cooking spray, 1 pound dried ziti pasta, 48 ounces marinara sauce, 1 (15-ounce) container whole milk ricotta cheese, 2 cups shredded low-moisture mozzarella cheese, divided.

Preparation: Coat a 6-quart or larger slow cooker with cooking spray. Add the ziti, marinara, ricotta, and 1 cup of the mozzarella cheese, and stir well to combine. Sprinkle with the remaining 1 cup of mozzarella.

Cover and cook until the pasta is cooked through and the cheese is melted, on the LOW setting for 3 to 4 hours or on the HIGH setting for 1 to 2 hours. Serve immediately.

Creamy Instant Pot Pasta: This recipe is a seriously creamy Instant Pot pasta recipe that you'll make again and again.

Ingredient: 1 1/2 cups water, 28 ounce can crushed fire roasted tomatoes (or best quality crushed tomatoes), 2 tablespoons olive oil, 1 tablespoon balsamic vinegar, 2 teaspoons garlic powder, 1 teaspoon dried oregano, 1 teaspoon kosher salt, 2 cups baby spinach leaves, tightly packed (or chopped spinach), 8 fresh basil leaves, 8 ounces penne pasta (regular, not whole wheat), 4 ounce goat cheese log

Preparation: Place the following ingredients into the Instant Pot: water, tomatoes, olive oil, balsamic vinegar, garlic powder, oregano, kosher salt, spinach, whole basil leaves, and penne. Cook on high pressure for 5 minutes: Press the Pressure Cook button, making sure the "High Pressure" setting is selected, and set the time. Note that it takes about 10 minutes for the pot to "preheat" and come up to pressure before it starts cooking. (During cooking, avoid touching the metal part of the lid.)

Quick release: Vent the remaining steam from the Instant Pot by moving the pressure release handle to "Venting", covering your hand with a towel or hot pad. Never put your hands or face near the vent when releasing steam. Open the pressure cooker lid.

Open the lid and crumble in the goat cheese; stir until a creamy sauce forms. The sauce will thicken even more as it cools.

Instant Pot Acorn Squash: This vegetarian stuffed acorn squash features a rice stuffing with toasted pecans.

Ingredient: 1 cup white basmati rice, 1/2 teaspoon dried sage, 1/2 teaspoon kosher salt, divided, plus more for sprinkling, 2 small acorn squash, 1 small yellow onion, 2 cloves garlic, 2 stalks celery, 1 tablespoon olive oil, plus more for drizzling, 1 teaspoon dried thyme, 1 teaspoon dried oregano, Fresh ground black pepper, 3 tablespoons unsalted butter, 3/4 cup raw pecan pieces, Feta or goat cheese crumbles, optional.

Preparation: Cook the rice: In an Instant Pot or digital pressure cooker, stir the rice, sage, 1/4 teaspoon kosher salt, and 1 cup of water. Pressure cook on high for 3 minutes. Then vent any remaining steam by moving the pressure release handle to "Venting", covering your hand with a towel or hot pad. (Never put your hands or face near the steam release valve when releasing steam.)

Prep the veggies: While the rice cooks, cut the squash in half and remove seeds, then cut it in half again (into quarters). Dice the onion and celery. Mince the garlic.

Toast the pecans: In a dry skillet over low heat, toast the pecans for about 3 minutes, stirring occasionally, until fragrant. Make the stuffing: Heat the olive oil in a skillet over medium heat. Sauté the onion and celery 5 to 7 minutes until tender and translucent. Add the garlic, thyme, and oregano, and sauté for an additional 2 minutes until fragrant. When the rice is cooked, stir it into the skillet. Stir in 1/4 teaspoon kosher salt, the fresh ground black pepper, butter, and pecans.

Cook the squash: Rinse the Instant Pot and place the steamer basket in the bottom with 1 cup of water. Rub the squash quarters with a bit of olive oil and sprinkle with a few pinches of dried oregano. Place the squash quarters in the pot, stacking as necessary. Pressure cook on high for 6 minutes. After the pot beeps, immediately do a Quick Release: vent the remaining steam by moving the pressure release handle to "Venting", covering your hand with a towel or hot pad.

Serve: Carefully remove the squash from the Instant Pot and sprinkle it with kosher salt. Spoon the stuffing over the squash quarters and serve immediately.

INSTANT POT VEGAN SATISFYING SIDES RECIPES.

Instant Pot 3-Cheese Macaroni and Cheese: This mac and cheese is decadent and over the top delicious. It makes a whole lot and is perfect to bring to a potluck or to serve a crowd.

Ingredient: 3 ¾ cups water, 16 oz. uncooked macaroni noodles, 3 Tbsp. butter, 2 tsp. kosher salt, ½ tsp. pepper, 2 tsp. ground mustard, 1 cup whole milk or half and half, 8 ounces grated sharp cheddar, 8 ounces grated Monterey jack cheese, 8 ounces grated Colby jack cheese, 1 cup panko breadcrumbs (optional).

Preparation: Pour the water into the Instant Pot. Add in the macaroni, butter, salt, pepper and ground mustard. Cover and secure the lid. Make sure the valve is set to sealing. Set the manual/pressure cook button to 4 minutes on high pressure. When the time is up let the pot sit for 5 minutes and then move the valve to venting. Remove the lid and stir in the milk. Then stir in the cheeses a couple of cups at a time until all the cheese is stirred in and creamy and smooth. Optional breadcrumb topping: Unplug your Instant Pot. Sprinkle the breadcrumbs on top of the macaroni and cheese. Place your Crisp Lid on top of the pot. Click the lid into place and set the temperature to 500 degrees and the timer to 4 minutes. When the time is up remove the lid and serve the mac and cheese. If you don't have a Crisp Lid then you can scoop the mac and cheese into a 9×13 inch pan. Sprinkle the breadcrumbs on top and broil in your oven until the breadcrumbs are toasted.

Instant Pot Tomato Basil Parmesan Rice: creamy rice with a punch of flavour from cherry tomatoes and fresh basil. This rice is made quickly in your electric pressure cooker and is a great summer dinner or side dish.

Ingredient: 1 Tbsp. olive oil, ½ cup diced onion, 1 Tbsp. minced garlic, 1 ¾ cups chicken broth or veggie broth, 1 ½ cups uncooked brown rice, 1 (8 oz.) can tomato sauce, 2 cups halved cherry tomatoes, ¼ cup chopped fresh basil, 1 cup shredded or grated parmesan cheese, Salt and pepper.

Preparation: Turn your Instant Pot to the sauté setting. When the display says HOT add in the oil and swirl it around. Add in the onion and sauté for 4 minutes. Add in the garlic and sauté for 20 seconds. Add in the broth and scrape the bottom of the pot. Add in the rice. Then dump the tomato sauce on top without stirring. Cover the pot and secure the lid. Make sure valve is set to sealing.

Set the manual/pressure cook button to 22 minutes. When the time is up let the pot sit for 10 minutes and then move the valve to venting. Remove the lid.

Stir in the tomatoes, basil and parmesan cheese. Salt and pepper to taste. Serve.

Instant Pot Spaghetti Squash Mac and Cheese: if you're looking for a lower calorie and lower carb way to enjoy mac and cheese this recipe is for you. Spaghetti squash is cooked quickly in your electric pressure cooker and then a cheesy sauce is stirred in with the squash strands to make a comforting meal.

Ingredient: 1 spaghetti squash (small enough to fit in your Instant Pot when cut in half), 1/4 cup butter, 1/2 tsp. salt, 1/2 tsp. pepper, 1/2 tsp. garlic powder, 2 cups grated cheddar (I like sharp), 1/2 cup grated Parmesan cheese.

Preparation: Use a paring knife to cut your spaghetti squash in half crosswise (not lengthwise). Use a spoon to scoop out all the seeds and gunk. Pour a cup of water into the bottom of your Instant Pot. Place the trivet in the bottom of the pot. Place the squash halves on top of the trivet. They can face up or down. You may have to manoeuvre them around to fit. Secure the lid on the Instant Pot and make sure the valve is set to "sealing." Set the manual (high pressure) timer to 7 minutes. Once the timer beeps remove the pressure quickly by moving the valve to "venting." Remove the lid and use a towel or hot pad to remove the squash. Use a fork to shred the flesh of the squash into long spaghetti-like strands. Dump the water out of your Instant Pot and remove the trivet. Turn your Instant Pot to the sauté setting. Melt the butter and add in the salt, pepper and garlic powder. Once butter is melted add in the flesh of the spaghetti squash. Coat the squash with the butter and seasonings. Then turn off the Instant Pot.

Stir in the cheeses until melted and creamy. Add additional salt and pepper to taste.

Instant Pot Lentil Stew: a comforting bowl of stew that can be make vegan or can be made with smoked sausage. Lentils cook so quickly in the electric pressure cooker! The leftovers make a great lunch the next day too.

Ingredient: 1 Tbsp. olive oil, 1 yellow onion, diced, 1 cup green or brown lentils, 3 cups chicken broth or vegetable broth, 2 tsp. garlic powder, 1 tsp. dried parsley, 1/2 tsp. dried basil, 1/2 tsp. dried oregano, 1/2 tsp. salt, 1/4 tsp. ground red pepper, 1 (14.5 oz.) can petite diced tomatoes, 1 Tbsp. tomato paste, 1 large carrot, diced

Optional: 10 ounces beef smoked sausage, sliced into quarter inch pieces.

Preparation: Turn your Instant Pot to the sauté function. When the display says HOT add in the oil. Swirl the pot around. Add in the onion and sauté for about 4 minutes. Add in the lentils, broth, garlic powder, parsley, basil, oregano, salt, red pepper, tomatoes, tomato paste, carrot, and sausage. Cover the pot and secure the lid. Make sure valve is set to sealing. Set the manual/pressure cook button to 5 minutes. Let the pot sit for 5-10 minutes and then move the valve to venting. Open the pot. Stir the stew and salt and pepper to taste. Ladle into bowls and serve.

Instant Pot/Slow Cooker Mexican Stuffed Peppers: bell peppers are stuffed with brown rice, black beans and salsa and cooked perfectly in your electric pressure cooker or your crockpot. You can make them vegetarian or with meat, it's up to you. Top with a dollop of sour cream and enjoy this healthy weeknight dinner.

Ingredient: 1 1/2 cups water (Instant Pot version only), 4 large green peppers or 5 medium green peppers, 1/2 cup uncooked instant brown rice, 2 cups picante sauce (I used mild), 1/2 tsp. salt, 1 tsp. cumin, 1 tsp. garlic powder, 1 (14 oz.) can black beans, rinsed and drained

Optional: 1 cup cooked and chopped chicken or 1 cup cooked ground beef or turkey

Grated cheddar and sour cream, for topping.

Preparation: Remove and discard the tops, seeds, and membranes of the bell peppers. In a bowl stir together the rice, picante sauce, salt, cumin, garlic powder, beans, and meat, if desired. Scoop the mixture into the hollowed out peppers. If using the Instant Pot: Pour 1 1/2 cups water in the bottom of your pot. Place a trivet in the bottom of the Instant Pot. Place the peppers on top of the trivet. You may have to arrange them to fit. Cover the pot and secure the lid. Make sure valve is set to sealing. Set the manual/pressure cook button to 6 minutes on high pressure. When the time is up let the pot sit for about 5-10 minutes before moving the valve to venting. Remove the lid. If using the slow cooker: arrange the filled peppers in the bottom of your slow cooker. Cover and cook on low for 5 hours or on high for 3 hours.

Serve the peppers topped with a bit of grated cheddar cheese and a dollop of sour cream, if desired.

Instant Pot Wheat Berry Salad: Instant Pot Wheat Berry Salad–The perfect summer salad for all picnics, potlucks and barbecues. Wheat berries with a lime dressing, black beans, avocados, grape tomatoes, red peppers, jicama, red onion and cilantro. It's got the crunch, the chewiness and the bright flavours all in one salad.

Ingredient: FOR THE WHEAT BERRIES— 1 cup wheat, 4 cups water, 1 tsp. salt.

FOR THE SALAD— 1 large avocado, diced, 1 1/2 cups cubed jicama, 1 small red onion, finely diced, red bell pepper, finely diced, 1 (15-ounce can) black beans, drained and rinsed, 2 cups grape or cherry tomatoes sliced in half, 1/2 cup lime juice, 1/3 cup chopped fresh cilantro, 1/4 cup extra-virgin olive oil, 1 teaspoon ground cumin, 1 tsp. salt, 1 teaspoon freshly ground black pepper.

Preparation: Cook the wheat berries. Place wheat berries, water, and salt into Instant Pot. Cover the pot and secure the lid. Make sure valve is set to sealing. Set the manual/pressure cook button to 30 minutes on high pressure. When time is up perform a quick release by moving the valve to venting. Pour the wheat into a sieve and run cold water over it. Set aside.

Toss it together. Combine the avocados, jicama, onion, bell pepper, wheat berries (cooked previously), black beans, tomatoes, lime juice, cilantro, olive oil, cumin, salt and pepper in a medium bowl and adjust seasonings to taste. Chill at least 30 minutes and up to overnight before serving.

Instant Pot Tomato Basil Parmesan Orzo: Instant Pot Tomato Basil Parmesan Orzo–orzo pasta is tossed with fresh basil, garlic, halved cherry tomatoes and parmesan cheese for a perfect side dish or meatless meal.

Ingredient: 1 Tbsp. olive oil, 1 yellow onion, diced, 4 garlic cloves, minced, 3 1/2 cup chicken broth (or vegetable broth), 2 1/3 cup uncooked orzo pasta, 1/2 tsp salt, 1/2 tsp pepper, 1/3 cup chopped fresh basil, 1 cup grated parmesan cheese, 1 pint cherry tomatoes, washed and sliced in half.

Preparation: Turn your Instant Pot to the sauté function. When the display says HOT add in the olive oil and swirl it around. Add in the diced onion and sauté for about 3-5 minutes. Add in the garlic and sauté for 30 seconds. Add in the chicken broth and scrape any bits off the bottom of the pot. Add in the orzo, salt and pepper. Turn off the sauté function.

Cover the pot and secure the lid. Make sure valve is set to sealing. Set the manual/pressure cook button to 1 minute on high pressure. When the time is up let the pot sit there for 5 minutes and then perform a quick release.

Remove the lid and stir in the basil, cheese and tomatoes. Scoop onto plates and enjoy!

Instant Pot Spinach Artichoke Mac and Cheese:

Instant Pot Spinach Artichoke Mac and Cheese–creamy, cheesy pasta with fresh spinach and chopped artichokes is a perfect way to indulge while sneaking in some greens.

Ingredient: 3 3/4 cups chicken broth (or water or vegetable broth), 16 ounces (1 pound) cavatappi, cellentani or macaroni pasta, uncooked,1/2 tsp. salt, 1 or 2 (14 oz.) cans artichoke hearts, drained and chopped, 10 oz. bag of fresh spinach, 8 ounces Monterey jack cheese, grated

1/2 cup grated or shredded parmesan cheese, 1/2 tsp. pepper, Red pepper flakes, optional.

Preparation: Pour chicken broth into Instant Pot. Add in the uncooked pasta and salt.

Cover and secure lid. Make sure valve is set to sealing. Set the manual/pressure cook button to 3 minutes on high pressure. When time is up let the pot sit there for 5-10 minutes and then move the valve to venting. Remove the lid.

Turn Instant Pot to sauté mode and add in the artichokes and spinach. Stir the spinach in until it is wilted and cooks down. Add in the Monterey jack cheese and the parmesan cheese and pepper. Stir until cheese is melted. Sprinkle in a bit of red pepper flakes, if desired.

Scoop onto serving dishes and enjoy.

Instant Pot Creamy Polenta With Roasted Tomatoes: Instant Pot Creamy Polenta with Roasted Tomatoes–easiest to make polenta ever, thanks to your electric pressure cooker! Creamy polenta is served hot with balsamic drizzled roasted tomatoes, mushrooms and garlic and then topped with tart goat cheese. A perfect meatless meal that will leave you feeling satisfied.

Ingredient: 5 cups water, 1 cup polenta/corn grits (not the instant kind), 1 tsp. salt, 10 ounces white mushrooms, sliced, 10 ounces cherry or grape tomatoes, halved, 2 Tbsp. olive oil, 1 Tbsp. balsamic vinegar, 1 Tbsp. minced garlic, Salt and pepper, 6 Tbsp. goat cheese, for serving.

Preparation: Add water, polenta and salt to your Instant Pot. Whisk. Cover the pot and make sure valve is set to sealing. Set the porridge button to 20 minutes (if you don't have a porridge button you can use the manual/pressure cook button for 20 minutes on high pressure).

Turn your oven to 400° F. While the polenta is cooking slice your vegetables. Add mushrooms, tomatoes, oil, balsamic vinegar and garlic to a large bowl. Toss to coat vegetables in the oil. Spread out the contents of bowl onto a sheet pan. Lightly salt and pepper. Cook in the oven for 15-20 minutes. Once the Instant Pot timer beeps, let the pressure release naturally for 10 minutes and then move the valve to venting to remove any remaining pressure. Carefully open the lid. Whisk the polenta until creamy.

Scoop into bowls and top with roasted veggies and top with 1 tablespoon of goat cheese.

Instant Pot Spinach Mushroom Pesto Pasta: Instant Pot Spinach Mushroom Pesto Pasta–an easy, tasty and fast meatless meal of your favourite type of pasta enveloped in a basil pesto sauce with plenty of sautéed mushrooms and spinach. Add bites of chicken if you prefer.

Ingredient: 1 Tbsp. canola oil, 8 oz. (1/2 lb.) white button mushrooms, chopped, 1/2 tsp. kosher salt, 1/2 tsp. black pepper, 8 oz. uncooked orecchiette pasta (or other pasta of your choice), 1 3/4 cups water, 5 oz. fresh spinach, 1/2 cup pesto, 1/3 cup grated mozzarella cheese or parmesan cheese (optional).

Preparation: Turn your Instant Pot to the sauté function. While it heats up, chop up your mushrooms. When the display reads HOT add in your oil. Then add in your mushrooms, salt and pepper and sauté for about 5 minutes. Add in your pasta and water. Cover and secure the lid into place. Make sure valve is set to sealing. Set the manual/pressure cook button to 5 minutes (if cooking with another type of pasta read my note below). When the time is up move the valve to venting. Remove the lid. Stir in the spinach. And then stir in the pesto and cheese. If there is too much liquid you can use a corn-starch slurry to thicken the sauce by mixing 1 Tbsp. of corn-starch with 1 Tbsp. of water and then stirring the mixture into the pot.

Scoop the pasta into serving dishes and enjoy! Store leftovers in an airtight container in the refrigerator for up to a week.

COMFORT FOOD FAVOURITE.

Instant Pot Vegan Quinoa Burrito Bowls: This Mexican-inspired dish features protein-rich quinoa and black beans mixed with spicy salsa.

Ingredient: 1 teaspoon extra-virgin olive oil, 1/2 red onion, diced, 1 bell pepper, diced, 1/2 teaspoon salt, 1 teaspoon ground cumin, 1 cup quinoa, rinsed well, 1 cup prepared salsa, 1 cup water, 1 1/2 cups cooked black beans, or 1 (15 oz.) can, drained and rinsed, Optional toppings: Avocado, guacamole, fresh cilantro, green onions, salsa, lime wedges, shredded lettuce.

Preparation: Heat the oil in the bottom of the Instant Pot, using the "sauté" setting. Sauté the onions and peppers until start to soften, about 5 to 8 minutes, then add in cumin and salt and sauté another minute. Turn of the Instant Pot for a moment. Add in the quinoa, salsa, water, and beans, then seal the lid, making sure that the switch at the top is flipped from venting to sealing. Press the "rice" button, or manually cook at low pressure for 12 minutes. Let the pressure naturally release once the cooking is over, to make sure the quinoa completely absorbs the liquid. (This takes 10 to 15 minutes.) Remove the lid, being careful to avoid any steam releasing from the pot, and fluff the quinoa with a fork. Serve warm, with any toppings you love, such as avocado, diced onions, salsa, and shredded lettuce.

Leftovers can be stored in an airtight container in the fridge for up to a week. You can quickly reheat on the stove top, or serve cold!

Curried Butternut Squash Soup: Sautéed onions and creamy coconut milk make this lightly spiced (and quintessentially fall) soup extra flavourful.

Ingredient: 1 teaspoon extra-virgin olive oil, 1 large onion, chopped, 2 cloves garlic, minced

1 tablespoon curry powder, 1 (3 pound) butternut squash, peeled and cut into 1-inch cubes (or use frozen), 1 1/2 teaspoons fine sea salt, 3 cups water, 1/2 cup coconut milk (coconut cream is fine, too)

OPTIONAL TOPPINGS: Hulled pumpkin seeds, dried cranberries.

Preparation: Hit the "sauté" button on the Instant Pot. Add in the olive oil and onion, and sauté until tender, about 8 minutes. Add in the garlic and curry powder sauté just until fragrant, about one minute. Turn the Instant Pot off for a moment, then add the butternut squash, salt, and water into the pot. Secure the lid and move the steam release valve to "sealing." Select the Manual or Pressure Cook button (this will vary by machine, but they do the same thing) and let the soup cook at high pressure for 15 minutes.

When the soup is done, wait 10 minutes before releasing the pressure. When the screen reads LO:10, you can move the steam release valve to "venting" to release any remaining pressure. When the floating valve in the lid drops, it's safe to open the lid.

Use an immersion blender to puree the soup directly in the pot, or transfer the cooked soup to a blender or food processor to blend until smooth. If using a blender, be sure to lightly cover the vent in your blender lid with a dish towel, to help the pressure from the steam release without splattering. (The pressure from hot liquids can blow the lid off your blender otherwise, and cause burns.)

Return the blended soup to the pot and stir in the coconut milk. (You can use coconut cream, if you don't mind a slightly creamier soup.) Adjust any seasoning to taste at this point, I usually add a touch more salt, and serve warm. Top with hulled pumpkin seeds and dried cranberries, if desired. For a sweeter soup, try adding a touch of maple syrup to taste.

Leftovers can be stored in an airtight container for up to a week in the fridge.

The Best Instant Pot Mac and Cheese: This dish is perfect for one of those snowy Sunday evenings after a day on the slopes or an afternoon reading by the fire.

Ingredient: 1 pound macaroni, 4 cups water, 2 teaspoons prepared yellow mustard, 1 teaspoon salt, 12 ounce can evaporated milk, 8 ounces Tillamook medium cheddar cheese grated, ¾ cup parmesan cheese grated, 2 Tablespoons butter, ¼ teaspoon nutmeg, Salt and pepper to taste.

Preparation: Mix the macaroni, water, mustard, and salt in your Instant Pot. Close and lock the lid of the Instant Pot. Press "Manual" and adjust the timer to 4 minutes (or half the time on the macaroni cooking directions). Check that the cooking pressure is on "high" and that the release valve is set to "Sealing". When time is up, open the Instant Pot using "Quick Pressure Release". Stir the pasta to break it up. Add the evaporated milk, cheese, butter and nutmeg; stir until completely incorporated and then, cheese has melted and coated the pasta.

Season to taste with salt and pepper, then serve immediately.

Instant Pot Cheesy South-western Lentils and Brown Rice: Simmered with diced tomatoes and green chili, this stew is chock full of flavour. Add in some melted sharp cheddar and mozzarella and you'll be good to go.

Ingredient: 1/2 red onion finely chopped, 1/2 red bell pepper finely chopped, 4 garlic cloves minced, 3/4 cup Bob's Red Mill brown rice, 3/4 cup Bob's Red Mill brown lentils, 2 1/2 cups vegetable broth, 1 can petite diced tomatoes 15 oz., 1 can diced green chillies 4 oz., 1 Tbsp. taco seasoning, 2 tsp. dried oregano, 1 tsp. kosher salt, 1/2 tsp. Black pepper, 2 cups shredded cheese I prefer mozzarella and sharp cheddar, 1/4 cup chopped fresh cilantro for topping.

Preparation: Add all ingredients, except cheese and cilantro, to your Instant Pot. Set to manual and cook on high pressure for 15 minutes. Allow pressure to naturally release for 15 minutes then release remaining pressure. Remove cover and stir in half of the cheese. Sprinkle remaining cheese over the top and replace the cover. Allow to stand for 5 minutes.

Sprinkle with cilantro and serve. Enjoy!

Cauliflower Tikka Masala: With a mix of Indian spices and a flavourful, creamy base, this vegan veggie stew will transform weeknight dinner forever.

Ingredient: 1 tbsp. vegan butter (or oil), 1 medium onion, diced, 3 cloves of garlic, minced, 1 tbsp. freshly grated ginger, 2 tsp. dried fenugreek leaves, 2 tsp. gram masala, 1 tsp. turmeric, 1/2 tsp. ground chili, 1/4 tsp. ground cumin, 1/2 tsp. salt, 1 28-ounce can diced tomatoes with their juice (about 3 cups), 1 tbsp. (15ml) maple syrup, 1 small cauliflower head, cut into florets (about 4 cups florets), 1/2 cup (118ml) non-dairy yogurt (or cashew cream)

Optional toppings: fresh parsley, roasted cashews.

Preparation: Set the Instant Pot to sauté mode for 7 minutes. Add the oil. Once hot, add the onion, garlic, and ginger. Cook for 3-4 minutes, or until the onions start to caramelize and become soft. Add the dried fenugreek leaves, gram masala, turmeric, chili, cumin, and salt. Continue to cook for another 2 minutes, stirring regularly to make sure it doesn't burn. Add a couple of tablespoons of water and scrape the bottom to make sure nothing is sticking to it, this will prevent the Instant Pot from giving you a "burn" message.

Add the crushed tomatoes, maple syrup, and cauliflower florets. Secure the lid and close the vent to Sealing. Press the Pressure Cook button and adjust the time to 2 minutes. The Instant Pot will take about 10 minutes to come to pressure, then cook under pressure for 2 minutes. Once the program is finished and you have heard the beeps, wait 1 minute and release the pressure. Stir in the non-dairy yogurt and stir to combine.

Serve hot with rice, Nan, or tofu, and top with fresh parsley and roasted cashews.

Instant Pot Sesame Basil Noodles with Roasted Veggies: Infused with nutty sesame oil and spicy ginger, this Asian-inspired noodle dish is perfect for a quick and easy dinner on the go (and it's great for leftovers the next day.).

Ingredient: ROASTED VEGGIES— 1 bell pepper, diced, 1 (about 300g) sweet potato, peeled and diced, 1 head broccoli, cut into florets, 1 tbsp. (15ml) olive oil, 1 tbsp. (15ml) soy sauce, 1/4 tsp. ground ginger, 1/4 tsp. ground chili powder.

NOODLES— 8 ounces (227g) linguine pasta, broken in half, 2 cups and 2 tbsp. (500ml) water, 3 tbsp. (45ml) soy sauce, 1 and 1/2 tbsp. sesame oil, 1 tbsp. (15ml) chili oil, 1 tbsp. (15ml) maple syrup, 1 tbsp. (15ml) white rice vinegar, 1 clove of garlic, minced, 1/8 tsp. five-spice powder (optional), 1/4 cup (6g) fresh basil, chopped.

For topping: sesame seeds, basil.

Preparation: Preheat oven to 400°F (200°C) and line a baking sheet with parchment paper.

Add the diced bell pepper, sweet potato, and broccoli to a large mixing bowl. Pour in the olive oil, and soy sauce and add the ground ginger and chili powder. Mix using your hands to coat the vegetables with the oil and spices. Transfer the veggies to the prepared baking sheet and spread into an even layer. Bake for 20-22 minutes, or until veggies are slightly browned. While the veggies are roasting, prepare the noodles.

NOODLES— add the noodles broken in half to the Instant Pot liner. Then add the water, soy sauce, sesame oil, chili oil, maple syrup, rice vinegar, minced garlic, five-spice powder if using, and fresh basil leaves.

479

Close the lid and pressure cook on manual for 8 minutes. Let the pressure release naturally for 3 minutes before doing a quick release of the steam.

Transfer the roasted veggies to the Instant Pot liner and mix until combined. Serve immediately topped with fresh basil and sesame seeds.

Lentil Sloppy Joes: For a healthier, veggie-based version of the traditional ground beef classic, try this innovative vegan recipe with a secret ingredient (liquid smoke!).

Ingredient: 1 tablespoon oil (Instant Pot or stovetop only, optional, see note below), 1 small, yellow onion diced, 3 garlic cloves minced, 2 teaspoons oregano, 1 teaspoon paprika, 1 tablespoon chili powder, 1 teaspoon salt, 1/2 teaspoon ground black pepper, 1 cup dry brown lentils, 1 1/2 cups vegetable broth or water, 1 28-oz can no salt added crushed tomatoes, 2 tablespoons tomato paste, 1 tablespoon yellow mustard, 3 tablespoons vegan Worcestershire sauce, 1/2 teaspoon liquid smoke (optional, see note below), 1-2 tablespoons pure maple syrup (optional).

Preparation: Set your Instant Pot to the Sauté function. Add oil. Once the oil is hot, add the onions and sauté for 2 minutes. Add the garlic. Sauté for another 2 minutes. Add the oregano, paprika, chili powder, salt, and pepper. Mix until spices have coated the onions and garlic. Cancel the sauté function. Add the brown lentils, the broth or water, crushed tomatoes, tomato paste, yellow mustard, and vegan Worcestershire sauce. Stir until everything has combined.

Lock the lid in place and make sure the steam release handle is closed. Set to manual high pressure for 12 minutes. Instant Pot will take roughly 10 minutes to build pressure, timer will start counting down after it has reached pressure. After the time has ended, let the pressure release naturally, this will take roughly 20 minutes. Once the pressure has been released naturally (you will know pressure has been released when the float valve has dropped back down), slowly unlock and remove the lid. Stir so everything combines.

If using, add the liquid smoke, stir and taste. If you find it too acidic, add maple syrup, starting with 1 tablespoon, to balance it out. Stir to combine and taste again. Add another tablespoon of maple syrup, if needed. Serve on rolls of your choice with toppings and sides of your choice (see above for suggestions).

Instant Pot Artichokes with Lemon Chive Butter: The Instant Pot isn't just for soups and stews. It's also an easy way to cook tough vegetables like steamed artichokes, which pair perfectly with a lemon and herb dipping sauce.

Ingredient: 3 large globe artichokes, 1/2 lemon, 2 tablespoons extra-virgin olive oil, 4 tablespoons butter, melted, 2 tablespoons lemon juice, 2 tablespoons minced fresh chives, 1/8 teaspoon kosher salt.

Preparation: Use a serrated edge knife to cut an inch off the top of the artichokes and cut off the stems. Rub the half lemon over the artichokes where they've been cut to prevent browning. Use scissors to trim any sharp tips from the tips of the leaves. Pour 1 1/2 cups water into the Instant Pot with the metal insert in place. Set the artichokes in the pot, stem-side-up. Cover and set to Manual/High for 13 minutes with the vent closed.

Release the steam with care and open the pot. Test to see if the artichokes are done by tasting a leaf or two and inserting the tip of a knife in the stem. It should slide in with relative ease. If they're not quite done, cook another 1 to 2 minutes. Whisk together the olive oil, melted butter, lemon juice, chives, and salt. Serve with the artichokes.

Instant Pot Broccoli Cheddar Quiche: Eggs are a mainstay ingredient for many vegetarians; they're filled with protein and a delicious foil to healthy veggies and tangy cheeses, like in this easy quiche recipe.

Ingredient: 6 large eggs, ½ cup whole milk, ½ teaspoon kosher salt, ¼ teaspoon freshly ground black pepper, 1 small head broccoli about 8 ounces, finely chopped, 3 green onions white and light green parts, sliced, 1 cup shredded Cheddar cheese 4 ounces.

Preparation: Butter a 1½-quart soufflé dish or a 7-cup round heatproof glass container. Fold a 20-inch-long sheet of aluminium foil in half lengthwise twice to create a 3-inch-wide strip. Centre it underneath the soufflé dish to act as a sling for lifting the dish into and out of the Instant Pot. Pour 1 1/2cups water into the pot and add the trivet. In a bowl, whisk together the eggs, milk, salt, and pepper. Stir in the broccoli, green onions, and cheese.

Pour the egg mixture into the prepared dish. Then, holding the ends of the foil sling, lift the dish and lower it into the Instant Pot. Fold over the ends of the sling so they fit inside the pot. Secure the lid and set the Pressure Release to Sealing. Select Manual setting and set the cooking time for 25 minutes at high pressure. Let the pressure release naturally for at least 10 minutes, then move the Pressure Release to Venting to release any remaining steam. Open the pot and, wearing heat-resistant mitts, grasp the ends of the foil sling and lift the quiche out of the Instant Pot. Let the quiche cool for at least 5 minutes, giving it time to reabsorb any liquid and set up.

Slice and serve warm or at room temperature.

Coconut Jasmine Rice: Rice is another ingredient that can be totally transformed using the Instant Pot. This vegan and gluten-free recipe is a great side dish for a veggie stir-fry or other hearty main course.

Ingredient: 2 cups Jasmine rice, 1 can reduced-fat coconut milk, (Lite coconut milk) 13.5 ounces, 1 cup water, 1 Tablespoon lime juice, 1 cup frozen peas, defrosted.

Preparation: Rinse the rice in a mesh strainer. Add the rice to the Instant Pot along with the coconut milk and water. Stir to combine. Close the lid and push the Rice function button. If you have a display, it will show as 12 minutes at low pressure. Note that the cooking time may adjust once the Instant Pot has come up to pressure.

After the rice is done cooking, allow the pressure to release naturally. After the pressure has released, remove the lid and add in the lime juice and peas. Use a rice paddle to gently fold all the ingredients together until well combined.

Let rest for a few minutes, then serve.

Cilantro Lime Quinoa: Ready in just 15 minutes, this bright side dish features lime juice and zest for added flavour.

Ingredient: 1 cup quinoa, (any colour) rinsed and drained, 1 1/4 cups vegetable broth, (for Instant Pot method) or 2 cups for stove top method, 2 Tablespoons lime juice, zest of one lime, 1/2 cup chopped cilantro, salt, to taste.

Preparation: Add the quinoa and 1 1/4 cup vegetable broth to the Instant Pot. Close the lid and select the manual button. Set the timer for 5 minutes.

When the 5 minutes is up, allow the pressure to release naturally.

Once the pressure has been released, remove the lid and stir in the lime juice, lime zest, and cilantro. Taste and add salt, as desired.

VEGAN LUNCH RECIPES BY INSTANT POT.

Smoky Sweet Pecan Brussels sprouts: a little bit sweet, a little bit smoky, with a nutty crunch. And they only take about 15 minutes to make!

Ingredient: 2 cups small baby Brussels sprouts - 176 g, as close to the same size as possible, ¼, cup water - 60 ml, 1/2 teaspoon liquid smoke

Sauté Ingredients— 1/4 cup chopped pecans - 28 g, 2 tablespoons maple syrup - 30 ml, salt - to taste.

Preparation: For the pressure cooker, add the Brussels sprouts, water and liquid smoke to your Instant Pot and mix well. Put the lid on and close the pressure valve. Cook on high pressure for 2 minutes. (Note: If you have very large Brussels sprouts, you may need to double the cooking time.) Once the cooking time is up, carefully move the pressure release valve to release the pressure manually.

For the sauté, switch to the sauté function and add in the pecans and maple syrup and reduce the liquid as you finish cooking the sprouts. Remove from the heat once tender and add salt to taste.

Instant Pot Stuffed Squash with Wild Rice: The key ingredient that makes this stuffed acorn squash healthy and filling is chickpeas. Canned chickpeas are one of my pantry staples. They are inexpensive, rich in fibre and protein, and incredibly versatile.

Ingredient: 1/2 cup uncooked wild rice — you can also use a brown and wild rice blend like this one, 1 teaspoon kosher salt — divided, 3 small — 1 pound each acorn squashes, halved lengthwise, stems trimmed, and seeded, 1 tablespoon olive oil, 1 medium shallot — finely chopped, or 1/2 small yellow onion, finely chopped, 3 large cloves garlic — minced (about 1 tablespoon), 8 ounces baby Bella — cremini mushrooms, finely chopped, 1/2 teaspoon black pepper, 1 can reduced-sodium chickpeas — (15 ounces) rinsed and drained, 1/3 cup reduced-sugar dried cranberries, 1/4 cup toasted pepitas — or chopped pecans, 1 tablespoon fresh thyme leaves — chopped.

Preparation: Bring 1 1/2 cups water to a boil in a small saucepan. Add the rice and 1/2 teaspoon kosher salt. Reduce heat to low, cover, and let simmer until the rice is tender, about 55 minutes. Drain off any excess liquid. Set aside. Pour 1/2 cup water into the bottom of an Instant Pot or electric pressure cooker. Place the steamer basket in the pot, then add the squash, cut sides up (they will overlap). Be sure not to exceed the max fill line. If your squash are larger and you exceed the line, cook the squash in two batches. Seal the lid, set pressure valve to sealing, and cook on HIGH (manual) for 4 minutes. Allow the pressure to release naturally for 5 minutes, then immediately vent to release any remaining pressure. Drain and arrange on a large serving plate or baking sheet.

Meanwhile, heat the olive oil in a large skillet over medium low. Add the shallot and cook until softened, about 4 minutes. Add the garlic and cook 30 seconds until fragrant, then add the mushrooms, black pepper, and remaining 1/2 teaspoon kosher salt. Increase heat to medium and cook until the mushrooms are softened and browned, about 5 to 7 additional minutes. Add the chickpeas, cranberries, pepitas, thyme, and cooked rice and stir to heat through, about 2 additional minutes. Taste and adjust seasonings as desired.

Spoon the hot filling into the squash halves. Serve immediately or keep warm in a 350 degree F oven.

Seasoned Black Beans: This Instant Pot Black Beans recipe makes a simple, tasty, healthy & budget friendly lunch. As well as being great on their own, they work equally as well as a base for other meals, so are perfect for meal prep!

Ingredient: 450g / 2½ cups dried black beans , no need to soak before using, 1 medium onion , chopped finely, 4 cloves garlic , chopped finely, 1 teaspoon chili flakes , or 1 fresh chili, (you can omit the chili if you prefer), 1 tablespoon ground cumin, 1 teaspoon ground coriander, 1 large bay leaf, 1 teaspoon dried mint , optional but recommended if you have it, 720 mls / 3 cups flavourful broth/stock, 1 lime, juice only, up to 1 teaspoon salt , plus more to taste if required.

Preparation: Add all ingredients except the lime to the Instant Pot and stir. Put the lid on the Instant Pot and seal the vent. Cook on high pressure MANUAL or PRESSURE COOK in newer models, for 25 minutes for tender, soft beans, (or 30 minutes of you prefer really soft slightly mushy beans) and leave the pressure to release naturally before opening the lid.

Please note that the beans continue to cook during the natural pressure release so if you skip this step and vent manually your beans will turn out much firmer. Add salt to taste then squeeze the juice of the lime into the beans and give them a quick stir before serving.

Instant Pot Maple Bourbon Sweet Potato Chili: A sweet and spicy soup with a kick, this Maple Bourbon Sweet Potato Instant Pot Chili is the perfect autumnal vegan and gluten-free family meal.

Ingredient: 1 tbsp. cooking oil, 1 small yellow onion, thinly sliced, 2-3 cloves garlic minced, 4 cups sweet potatoes, peeled and cubed into 1/2 pieces, 2 cups vegetable broth, 1 1/2 tbsp. chili powder, 2 tsp. cumin, 1/2 tsp. paprika, 1/4 tsp. cayenne pepper, 2 (15) ounce cans kidney beans, drained and rinsed, 1 (15) ounce can diced tomatoes, 1/4 cup bourbon, 2 tbsp. maple syrup, salt and pepper, to taste, a few fresh springs of cilantro, 2 green onions, diced, 3 small corn tortillas, toasted and sliced (optional).

Preparation: Turn your Instant Pot to sauté, add oil, and let it heat up for 30 seconds. Once the oil is hot, add onions and sauté for about 5 minutes, stirring occasionally, until onions are translucent and fragrant. Add garlic and sauté for another 30 seconds. Add cubed sweet potatoes, chili powder, cumin, paprika, and cayenne pepper, stirring until vegetables are well coated. Add vegetable broth, beans, tomatoes, maple syrup, and bourbon. Secure the lid on the Instant Pot and set the mode to "soup". Set a timer for 15 minutes. Once the timer goes off, lid should release itself. If it doesn't, turn the air valve to "venting" until the pressure has been released. Remove lid and check to make sure the sweet potatoes are tender. If using tortillas, lightly oil a cast iron skillet and pan-fry the tortillas on each side for 2-3 minutes until crispy. Remove from heat and let cool before cutting into thin strips.

Serve with cilantro, green onions, and toasted tortillas.

Instant Pot Walnut Lentil Tacos: I love these most wrapped in a flour tortilla with lots of shredded lettuce and salsa, but they also taste great over a loaded salad with crunchy tortilla chips. Either way, it's a healthy, protein-packed weeknight meal that you are sure to love.

Ingredient: 1 white onion, diced, 1 tablespoon olive oil, 1 garlic clove, minced, 1 tablespoon chili powder, 1/2 teaspoon garlic powder, 1/4 teaspoon onion powder, 1/4 teaspoon red pepper flakes, 1/4 teaspoon oregano, 1/2 teaspoon paprika, 1 1/2 teaspoon ground cumin, 1/2 teaspoon kosher salt, 1/4 teaspoon freshly ground pepper, 2 1/4 cups vegetable broth, 1 15 ounce can fire-roasted diced tomatoes, 3/4 cup chopped walnuts, 1 cup dried brown lentils, Taco toppings of choice: shredded lettuce, tomato, jalapenos, Flour or corn tortillas.

Preparation: Turn the Instant Pot on and press the Sauté button. Add the olive oil, onion and garlic clove and sauté until onion is tender and cooked through, stirring often, about 3-4 minutes. Add the spices and stir together. Hit cancel and add the vegetable broth, tomatoes, walnuts and lentils and stir to combine. Place the top on and cook on high manual pressure for 15 minutes. Let pressure come down naturally for 4 minutes, then quick release. Remove the lid and stir lentils, seasoning to taste if needed.

Serve lentils on tortillas of choice with toppings. The lentil mixture will thicken as it cools.

Instant Pot Quinoa Enchiladas: What do we call this? It's got all the flavours of enchiladas, but it's definitely not enchiladas. No rolling, no filling, no baking. Just throwing all of the ingredients in the pressure cooker and in 25 minutes, lunch is served.

Ingredient: 3 tablespoons oil (use canola), 3 tablespoons all-purpose flour (see notes for GF version), 1 tablespoon chili powder, 1 1/2 teaspoons cumin, 1/2 teaspoon oregano, 1/2 teaspoon garlic powder, 1/4 teaspoon salt, 1/8 teaspoon cinnamon, 1/4 teaspoon cayenne pepper, 1 (15 ounce) can crushed tomatoes, 1 cup water (or vegetable broth).

Enchilada Ingredients: 2 bell peppers, chopped, 1 medium onion, chopped, 1 cup enchilada sauce, 1 medium zucchini, chopped, 1 cup uncooked quinoa, 3/4 cup water, 1 (15 ounce) can black beans, drained and rinsed, 1 (15 ounce) can corn, drained and rinsed, 1 (4 ounce) can diced jalapeños, 1/4 cup fresh cilantro, 4 corn tortillas, cut into strips, 1 cup shredded cheddar cheese

Preparation: Make the enchilada sauce: heat the oil in a medium saucepan over medium heat. Stir in the flour and cook until golden brown, about 3-4 minutes stirring often. Add in the rest of the spices: chili powder, cumin, garlic powder, oregano, salt, cinnamon, and cayenne and stir another minute until toasted. Whisk in the crushed tomatoes and water and stir until thickened, about 5-7 minutes. Remove 1 cup of the sauce and set the rest aside for drizzling over finished dish or for later. (This sauce freezes beautifully!) Turn the Instant Pot on and hit the sauté button. Add the bell peppers, onion, zucchini and a drizzle of olive oil and pinch of salt. Cook, stirring often, until vegetables are soft. Add in the uncooked quinoa and cook another minute or two until just toasted. Press the cancel button on the Instant Pot and add in the water and 1 cup of the enchilada sauce. Cover and cook at high pressure for 1 minute, then let the pressure come down naturally.

Remove the lid and immediately once pressure has subsided (about 15 minutes) then stir in the black beans, corn, jalapeno, cheese, and cilantro and corn tortillas. Serve hot, with extra enchilada sauce if desired

Instant Pot Apple Spice Steel Cut Oats: Substitute almond milk for cow's milk and you've got one heck of a vegan lunch.

Ingredient: 1 cup steel cut oats, 1/2 cup unsweetened plain applesauce, 1 teaspoon ground cinnamon, 1/2 teaspoon ground nutmeg, 1/4 teaspoon salt, 3 cups water, 1 small apple, chopped, 1/2 cup raisins (optional), chopped nuts, or fresh diced or sliced apples for garnish (optional), milk (enough to reach desired consistency), sweetener, to taste (optional).

Preparation: Add steel cut oats, applesauce, ground cinnamon, ground nutmeg, salt, and water to your Instant Pot. Stir to combine all the ingredients. Lock the lid in place and make sure the steam release handle is closed. Set to manual high pressure for 10 minutes. Instant Pot will take roughly 10 minutes to build pressure, timer will start counting down after it has reached pressure. After the time has ended, let the Instant Pot naturally release the pressure. This will take roughly 20 minutes.

Once the pressure has been released naturally (you will know pressure has been released when the float valve has dropped back down), slowly unlock and remove the lid. Stir the oats so everything recombines. Add the apples and, if using, raisins, and stir. Let sit for a minute or two so apples (and raisins) can warm up. Add desired amount of milk and stir. Add sweetener, to taste. Sprinkle nuts and/or fresh fruit on top for garnish.

Instant Pot Vegan Lentil Chili: Thick, hearty and packed with plant-based protein. You're going to love this Instant Pot vegan lentil chili.

Ingredient: 1 tablespoon olive oil, 1 onion, chopped, 4 cloves minced garlic, 2 carrots, chopped, 1–2 jalapeños, chopped, 1 1/2 tablespoons chili powder, 1 tablespoon cumin, 1/2 teaspoon ground coriander, 1 teaspoon dried oregano, 1/2–3/4 teaspoon salt, 1 (15 ounce) can crushed tomatoes, 1 (28 ounce) can fire roasted diced tomatoes, 2 cups brown or green lentils (I used French green lentils for this, I find they hold their shape best), 4 cups vegetable broth, 1 teaspoon fresh lime juice, 1/2 cup chopped fresh cilantro

Preparation: Press the sauté button on the Instant Pot. Heat the olive oil in the pot, then add the onion, garlic, carrots and jalapeños and sauté until soft, about 3-4 minutes.

Add the spices and remaining ingredients except for lime juice and cilantro, then cover. Cook on high pressure for 15 minutes, then quick-release.

Stir in lime juice and cilantro, and serve.

Instant Pot Vegan Butter Chicken: The garnish of fresh minced ginger and chili and some dried fenugreek takes this dish to an amazing flavour level. Make it!

Ingredient: 3 large ripe tomatoes or 1 15 oz. can diced tomatoes, 4 cloves of garlic, 1/2 inch (0.5 inch) cube of ginger, 1 hot or mild green chili , I use Serrano, 3/4 cup (250 ml) water , use 1, cup if the tomatoes aren't very juicy, ½ to 1 tsp. (1/2 to 1 tsp.) garam masala, ½ tsp. (0.5 tsp.) paprika or Kashmiri chili powder, ¼ to ½ tsp. (1/4 to 1/2 tsp.) cayenne, 3/4 tsp. (0.75 tsp.) salt, 1 cup (55 g) soy curls (dry, not rehydrated), 1 cup (5.78 oz.) cooked chickpeas, Cashew cream made with ¼ cup soaked cashews blended with ½ cup water, 1/2 tsp. (0.5 tsp.) or more garam masala, 1/2 tsp. (0.5 tsp.) or more sugar or sweetener, 1 tsp. kasoori methi - dried fenugreek leaves or add a 1/4 tsp. ground mustard, 1/2 (0.5) moderately hot green chili finely chopped, or use 2 tbsp. finely chopped green bell pepper, 1/2 tsp. (0.5 tsp.) minced or finely chopped ginger, 1/4 cup (4 g) cilantro for garnish.

Preparation: Blend the tomatoes, garlic, ginger, chili with water until smooth.

Add pureed tomato mixture to the Instant pot or pressure cooker. Add soy curls, chickpeas, spices and salt. Close the lid and cook on Manual for 8 to 10 minutes. Quick release after 10 minutes. Start the IP on sauté (medium heat for stove top pressure cooker). Add the cashew cream, garam masala, sweetener and fenugreek leaves and mix in. Bring to a boil, taste and adjust salt, heat, sweet. Add more cayenne and salt if needed. Fold in the chopped green chili, ginger and cilantro and press cancel (take off heat).

At this point you can add some vegan butter or oil for additional buttery flavour. Serve hot over rice or with flatbread or Naan.

Fluffy Mashed Potatoes with Vegan Gravy: Mashed Potatoes don't need an introduction. They are used is many cuisines in many different ways. These are basic mashed potatoes that you can amp up to preference.

Ingredient: 5 to 6 potatoes cubed into large pieces Yukon gold or baking potatoes, peeled if desired, 5 cloves of garlic, 1/2 tsp. (0.5 tsp.) salt, 1 tbsp. extra virgin olive oil or vegan butter, a good dash of black pepper, dash of parsley or thyme, pinch of nutmeg, 1 cup (226 ml) full fat coconut milk, fresh chives for garnish.

preparation: Pressure cook the cubed potatoes, garlic cloves, 1/4 tsp. salt with 1.5 cups water at high pressure for 4 minutes in Instant pot (manual 4 mins) or 2 minutes in stove top pressure cooker. Release the pressure after 5 minutes. (You can also boil them in a saucepan. Put the potatoes into a large pot, adding enough water to cover them. Bring to a boil and simmer for 10-15 mins, until they're fork-tender. Transfer to a colander to drain.)

Drain really well. Transfer to a bowl, let sit for a few minutes to dry out. Mash lightly and let sit for a minute for the steam to escape. Make sure to mash the cooked garlic. Mix in salt, the rest of the ingredients and half cup coconut milk. Mix and whip lightly, just enough to add air and still have some texture. Let sit for a minute for the milks to incorporate and absorb.

Taste and adjust. Add 1/4 tsp. or more salt as needed. Add more coconut milk for creamier consistency to preference if needed and mix in. Add 1-2 tbsp. nutritional yeast for cheesy potatoes. Garnish with chives.

Instant Pot Artichokes: Easy, Fast, Fool proof Artichokes Recipe in 20 mins! Super food nutrient powerhouse with delicious delicate flavours.

Ingredient: 2 artichokes (1/2lb, 250g each, 11" circumference), 4 cloves (13g) garlic, minced, 2 tablespoons (30g) unsalted butter, Kosher Salt to taste (about 2 pinches) Optional: lemon juice from 1 lemon.

Preparation: Wash   Artichokes: Submerge artichokes in cold water for 5 minutes.

Optional - Prep Artichokes: Cut stem off and trim about 1 inch off the tip of the artichokes.

Place Artichokes in Pressure Cooker— Place 1 cup of cold water and a steamer rack in the Instant Pot pressure cooker. Place 2 whole artichokes on the steamer rack, and close the lid.

Optional: If you like, squeeze some lemon juice on the artichokes to slow the rate of oxidation.

Pressure Cook Artichokes: Pressure cook

a) Trimmed Artichokes: High Pressure for 8 minutes (using the Manual Button/Pressure Cook) + Quick Release OR

b) Uncut Whole Artichokes: High Pressure for 9 minutes (using the Manual Button/Pressure Cook) + Quick Release

c) For Large Artichokes: Increase the pressure cooking time accordingly.

Open the lid carefully.

Prepare Garlic Butter: While the artichokes are cooking in the pressure cooker, heat a sauce pan over medium low heat. Melt 2 tbsp. (30g) unsalted butter and add in the minced garlic. Sauté garlic until golden brown. Do not let the garlic burn. Set aside to cool it down slightly. Season with kosher salt and adjust to taste (about 2 pinches).

Serve: Serve artichokes with Garlic Butter Sauce.

Note: use olive oil in place of unsalted butter for dipping sauce.

CILANTRO LIME BROWN RICE: The flavour of this rice is so spot on, and using brown rice made it feel way less guilty going back for seconds.

Ingredient: 1 cup Uncooked Long-grain Brown Rice, 1 teaspoon Butter, 2 cloves Garlic, Minced, 5 teaspoons Fresh Lime Juice, Divided, 1 can (15 Oz. Size) Vegetable Broth, 1 cup Water, 4 Tablespoons Fresh Cilantro, Chopped.

Preparation: In a saucepan add the rice, butter, garlic, 2 teaspoons of lime juice, broth and water; stir to combine. Bring the rice mixture to a boil, then reduce heat to low, cover and cook for 40 minutes, until rice is tender. While rice is cooking, whisk the remaining 3 teaspoons (or 1 tablespoon) lime juice and cilantro together in a small bowl. When rice is ready, remove it from the heat and pour the lime/cilantro mixture over the rice, mixing it in as you fluff the rice. Serve immediately.

VEGAN BREAKFAST RECIPES BY INSTANT POT.

Start your day with one of these Easy Instant Pot vegan breakfast recipes and you'll be surprised at good you feel. When you start off your day right it's so much easier to eat right all day long.

Stuffed sweet potatoes: These Instant Pot Breakfast Stuffed Sweet Potatoes are an easy, healthy, vegan way to start your day! They're quickly cooked in a pressure cooker, then stuffed with almond butter, maple syrup, and blueberries!

Ingredient: 1 cup water, 1 sweet potato, 1 tablespoon pure maple syrup, 1 tablespoon almond butter, 1 tablespoon chopped pecans, 2 tablespoons blueberries, 1 teaspoon chia seeds.

Preparation: Place the steamer rack in your instant pot and add one cup of water. Place the sweet potato on the rack and seal the lid, making sure the release valve is in the proper position. Set the Instant Pot to manual high pressure for 15 minutes. It will take a few minutes to come up to pressure.

Once the time is up, allow the pressure to release naturally for ten minutes. Turn the release valve to release any leftover pressure. Once the float valve has dropped, open the lid and remove the sweet potato. When it is cool enough to handle, cut the sweet potato and mash the flesh with a fork. Drizzle with maple syrup and almond butter, then sprinkle with pecans, blueberries, and chia seeds.

Uttapams savoury Indian pancakes: It's a savoury Indian pancake that's easy to make and actually is inexpensive too. My whole foods recipe uses healthy grains and lentils that ferment into a flavourful batter overnight.

Ingredient: 1 cup urad dal, 1 cup brown rice, 1 cup millet, 1 cup quinoa, washed well to remove the seed coating, 5 cups water.

Preparation: Mix the urad dal, rice, millet, quinoa and water in a large bowl. Cover and let soak to soften for 8 hours. After the soak, puree the mixture (including the soaking water) in your blender in batches and add to your Instant Pot liner. Place the liner in your Instant Pot, cover and press the yogurt setting. Leave it at the default 8 hours for it to ferment.

Note: You can store the fermented mixture in your fridge for up to 1 week or you can cook up all the pancakes at once and freeze them to heat for later.

Heat a non-stick skillet over medium heat. Once hot, add ½ cup (120 ml) of the batter per pancake and shape into a circle. Cook until bubbles begin to form. Sprinkle the topping you choose over the top of the pancake and press in a little with your spatula. Flip the pancake and cook until both sides are browned. Place on a plate and cook the next one. You could also have more than one skillet going at a time.

INSTANT POT BREAKFAST POTATOES: Instant Pot breakfast potatoes are prepared ahead of time for a quick breakfast, brunch or even dinner. Season this savoury side in the IP then brown and crisp them on a skillet. They're easy to make and full of flavour!

Ingredient: 6 yukon gold or red potatoes, or 4 russets (roughly 2lbs), diced into 1/2-inch cubes, 2-3 Tablespoons refined coconut oil, or neutral oil of choice, 3/4 cup of water or vegetable broth, 1 Tablespoon nutritional yeast, 2 teaspoons garlic powder, 1 teaspoons onion powder, 1/4 teaspoon paprika, Himalayan pink salt to taste (I use about 3/4 teaspoon), Pepper to taste, neutral oil for sautéing, I use refined coconut oil, 1 small onion, 1 green bell pepper.

Preparation: In a small bowl combine the seasonings and set aside. Dice the potatoes into evenly sized cubes. Dry the cubed potatoes with a kitchen/paper towels to remove excess moisture.

Add the potatoes and oil to the IP and press the sauté feature. Sauté the potatoes just until they begin to change texture (about 5 minutes). The potatoes may stick so be sure to frequently stir them. Don't worry, any sticking will come up after pressure cooking and add extra flavour to the potatoes. Halfway through cooking mix-in the seasonings. Once the potatoes have started to change texture, press the cancel button on the IP. You don't want to over sauté them since they will be pressure cooked as well.

Pour in the water or broth, but don't mix. Secure the lid and make sure the steam vent is sealed. Set the IP to low pressure for 1 minute. Once done, carefully, quick release the steam vent. The potatoes may be undercooked, but they will fully cook when reheated in the skillet. Gently mix the potatoes to prevent mashing while scraping up any browning on the bottom of the pot. Let cool, then refrigerate for the next morning, or at least 2 hours.

Instant Pot Vegan Quinoa Breakfast Recipe: instant Pot Vegan Quinoa Breakfast Recipe is super yum & easy to put together. Vegan Quinoa Porridge is a quick make ahead recipe for breakfast or brunch.

Ingredient: 1 Cup Quinoa, 3 Cups Almond Milk, unsweetened, Toppings & Garnishes, 1/4 cup Maple Syrup, original, 1 Tbsp. Walnuts chopped, plain, 1/2 Tbsp. Pistachio chopped, plain, 1 Tbsp. Resins, and 2 Tbsp. Almonds chopped, plain, 1/2 Cup Fresh Berries of Choice.

Preparation: Place the inner pot inside the Instant Pot. Plug it in. Wash the quinoa under running cold water till water runs clear. Set aside. Place the washed quinoa and 3 cups of Almond Milk inside the Inner Pot. If you want slightly more liquid consistency, then add 5 cups of almond milk. You can also add more milk later once it is cooked to adjust the consistency to your liking. Place the Lid and lock it to SEALING. Select the Pressure Cook/Manual Mode and set it on HIGH for 2 MINUTES.

Once the timer goes off, follow NPR. Once the safety valve drops down, open the lid carefully. You will get the porridge of THICK CONSISTENCY. I liked this consistency. If you like little more runny porridge, then add more almond milk to it. Just warm the almond milk and add and stir. Use as required. Top your Quinoa Porridge with Maple Syrup, Fresh Berries and Dry Nuts. Enjoy a hearty Breakfast. It is a perfect example of Dessert for Breakfast too.

Pumpkin Coffeecake Steel-cut Oatmeal: This recipe for Instant Pot Vegan Pumpkin Coffeecake Steel-cut Oatmeal makes a ton. It's a departure from my usual recipes for two servings. You actually get 6 to 8 servings – enough to make once and grab breakfast from the fridge or freezer all week long.

Ingredient: 4 1/2 cups water, 1 1/2 cups steel-cut oats, 1 1/2 cups pumpkin puree or 1 15 oz. can, 2 teaspoons cinnamon, 1 teaspoon allspice, 1 teaspoon vanilla, 1/2 cup coconut sugar or brown sugar or sweetener of choice, to taste, 1/4 cup pecans or walnuts chopped, 1 tablespoon cinnamon.

Preparation: Add all the instant pot ingredients to your stainless steel insert and put it into the base. Secure the lid and make sure the valve is closed. Set on manual and cook for 3 minutes. While the oats are cooking, mix all the topping ingredients together and store in an airtight container.

Once the oats are cooked, allow the pressure to come down naturally. Once the silver pressure indicator goes down you can open the lid.

Serve sprinkled with topping and/or your favourite non-dairy milk!

Instant Pot Steel Cut Oats Cooked with Earl Grey Tea: Earl Grey tea is the perfect cooking liquid for your morning oats. It adds the unique punch of flavour in my Instant Pot Earl Grey Steel Cut Oats. I suggest adding some rosewater, vanilla, or a little lavender extract to customize your steel cut oats even more!

Ingredient: 1 ½ cups brewed Earl Grey Tea, you can use black, decaf or rooibos, ½ cup steel- cut oats, ½ teaspoon rosewater, vanilla, or a few drops of lavender extract, sweetener of your choice, to taste.

Preparation: Add the brewed tea and oats to your Instant Pot. Put your lid on and make sure the vent is closed. Select the manual/pressure cooker setting and set to cook for 3 minutes.

Allow the pressure to release naturally. Open and mix in your choice of sweetener and extra flavouring. Serve topped with non-dairy milk.

Sprouted Lentils Bowl: Sprouted Lentils Breakfast Bowl – A perfect make-ahead, meatless breakfast with protein-rich sprouted brown lentils, lightly spiced with freshly grated ginger, turmeric, mild red Kashmiri chili powder, and cumin!

Ingredient: 1 tablespoon cooking oil, 1 medium onion finely chopped, 1/2 tsp. turmeric, 1 teaspoon ginger grated, 1 teaspoon mild red chili powder, 1 teaspoon cumin powder, 1 teaspoon salt, 3 cups whole brown lentils sprouted.

Optional Toppings: 1 plum tomato diced, 2 tablespoon cilantro chopped, 1 tablespoon fresh coconut grated, Egg cooked sunny side up, salt & pepper to taste.

Preparation: Turn Instant Pot to Sauté mode. Once the 'hot' sign displays, add oil. Add onions and cook for a minute. Cook covered with a glass lid on for another minute or until the onions become translucent stirring frequently. Add turmeric, ginger, red chili powder, salt and cumin powder. Mix well and add sprouted lentils. Add 1/3 cup of water and mix well. Close Instant Pot with the pressure valve to sealing. Cook on Manual for 1 min followed by Natural Pressure Release. Open Instant Pot, Garnish with tomatoes and cilantro. Add additional toppings - fresh grated coconut or eggs. Add salt and pepper to taste. Enjoy hot or cold.

Healthy Chocolate Instant Pot Steel Cut Oats:
Satisfying & nourishing Healthy Chocolate Instant Pot
Steel Cut Oats. Quick to make, simple & naturally
sweetened with banana only. There is no added sugar
at all! Just perfect for a hearty breakfast.

Ingredient: 1 cup / 176g / 6.2 oz. steel cut oats, 3
medium bananas, don't use large bananas as it will
make the mixture too thick for the IP to handle, 3
tablespoons cocoa, 3½ cups / 840 mls / 28 FL oz. water
, or use half non-dairy milk, half water.

Preparation: Add the oats, water and cocoa to the
Instant Pot and stir well. Mash the bananas with a fork
until a puree. A few small chunks are ok. Add them on
top of the other ingredients and DO NOT stir. Put the lid
on, make sure the steam vent is sealed and set to
manual, high pressure, for 9 minutes. Then leave the
pressure to release naturally. Once the pressure has
been released and the pin has dropped, remove the lid
and stir the oatmeal really well before serving. It will
thicken up as it cools. You can add more water or milk
before serving for a looser texture if you want.

Instant Pot Steel Cut Oats: Oatmeal is one of my favourite winter meals and Instant Pot Steel Cut Oats make it easier to have them every day. You can set them up the night before and wake up to a steaming hot bowl of oats. Plus you can make them sweet or savoury depending on how you choose to top them.

Ingredient: 1 1/2 cups water, 1/2 cup steel-cut oats.

Preparation: Add the water and oats to your Instant Pot. Put your lid on and make sure the vent is closed. Plug it in and select the manual setting and set to cook on high pressure for 3 minutes. The Instant Pot timer will begin counting down the time once it gets up to pressure. Allow the pressure to release naturally. You'll know when it's ready because the round silver pressure gauge will drop down. This will take about 5 to 10 minutes.

Homemade Instant Pot Almond Milk: While you do not need an Instant Pot to make a plant-based milk, this recipe does use one. It's the last minute plant based milk recipe that you'll have when you need it. (This is not raw almond milk.)

Ingredient: 2 cups water, 1 cup almonds, 4 cups water.

Preparation: Add the water and almonds to your Instant Pot and cook on high pressure for 10 minutes. Carefully manually release the pressure. Drain the almonds. Add the almonds and the 4 cups (946 ml) water to your blender and blend well. Strain through a nut milk bag and store in the refrigerator. The recipe makes an unsweetened plain non-dairy milk.

SOUPS, STEWS AND CURRIES BY INSTANT POT.

Thai Curried Butternut Squash Soup: Excited to have a warm bowl of creamy soupy goodness? This Thai Butternut Squash Soup made in the Instant Pot is what you have been waiting for. It is creamy, flavourful, healthy and vegan!

Ingredient: 1 tbsp. Oil, 1 cup Yellow Onion diced, 3 cloves Garlic minced, 1 tbsp. Ginger minced, 2 lbs. Butternut Squash peeled, seeded and cut into pieces, about 6 cups, 1 tbsp. Red curry paste adjust more to taste. 1.5 cups Vegetable broth, 1/2 can Coconut milk 14oz canned full fat, 1/2 tsp. Salt adjust to taste, Black Pepper add to taste (optional), 1/2 Lime juice, 2 tbsp. Roasted peanuts chopped, 2 tbsp. Coconut milk, 2 tbsp. Cilantro chopped, Red Chili flakes (optional)

Preparation: Start the instant pot in sauté mode and heat oil in it. Add diced onions, ginger and garlic and sauté for about 3 minutes. Add butternut squash, red curry paste, and broth and stir to combine. Press Cancel and close lid with vent in sealing position. Change the instant pot setting to manual or pressure cook mode at high pressure for 8 mins. After the instant pot beeps, let the pressure release naturally for 10 minutes then release the pressure manually. Use an immersion blender to blend the soup to a creamy texture. You can also transfer to a blender to blend the soup. Be careful while blending to avoid hot splatters. Add coconut milk, lime juice and stir well. Add salt, pepper and chili flakes to taste. Garnish the soup with cilantro, coconut milk and peanuts. Serve hot with a side of crusty bread!

Instant Pot Potato Soup: If you're looking for a delicious soup recipe for your Instant Pot, try this hearty and delicious Instant Pot Potato Soup. It comes together in just a few simple steps.

ingredient: 2 tbsp. olive oil, 3 leeks trimmed, thinly sliced, washed and drained, 1 lb. (450g) potatoes peeled and cubed, 4 cups (1 litre) vegetable stock hot, 0.5 tsp. ground nutmeg, Salt, Ground black pepper, 0.5 cups (125 ml) almond milk, or to taste.

Preparation: Press the sauté button on the Instant Pot. When the display reads Hot, add the oil. When hot add the leeks and sauté for about 5 mins till soft. Add the potatoes and cook for a couple of mins. Mix in the vegetable stock, nutmeg and seasoning. Put the lid on the Instant pot make sure the steam release part is pointing to sealing. Press the manual button and set the timer to 10 mins. Cook and once done release the pressure naturally over 10- 15 mins. Add the almond milk and blend the soup into a puree using an immersion blender (or using a regular blender) Adjust seasoning and serve in bowls topped with toasted seeds or chilli oil.

Hearty Brown Lentil Soup: Hearty Brown Lentil & Vegetable Soup in the Instant Pot or Pressure Cooker. Make this warm soup on a cold & rainy (or snowy) day. Get cosy with this nutritious and easy to make vegan soup.

Ingredient: 1 cup Brown lentils (Whole Masoor Dal) rinsed, 2 tbsp. Olive Oil, 1 Onion small, diced (about 1 cup), 1 tbsp. Garlic minced, 2 Carrot cut into small pieces, 2 stalks Celery cut into small pieces, 3 cups Vegetable Broth or Water, 2 cups Baby Spinach packed, 1 tbsp. Lemon juice, 1/4 tsp. Sugar (optional), 1/2 tsp. Red Chili flakes (optional). 1 tsp. Ground Cumin, 1 tsp. Coriander powder, 1/2 tsp. Sumac (optional), 1/2 tsp. Ground Turmeric, 1 tsp. Salt, 1/2 tsp. Thyme dried (optional)

Preparation: Start the instant pot in SAUTE mode and heat oil in it. Add onions and garlic. Mix and sauté for 1 minute. Add carrots, celery and all spices along with thyme. Add the lentils and broth. Stir it all up. Press Cancel and close the lid with vent in sealing position. Set the instant pot to SOUP mode for 20 minutes. When the instant pot beeps, release the pressure naturally. Press Cancel. Add in spinach, lemon juice and sugar. Add some red chili flakes if you like. Stir it all up. Brown Lentil Soup is ready to enjoy!

Sweet Potato Kale Soup: Adding to my soup obsession, and wanting to make something special with my sweet potatoes, I created this lovely healthy soup that will be a friend to you, in the resolution keeping.

Ingredient: 2 Tbsp. Olive Oil, 1 small Onion, diced, 2 small Bay Leaves, 2 medium Sweet Potatoes, peeled and cubed (about 1 1/2 lbs.), 1/2 tsp. Coriander Powder, 1/2 tsp. Cumin, 1/8 tsp. Cinnamon, 1 tsp. Turmeric, 1 tsp. Kosher Salt (or 3/4 tsp. table salt), 1 3-4" sprig Fresh Rosemary (don't use dried), 3 cloves Garlic, pressed or minced, (1) 15 oz. can Diced Tomatoes, with juice, 1 tsp. Paprika, sweet, (1) 14 oz. can Coconut Milk (use light for fewer calories), 1 1/2 cups Water, 5 oz. Kale, chopped (1/2 of a 10 oz. bag).

Preparation: Turn on pressure cooker to the Sauté function. When the display reads "Hot" add the oil. Add the onion, and bay leaves. Cook, stirring occasionally, until onion starts to turn translucent. Add the sweet potatoes, coriander, cumin, cinnamon, turmeric, salt, rosemary, and garlic. Stir well and cook for about 1 minute. Add the tomatoes and paprika. Cook, stirring, for 2 minutes. Stir in the coconut milk, incorporating it well, and then add the water and stir well. Place the lid on the pressure cooker and lock in place. Turn the steam release knob to the Sealing position. Cancel the Sauté function and set to Pressure Cook (or Manual), and use the + or - button (or dial) to choose 5 minutes.

When cooking cycle has ended, let the pot sit undisturbed for 10 minutes (10 minutes of Natural Release). Then manually (Quick Release) the remaining steam by turning the steam release knob to the Venting position. When the pin in the lid drops down, open the lid carefully. Don't stir the soup yet. Add the kale to the soup and very gently fold it into the soup (Do this gently so the sweet potatoes don't all break up. You do want some of them to as this naturally thickens it. Use your own judgement on this). Let the soup sit for a couple of minutes so the kale can wilt. Then taste and adjust salt, if desired. Serve nice and hot. Garnish with some extra coconut milk, or heavy cream if you are not dairy-free. Enjoy!

Cream of Broccoli Soup: Enjoy this healthy Cream of Broccoli soup made in the Instant Pot (Pressure Cooker) in less than 30 minutes. This delicious comfort food can be enjoyed guilt free now, with this plant based vegan & gluten free recipe. Perfect for a quick satisfying lunch or dinner.

Ingredient: 1 tbsp. Oil, 1 cup Onion diced, 3 cloves Garlic minced, 1 lb Broccoli cut into small florets, about 5 cups, 1 cup Carrots cut into pieces, 1/3 cup Cashews, 2 cups Broth, 3/4 cup Coconut milk, 1 tbsp. Lemon juice (optional), Salt to taste, Black pepper to taste (optional). Basil (optional), 2 tbsp. Parsley chopped.

Preparation: Start the instant pot in sauté mode and heat oil in it. Add diced onions and garlic and sauté for about 3 minutes. Add broccoli, carrots, cashews and broth. Stir it all up. Press Cancel and close lid with vent in sealing position. Change the instant pot setting to manual or pressure cook mode at high pressure for 3 mins. After the instant pot beeps, let the pressure release naturally for 10 minutes then release the pressure manually. Add coconut milk. Use an immersion blender to blend the soup to a creamy texture. You can also transfer to a blender to blend the soup. Be careful while blending to avoid hot splatters. Season the soup with salt, pepper and lemon juice. Top with parsley and basil to garnish. Enjoy with toasted bread!

Instant Pot Lasagna Soup: LASAGNA SOUP is totally a thing, you wouldn't believe how much savoury this dish can give you— unless, of course you try.

Ingredient: 32 oz. Rao's Marinara Sauce, 32 oz. Rao's Arrabbiata Sauce, 3 cups Mafalda Pasta or Campanile (Or broken Lasagne Noodles), 2 Serrano's, diced small, 4 garlic cloves, minced/grated, 3-4 Cups Spinach Leaves (fresh not frozen), 1 green bell pepper, diced small, 1 onion, diced small, 1/4 cup cilantro chopped, 1/4 cup parsley chopped, 1/4 cup scallions, sliced, 1/2 tsp. fresh oregano, finely minced, 4 cups Vegetable broth (I prefer Pacific Foods), 2 cups water, 1 cup parmesan cheese, 1 cup ricotta cheese, 1 cup mozzarella cheese, shredded, 1 Bay Leaf, 2 tbsp. oil.

Preparation: Set your IP to sauté mode and add two tablespoons of oil. Once the oil is hot, add the Serrano chillies and oregano and let splutter for a few moments. Add the onions and peppers and continue to cook for 3-4 minutes. Add garlic- stirring continuously so the garlic does not brown. Once the onions and peppers have softened a bit- add in the Rao's sauce, spinach, vegetable broth, 1 cup water, bay leaf, scallions, cilantro, and parsley. Stir well for a few minutes until all the ingredients are incorporated. Add in the pasta. Hit cancel on the IP and switch it to Pressure Cook on High Mode- for 3 minutes (If you use a different pasta than I did- just cut the cooking time on the box in half for the pressure cook time- my box said 6 minutes to al dente- so I cooked the pasta for 3 minutes). After 3 minutes- do a manual release (use a towel to protect your hands). Once the silver pin drops- open the IP.

The consistency should be soupy- if it is too thick- add water in one cup increments until you reach the desired consistency. If your pasta is undercooked- just set it on sauté mode and let it simmer until the pasta cooks. Add in the parmesan, mozzarella and ricotta. Add more or less cheese as you like- add salt per your taste (I did not add any salt in my recipe).

Vegan Instant Pot Cauliflower Soup: A healthy and healing Turmeric Cauliflower Soup made in the Instant Pot. This vegan & gluten free soup is so easy to make, and the result is creamy, satisfying goodness you will not want to stop eating!

Ingredient: 1 tbsp. Olive Oil, 3/4 cup Onion diced, 4 cloves Garlic minced, 1 head Cauliflower about 5 cups or 1.6lbs, cut into 2 inch florets, 1/2 cup Cashews, 1/2 tsp. Ground Turmeric, 1/2 tsp. Ground Cinnamon, 3 cups Vegetable broth, 1 tsp. Salt adjust to taste, 1 tbsp. Lemon juice, Parsley, Red Chili flakes (optional).

Preparation: Start the instant pot in sauté mode and heat oil in it. Add diced onions and garlic and sauté for about 3 minutes. Add cauliflower, cashews, turmeric, cinnamon, broth and salt. Stir it all up. Press Cancel and close lid with vent in sealing position. Change the instant pot setting to manual or pressure cook mode at high pressure for 3 mins. After the instant pot beeps, let the pressure release naturally for 10 minutes then release the pressure manually. Add the lemon juice. Use an immersion blender to blend the soup to a creamy texture. You can also transfer to a blender to blend the soup. Be careful while blending to avoid hot splatters. Top with parsley and some chili flakes (optional). Enjoy with toasted bread!

Instant Pot Vegetable Quinoa Soup: Ready for the easiest soup recipe of your life? You won't believe the flavours in this easy-to-make Instant Pot Vegetable Quinoa Soup!

Ingredient: 2 1/2 Tbsp. olive oil, 1Tbsp Italian seasoning, 1 cup chopped onion, 1 cup peeled and chopped carrots, 1 cup chopped celery, 6 cups low-sodium organic vegetable broth, 1 cup Quinoa, 1-1/2 cup tomatoes puree, Salt and freshly ground black pepper to taste, 1/2 cup chopped fresh green beans or Asparagus, 1 chopped zucchini, 3 cups baby spinach.

Preparation: Heat oil in pressure cooker set to Sauté on Normal. Cook onion, carrots, zucchini, asparagus, celery and baby spinach in hot oil and give it a quick stir. Add in the tomato puree, add the quinoa and vegetable stock, add Italian seasoning, salt, pepper to taste. Lock pressure cooker lid in place and set steam vent to Sealing. Select Soup/Stew and cook for 3 minutes on High pressure. Once the cooking cycle has completed, set steam vent to Venting to quick-release pressure. Stir the soup and season with salt and pepper to serve.

Minestrone Soup: A perfect soup that is a complete meal in itself – Beans, loads of veggies and pasta, topped with cheese and a side of bread. Vegetarian friendly and can easily be made gluten-free and vegan.

Ingredient: 2 tbsp. Olive Oil, 1 Onion diced, 1 tbsp. Garlic minced, 4 Tomato diced, 2 Celery Stalks chopped, 2 Carrot chopped, 1 Zucchini chopped, 1/2 cup Pasta (I used elbow macaroni), 32 oz. Vegetable Broth, 1 can White Kidney Beans 15oz (cannellini), 2 cups Spinach (Palak) chopped, 1/4 cup Parmesan cheese freshly grated (optional).

Preparation: Start the instant pot in SAUTE mode and heat olive oil in it. Add diced onions and minced garlic. Stir and sauté for 2 minutes. Add diced tomatoes and chopped celery, carrots and zucchini. Add in the Italian seasoning, salt, pepper and paprika. Add in the pasta, veggie broth and white kidney beans. Stir it all up. Make sure the pasta is under the broth. Press Cancel and set to SOUP setting (high pressure) for 20 minutes. (For firmer pasta, only cook for 10 minutes on SOUP setting) When the instant pot beeps, let the pressure release naturally for 5 minutes. Then manually release the pressure. If you have time, you can also allow a NPR. Stir in the chopped spinach and let it sit for 5 minutes. Garnish with parmesan cheese and minestrone soup is ready to serve.

Instant Pot Pumpkin Soup: This Instant Pot pumpkin soup is thick, creamy and perfectly seasoned with fall spices. Quick and easy to make, this soup recipe will fill you with warmth and comfort on those cold fall and winter days.

Ingredient: 4 tablespoons unsalted butter, 2 cups sweet onion chopped, 2 cloves garlic minced, 1 teaspoon ground cinnamon, ½ teaspoon ground nutmeg, ¼ teaspoon ground ginger, 4 cups unsalted vegetable stock, 2 tablespoons dark brown sugar, 1 teaspoon kosher salt or to taste, 1 can pumpkin puree 29 ounce, ½ cup heavy whipping cream.

preparation: Turn on the Instant Pot to 'Sauté' and using the 'Adjust' button, adjust the sauté heat level to 'Normal' and allow it to heat up for a few minutes so that the panel reads 'Hot' before adding the butter. Add the butter to the pot and, using a spoon or spatula, move it around the bottom of the hot liner to help it melt more quickly. Once the butter has melted and started to get hot, add the onion and cook, stirring occasionally until it becomes soft and translucent, 4 to 5 minutes. Do not allow the onions to brown. Add the garlic, stir into the onions and continue to sauté for another 1 to 2 minutes. Add the cinnamon, nutmeg, and ginger to the pot and mix them into the onions. Allow the spices to cook in the onions until they start to release their aroma, approximately 1 minute.

Turn off the 'Sauté' function and add the vegetable stock, brown sugar, and salt then mix everything together well. Add the pumpkin puree, just spooning it into the centre of the pot. Do not mix it into the stock. Close the pot and set the pressure release valve to 'Sealing'. Select the 'Soup' function and set the cook time to 10 minutes. Once the 10 minute cook time has completed, perform a 5 minute NPR (natural pressure release). As soon as all of the pressure has been released, open the Instant Pot. Turn off the Instant Pot and allow the soup to cool for a few minutes. Using an immersion blender, puree all of the ingredients and then mix in the heavy whipping cream.

Serve and enjoy!

Instant Pot Creamy Tomato Soup: Instant Pot Creamy Tomato Soup is delicious and nutritious with lots of veggies. Made with fresh tomatoes along with carrots, celery, onion and a hint of garlic, topped with some cream and cheese. Oh so creamy...you will love it!

Ingredient: 1 tbsp. Butter or Oil, 7 cloves Garlic, 1/2 Onion chopped, 5 Carrot chopped (I used small thin carrots), 3 stalks Celery chopped, 5 Tomato chopped, 3/4 cup Broth or water, 1/4 cup Romano Cheese grated (optional), 1/4 cup Cream heavy whipping, use coconut milk for vegan, 2 tbsp. Cilantro to garnish, Salt & Pepper to taste.

Preparation: Start the instant pot in Sauté mode and wait till it displays HOT. Add butter and let it melt. Add chopped onions, garlic and cook for a minute. Add in carrots and celery to instant pot. Add in the chopped tomatoes. Add broth to instant pot and stir it with all the veggies making sure nothing is stuck to the bottom of the pot. Press cancel and close the lid with vent in sealing position. Start instant pot in manual or pressure cook mode at high pressure for 6 minutes. When the instant pot beeps, let the pressure release naturally.

Open the lid and use an immersion blender to puree the mixture until it is smooth. Or transfer to a blender and carefully blend the soup in batches. (If you like your tomato soup to be very smooth, you can strain it over a fine mesh strainer) Stir in the cream and cheese. Simmer for another 2 minutes on sauté mode until the cheese mixes well. Add salt and pepper to taste. Give the soup a taste and adjust broth or seasoning to taste, adding any extra of whatever you prefer to get your ideal thickness and flavour. Garnish with cilantro and grated cheese (optional). Creamy Tomato Soup is ready to be served with garlic bread or your favourite side.

Tuscan Vegetable Soup: Tuscan Vegetable Soup Instant Pot Recipe is an easy + delicious + nutritious recipe. It is loaded with seasonal vegetables and cannellini beans and mildly flavoured with seasonings. The soup is light in calories but very filling. Add some shell pasta in it or put some bread on the side and make it a complete meal.

Ingredient: 1 Tbsp. Olive Oil, 3 Cloves Garlic chopped fine, 1 Medium Onion, red or white cut into chunky pieces, 2 Large Tomatoes cut into chunky pieces, 4 Sticks Celery cut into chunky pieces, 1 Medium Zucchini cut into chunky pieces, 1 Large Carrot cut into chunky pieces, 1 Cup Spinach, 1 Can Cannellini Beans drained, 2 Tbsp. Tomato Paste, 1 Tsp. Rosemary, dry, To Taste Salt and Black Pepper, 5 Cups Water, 1/2 Tsp. Cayenne Pepper or Fancy Paprika this is optional but elevates the taste to another level.

Preparation: Set the instant pot to sauté mode on MORE. When it displays HOT, add olive oil to it. After 30 seconds, add onions and garlic to the hot oil. Sauté for 2 minutes till onions become soft. Now add celery and carrots to the pot. Cook for 1 minute and then add cannellini beans + all the remaining vegetables + tomato paste + seasonings + herbs to the pot. Give it a good stir. Add 5 cups of water. Stir again. Place the lid and Switch off the sauté mode. Place the floating vent to CLOSE. Set the SOUP / BROTH MODE to NORMAL for 6 minutes. After the cooking is done and you hear the beep. There are 2 things you can do- 1). Release the pressure immediately and serve the soup while warm. IT is fully cooked and does not need Natural Pressure Release for further cooking. OR 2). If you are making it in the morning and coming back in the evening for a hearty soup, then, do not worry about releasing the pressure. Little over cooking will make vegetables slightly soft that's it but will still taste awesome.

Easy Jackfruit Curry: Young green Jackfruit makes a great shredded meat sub. Easy, Vegan, Soy-free Gluten-free Grain-free Indian curry. Simple spices, amazing flavour.

Ingredient: 1 tsp. oil, 1/2 tsp. (0.5 tsp.) cumin seeds, 1/2 tsp. (0.5 tsp.) mustard seeds, 1/2 tsp. (0.5 tsp.) nigella seeds, 2 bay leaves, 2 dried red chilies, 1 small onion chopped, 5 cloves of garlic chopped, 1 inch ginger chopped, 1 tsp. coriander powder, 1/2 tsp. (0.5 tsp.) turmeric, 1/4 tsp. (0.25 tsp.) black pepper, 2 medium tomatoes pureed or 1.5 cups puree, 20 oz. (566 g) can green Jackfruit, drained, rinsed and squeezed to remove excess brine. Also chop into smaller pieces if too big. 1/2 to 3/4 tsp. salt or to taste, 1 to 1.5 cups (235 to 353 ml) water.

Preparation: Heat oil in a skillet over medium heat. When hot, add cumin, mustard and nigella seeds and let them start to sizzle or pop. 1 minute. Add bay leaves and red chilies and cook for a few seconds. Add in the onion, garlic and ginger and a pinch of salt. Cook until translucent. 5 to 6 minutes. Stir occasionally. Add coriander, turmeric, black pepper and mix well. Add pureed tomato, salt and Jackfruit. Mix. Cover and cook for 15 minutes. Add tomato puree and cook for 2 minutes, then add jackfruit, salt and 1/2 to 1 cup water. Close the lid and pressure cook for 7 to 8 minutes once the cooker comes to pressure (manual 8 mins on IP). Wait for natural release.

DESSERT RECIPES.

New York-Style Instant Pot Cheesecake: The cheesecake is an ideal make-ahead dessert—it's better after a rest in the fridge and will knock your dinner guests' socks off. Plus, since the decadent dessert comes together rather effortlessly in the Instant Pot, there's no reason not to make one. Serve with classic cherries or strawberries, or drizzle with chocolate or caramel (or both!).

Ingredient: 3 tablespoons sugar, 5 tablespoons butter, 9 large graham crackers, pulsed into crumbs, 2 tablespoons ground pecans, 1/4 teaspoon cinnamon, 12 ounces cream cheese (or 1 1/2 packages), 1/4 teaspoon kosher salt, 2 teaspoons lemon zest, 2 teaspoons vanilla extract, 1 tablespoon corn-starch, 1/2 cup + 2 tablespoons granulated sugar, 2 large eggs + 1 egg yolk, 1/2 cup sour cream.

Preparation: Position a rack in the centre of the oven and preheat the oven to 350ºF if you plan on baking the crust. If you're freezing it, you can skip this step. Regardless of which method you use, wrap your 6 or 7-inch spring form pan tightly in foil and spray the inside of the pan with non-stick cooking spray.

CRUST: combine the butter and sugar in a microwave-safe bowl and zap until the butter melts, about 30-40 seconds. In a medium bowl, combine the cracker crumbs, pecans, and cinnamon. Pour the melted butter on top and using a rubber spatula mix until the crumbs are covered in the butter. Press the crumb mixture into the bottom of the prepared pan and about 1-inch up the sides. Place the pan in the freezer for 15-20 minutes or bake for 10 minutes. If baking, allow the crust to cool to room temperature before proceeding.

CHEESECAKE FILLING: In the bowl of a stand mixer fitted with the paddle attachment, beat the cream cheese, salt, vanilla, lemon zest, and corn-starch until smooth, about 1-2 minutes. Add the sugar and let it mix in completely before adding the eggs one at a time. Add the sour cream and mix until just combined. Pour the batter into the crust. Cover the top of the spring form pan with a piece of foil and wrap it tightly around the rim.

PRESSURE COOK: Pour 1 1/4 cups of water into the base of the instant pot and place the steaming rack on the bottom. Place the spring form pan on the rack. Lock the lid in place and seal the vent. Cook the cheesecake on manual high pressure for 37 minutes and allow the Instant Pot to naturally release its pressure for 25 minutes afterward (the 'keep warm' setting should still be on, you don't want to turn your IP off completely).

LET COOL: carefully remove the spring form pan from the IP then remove the foil. Using a piece of kitchen towel, gently wipe the surface of the cheesecake if there is any moisture on the surface of the cake. Allow the cheesecake to cool to room temperature, about 3 hours before placing it in the refrigerator to cool overnight. Cheesecake can be prepared 24-48 hours in advance. Top with whipped cream, berries, or apple or cherry pie filling before serving!

Instant Pot Banana Bread: This pressure cooker banana bread is a moist, dense bread, so making it in the instant Pot is perfect!

Ingredient: 3 Ripe Bananas, mashed, 1/2 cup Butter, softened, 1/2 cup Brown Sugar, 1/2 cup White Sugar, 2 Eggs, beaten, 1 tsp. Vanilla, 1/4 cup Buttermilk (or Sour Cream), 2 cups All Purpose Flour, sifted, 1 tsp. Baking Soda, 1 tsp. Baking Powder, 1/4 tsp. Cinnamon, 1/2 tsp. Salt, 6 qtr. or 8 qtr. Electric Pressure Cooker, Trivet with handles, Mixing Bowls, Hand Mixer

6 cup Bundt or Cake Pan (7" is ideal), Baking Spray, Foil.

Preparation: Add 1 1/2 cups of water to the inner liner of the pressure cooker (2 cups if using the 8 qtr.). Spray the cake pan with baking spray and set aside. In a mixing bowl, mash the ripe bananas using a fork. In another mixing bowl, use a hand mixer to cream the butter and sugars together. Add the beaten eggs and vanilla to the creamed butter/sugar mixture. Use a spoon to mix well. Stir the bananas and sour cream/buttermilk into the butter/sugar mixture and mix well. In another mixing bowl, sift together the flour, baking soda, baking powder, cinnamon and salt. Add the dry ingredients to the wet ingredients and gently stir by hand, until just moistened. Spoon the batter into prepared cake/Bundt pan and cover with foil, leaving some room for the bread to rise a little. Gently crimp the edges. Set the trivet on the counter, and put the cake/Bundt pan on it. Carefully place it in the pot using the handles. Close the lid and set the steam release knob to the Sealing position. Press the Pressure Cook/Manual button or dial, then the +/- button or dial to select 50 minutes for a Bundt style pan, and 55 minutes for a regular 7" pan. High pressure.

After the cook time is finished, let the pot sit undisturbed for 15 minutes (15 minute natural release). Then turn the steam release knob to the Venting position to release the remaining steam/pressure. After all of the pressure is out and the pin in the lid drops down, open it and use silicone mitts or pot holders to very carefully remove the cake/bundt pan from the pressure cooker, using the trivet handles. Carefully remove the foil, and let the banana bread sit for 10-15 minutes to cool a bit. Then release the bread from the pan onto a plate. Either invert the pan, or with a push pan, set it on a can and gently push the pan down.

Serve the banana bread warm, slathered in butter, or let it cool and drizzle with my Vanilla Icing Glaze.

Pressure Cooker Applesauce: You'll love how quickly and easily you can make applesauce in a pressure cooker. It truly takes mere minutes to cook and yields delicious tender-yet-chunky results. Use a combination of tart and sweet apples, or adjust the amounts of brown sugar and lemon juice in this applesauce recipe to achieve the perfect sweet-sour flavour.

Ingredient: 2 1/2 pounds apples, 1/4 cup brown sugar, 1 teaspoon cinnamon, 3/4 cups apple juice (or apple cider), 1 tablespoon lemon juice, Pinch salt.

Preparation: Peel and core the apples and cut them into equally sized wedges. In a pressure cooker, combine the apples, brown sugar, cinnamon, apple juice or cider, lemon juice, and salt. Cover the cooker and lock it into place, then place the cooker on the stove over high heat. Bring the pressure cooker up to high pressure, then immediately start the timer for 4 minutes and reduce the heat to maintain pressure.

After 4 minutes, remove the pressure cooker from the heat and release pressure using the natural method (in other words, just let the closed pressure cooker rest until the pressure gauge indicates the steam pressure has been released, about 10 minutes). Carefully open lid, angling it away from you to avoid getting burned by the steam. With a wooden spoon, stir the apples, breaking them up large chunks, until you've achieved the desired consistency. If you like a very smooth applesauce, you can put the mixture in a food processor and pulse it a few times, or put it through a food mill.

Instant Pot Arroz Con Leche: Arroz con Leche is a traditional Hispanic rice pudding that's sweet, rich, and creamy and served with a dash of cinnamon. A warm bowl of this dessert is guaranteed to comfort your soul and satisfy your sweet tooth.

Ingredient: 1 cup long grain rice white, I use the rice measuring cup provided with the Instant Pot, 1 ¼ cups water, 2 cups whole milk, ⅛ teaspoon kosher salt, 1 can sweetened condensed milk 14 oz., 1 teaspoon vanilla extract, ground cinnamon.

Preparation: Rinse the rice using a mesh strainer until the water runs clean. I like the brand Mahatma. Add the milk, water, rice and salt to the Instant Pot and stir. Set the Instant Pot on the Porridge setting (20 minutes). Allow for a 10 minute NPR (natural pressure release) and then release the remaining pressure and open the pot. Add the can of condensed milk and the teaspoon of vanilla extract to the rice. Mix it all together.

Serve warm and enjoy!

Pressure Cooker Chocolate Pots De Crème: Chocolate Pots de Crème is a decadent and creamy chocolate custard dessert. Baked chocolate custard made in an Instant Pot is effortless and quick. This Pressure Cooker Chocolate Pots de Crème recipe is elegant enough for entertaining, but simple enough for a casual weeknight dessert.

Ingredient: 1 1/2 cups heavy cream, 1/2 cup whole milk, 5 large egg yolks, 1/4 cup sugar, pinch of salt, 8 ounces bittersweet chocolate, melted, whipped cream and grated chocolate for decoration, optional.

Preparation: In a small saucepan, bring the cream and milk to a simmer. In a large mixing bowl, whisk together egg yolks, sugar, and salt. Slowly whisk in the hot cream and milk. Whisk in chocolate until blended. Pour into 6 custard cups. (I used 1/2 pint mason jars.) Add 1 1/2 cups of water to the pressure cooker and place the trivet in the bottom. Place 3 cups on the trivet and place a second trivet on top of the cups. Stack the remaining three cups on top of the second trivet. Lock the lid in place. Select High Pressure and set the timer for 6 minutes. When beep sounds, turn off pressure cooker and use a natural pressure release for 15 minutes and then do a quick pressure release to release any remaining pressure. When valve drops carefully remove lid.

Carefully remove the cups to a wire rack to cool uncovered. When cool, refrigerate covered with plastic wrap for at least 4 hours or overnight.

2-ingredient Cheesecake (Instant Pot Indian Cheesecake): You only need two ingredients to make this Instant Pot Cheesecake.

Ingredient: 1 (14 ounce) can condensed milk (sweetened), 1 cup whole milk yogurt (full-fat yogurt or full-fat Greek yogurt), Oil or butter, for greasing ramekins or cheesecake pan.

Preparation: Add the condensed milk and yogurt to a bowl and mix well. Pour this mixture into 4 (6 ounce) greased ramekins or into a cheesecake pan and cover the pan(s) with foil.

Add 2 cups water into the steel inner pot, then place the trivet/wire rack that came with your pressure cooker into the pot. Place the ramekins or the cheesecake pan on top of the rack. Secure the lid, close the pressure valve and cook for 25 minutes at high pressure if using ramekins or 30 minutes at high pressure if using a cheesecake pan. Naturally release pressure for 20 minutes, then release any remaining pressure (do not leave the cheesecake sitting in the pot). The cheesecake should be set (it shouldn't wiggle). Stick a toothpick into the cheesecake and if it comes out clean, it's done. Allow the cheesecakes to cool down on a wire rack. I find it easiest to unmould the cheesecake while slightly warm. (To unmould the cheesecake from ramekins, use a paring knife to loosen the sides of the cake from the ramekin if needed and then flip it out onto a plate. To unmould the cheesecake from a cheesecake pan, use a paring knife to loosen the sides of the cake from the pan – then I suggest watching this video to get a better idea of how I remove the cake).

Put the cheesecake in the fridge to chill for 4-6 hours.

Instant Pot Vegan Borscht: It's very easy to make: Just cut and prepare the veggies, put them into the pot, and start the Soup program.

ingredient: 1 tablespoon canola oil, or as needed1/2 large onion, diced8 cups water, divided1/2 medium head cabbage, finely shredded3/4 pound beets, grated1/2 pound potatoes, cut into small cubes2 carrots, grated1 green bell pepper, chopped (optional)3 bay leaves-salt and ground black pepper to taste.

Preparation: Turn on a multi-functional pressure cooker (such as Instant Pot(R)) and select sauté function. Add oil and onion. Cook, stirring often, until translucent, 3 to 5 minutes. Add a splash of water to stop cooking. Add 8 cups water, cabbage, beets, potatoes, carrots, bell pepper, bay leaves, salt, and pepper to the pot. Close and lock the lid. Select high pressure according to manufacturer's instructions; set timer for 40 minutes. Allow 10 to 15 minutes for pressure to build. Release pressure carefully using the quick-release method according to manufacturer's instructions, about 5 minutes. Unlock and remove the lid.

Instant Pot Vegan Apple Cake: Easy Instant Pot vegan apple cake is so moist and delicious, this cake is vegan gluten-free, oil-free. This flavourful apple crumb cake is loaded with fresh apples and a hint of spice. Serve it as a snack, breakfast cake, or dessert.

Ingredient: 1 medium apple, peeled and finely cubed, 1 medium ripe banana, peeled and mashed, 2 tablespoons almond flour, 1 tablespoon sugar, 1/4 teaspoon cinnamon, 1 cup almond milk, 2 tablespoons ground flaxseeds, 2 teaspoons vanilla, 1 cup brown rice flour, 1/2 cup rolled oats, 1/2 cup almond flour, 3/4 cup sugar, 1 tablespoon baking powder, 1/2 teaspoon cinnamon

1/4 teaspoon nutmeg, 1/4 teaspoon salt.

Preparation: Line the 6-inch cake pan with parchment paper and spray or lightly brush with oil and set aside. To prepare crumb topping mix almond meal or flour, sugar, and cinnamon in a bowl and set aside. In a medium bowl mix the almond milk, ground flaxseeds, banana, and vanilla. Set aside In a large bowl, add brown rice flour, rolled oats, almond flour, sugar, ground flaxseed, baking powder, cinnamon, nutmeg, and sea salt. Add the almond milk mixture and stir to combine. Fold in mashed banana and apple pieces. Scoop batter in cake pan. Sprinkle crumb topping mix on top of the batter. Cover the pan with the lid or foil if using another 6-inch cake pan. Place the covered container with your cake batter on the trivet. Lower the trivet in the inner pot of the Instant Pot using the sling handle. Seal the Instant Pot on Manual High Pressure for 50 minutes, when cooking is complete Natural Pressure Release for 10 minutes after complete then turn the knob to venting to release the remaining steam. Open the lid, and carefully remove the baking pan using the sling handle.

Allow the cake to cool in the pan for 10 minutes then gently remove the cake from the pan onto a cooling rack to completely cool. Delicious topped with vegan vanilla ice cream or coconut whipped cream, or served as a breakfast cake.

Instant Pot Apple Crisp: This Instant Pot apple crisp made with organic granola is quick and delicious! It's a cosy vegan dessert recipe that cooks in minutes in a pressure cooker.

Ingredient: 1 1/2 cups One Degree Organic Sprouted Oat Vanilla Chia Granola, 1/4 cup coconut oil, 1/4 cup organic brown sugar, 4 large or 6 small tart apples (like Granny Smith), enough for 5 cups sliced, 2 tablespoons maple syrup, 1 teaspoon cinnamon, plus 1/8 teaspoon for serving, 1/2 teaspoon ground ginger, 1 teaspoon vanilla extract, 2/3 cup water, Zest of 1/2 lemon, for serving.

Preparation: In a small bowl, mix together the granola, room temperature coconut oil and 2 tablespoons brown sugar; you may need to use your hands to bring everything together. (Note: The granola we used was lightly sweet. If using a very sweet granola, you can lessen the sugar in the topping.) Peel and slice the apples into about 1/4 slices, enough for 5 cups, and place them in the bowl of the Instant Pot. Stir in 2 tablespoons brown sugar, then the maple, cinnamon, ginger, vanilla and water. Smooth the apples into an even layer and pour the granola mixture over the top, covering the apples. Lock the top of the Instant Pot. Pressure cook on high for 2 minutes. (Note: It takes about 5 minutes for the pot to "preheat" before it starts cooking. During cooking, avoid touching the metal part of the lid.) After the pot beeps, immediately do a Quick Release: vent the remaining steam by moving the pressure release handle to "Venting", covering your hand with a towel or hot pad. (Never put your hands or face near the steam release valve when releasing steam.)

While the crisp is cooking, prepare the garnish: Zest 1 lemon. Mix it together with 1/4 teaspoon cinnamon. After the Quick Release, remove the lid. Turn off the pot and let the crisp sit uncovered for 5 minutes (make sure Keep Warm feature is turned off). This lets the sauce thicken; the oats will be intentionally chewy, not crunchy. Scoop the crisp into bowls and add a pinch of the lemon zest garnish. If desired, serve with vegan vanilla ice cream or Coconut Whipped Cream.

SUMMARY.

I am certain that you have enjoyed most, if not all of our instant pot recipes as they are some of the finest dishes across the continents. We are committed to making your vegan journey an absolute treat and would welcome any inquiries that you may have; we'd be glad to give our suggestions.